Pulmonary Defences

Pulmonary Defences

Edited by

ROBERT A. STOCKLEY

Queen Elizabeth Hospital, Birmingham, UK

JOHN WILEY & SONS

Chichester • New York • Weinheim • Brisbane • Singapore • Toronto

Other Wiley Editorial Offices

John Wiley & Sons, Inc., 605 Third Avenue,
New York, NY 10158-0012, USA

VCH Verlagsgesellschaft mbh, Pappelallee 3,
D-69469 Weinheim, Germany

Jacaranda Wiley Ltd, 33 Park Road, Milton,
Queensland 4064, Australia

John Wiley & Sons (Asia) Pte Ltd, 2 Clementi Loop #02-01,
Jin Xing Distripark, Singapore 129809

John Wiley & Sons (Canada) Ltd, 22 Worcester Road,
Rexdale, Ontario M9W 1L1, Canada

Library of Congress Cataloging-in-Publication Data

Pulmonary defences / edited by Robert A. Stockley.
     p. cm.
     Includes bibliographical references and index.
     ISBN 0-471-97000-X (cased : alk. paper)
     1. Lungs — Immunology.   2. Lungs — Diseases — Immunological aspects.
  I. Stockley, Robert A.
     [DNLM: 1. Lung — immunology.   2. Lung Diseases — immunology.
  3. Immunity, Cellular.   WF 600   P98249   1997]
  QP121.P775   1997
  616.2′4079 — dc20
  DNLM/DLC
  for Library of Congress   96–35098
                                                                          CIP

British Library Cataloguing in Publication Data

A catalogue record for this book is available from the British Library

ISBN 0-471-97000-X

Typeset in 10/11.5 pt Times by Laser Words, Madras, India
Printed and bound in Great Britain by Biddles Ltd, Guildford and King's Lynn
This book is printed on acid-free paper responsibly manufactured from sustainable forestation, for which at least two trees are planted for each one used for paper production.

Contents

Contributors

Dr David H. Adams
Liver Research Laboratories, Clinical Research Block, Queen Elizabeth Hospital, Edgbaston, Birmingham B15 2TH, UK

Dr Peter B. Bitterman
Pulmonary and Critical Care Medicine, University of Minnesota, Box 132 UMHC, 420 Delaware Street SE, Minneapolis, MN 55455, USA

Professor L. K. Borysiewicz
University of Wales College of Medicine, Heath Park, Cardiff CF4 4XN, UK

Dr David Burnett
Micropathology Ltd, Institute of Research and Development, University of Birmingham Research Park, Vincent Drive, Birmingham B15 2SQ, UK

Professor Martin K. Church
Immunopharmacology Group, Centre Block, Southampton General Hospital, Southampton SO16 6YD, UK

Dr Craig A. Henke
Pulmonary and Critical Care Medicine, University of Minnesota, Box 276 UMHC, 420 Delaware Street SE, Minneapolis, MN 55455, USA

Dr P. Howarth
University Department of Medicine, Southampton General Hospital, Tremona Road, Southampton SO16 6YD, UK

Professor R. Jefferis
Department of Immunology, The Medical School, University of Birmingham, Edgbaston, Birmingham B15 2TT, UK

Dr R. J. Moots
Department of Rheumatology, University of Birmingham, Edgbaston, Birmingham B15 2TT, UK

Dr Yoshimichi Okayama
Immunopharmacology Group, Centre Block, Southampton General Hospital, Southampton SO16 6YD, UK

Professor R. Pabst
Zentrum Anatomie 4120, Medizinsche Hochschule Hannover, D-30623 Hannover, Germany

Professor L. W. Poulter
Department of Clinical Immunology, Royal Free Hospital, Pond Street, London NW3 2QG, UK

Dr D. I. Pritchard
Reader in Parasitology Immunology, Department of Life Science, University of Nottingham, Nottingham NG7 2RD, UK

Dr Charlotte F. J. Rayner
Host Defence Unit, Department of Thoracic Medicine, Imperial College of Science, Technology and Medicine, National Heart and Lung Institute, Emmanuel Kaye Building, Manresa Road, London SW3 6LR, UK

Dr S. I. Rennard
Pulmonary and Critical Care Medicine Section, University of Nebraska Medical Center, 600 South 42nd Street, Omaha, NE 68198-5300, USA

Professor Richard A. Robbins
Departments of Medicine and Physiology, LSU Medical Center, ACOS for Research and Development, Overton Brooks VA Medical Center, 510 E. Stoner, Shreveport, LA 71101, USA

Dr R. L. Smyth
Respiratory and Infectious Diseases, Royal Liverpool Children's Hospital, Alder Hey, Eaton Road, Liverpool L12 2AP, UK

Dr Robert A. Stockley
Department of Medicine, Queen Elizabeth Hospital, Birmingham B15 2TH, UK

Professor Galen B. Toews
Division of Pulmonary and Critical Care Medicine, Department of Internal Medicine, University of Michigan Medical Center, 3916 Taubman Center, 1500 E Medical Center Drive, Ann Arbor, MI 48109-0360, USA

Dr Robert G. Townley
Creighton University Allergic Diseases Center, 2500 California Plaza, Omaha, NE 68178, USA

Dr V. A. Varney
Department of Respiratory Medicine, St Helier Hospital, Wrythe Lane, Carshalton, Surrey SM5 1AA, UK

Dr G. M. Walsh
Department of Respiratory Medicine, Leicester University Medical School, Glenfield Hospital, Groby Road, Leicester LE3 9QP, UK

Dr A. J. Wardlaw
Department of Respiratory Medicine, Leicester University Medical School, Glenfield Hospital, Groby Road, Leicester LE3 9QP, UK

Dr W. W. West
Pathology/Microbiology, University of Nebraska Medical Center, 600 South 42nd Street, Omaha, NE 68198-5300, USA

Professor John Widdicombe
Department of Physiology, St George's Hospital Medical School, Cranmer Terrace, London SW17 0RE, UK

Professor R. A. Wilson
Department of Biology, The University of York, York YO1 5DD, UK

Dr Robert Wilson
Host Defence Unit, Department of Thoracic Medicine, Imperial College of Science, Technology and Medicine, National Heart and Lung Institute, Emmanuel Kaye Building, Manresa Road, London SW3 6LR, UK

Dr Stephen P. Young
Department of Rheumatology, University of Birmingham, Edgbaston, Birmingham B15 2TT, UK

1

Physical Defences of the Lung

JOHN WIDDICOMBE

St George's Hospital Medical School, London, UK

INTRODUCTION

The physical defences of the lungs have a double role: they act to prevent airway and pulmonary damage from inhaled intruders, and they can deal with any physical material that arises endogenously in the airways and alveoli. Thus inhaled material may be kept out or removed by cough and, if this process is not effective, will be trapped by mucus and removed by mucociliary transport. Debris in the lungs, for example infected mucus and the products of epithelial damage in the airway lumen, will promote additional mucus secretion and will be cleared from the airways by mucociliary transport and coughing. If these two defensive systems fail, the epithelium itself constitutes a further barrier against invasion of the mucosa.

COUGH

The classical description of cough is a deep breath, followed by a forced expiration against a closed glottis, which opens suddenly to produce the expulsive phase of the cough[1-4]. While this description is generally true, there are many different patterns of cough. To some extent, the pattern depends upon the site of the origin of the cough. Mechanical stimulation of the larynx or vocal folds usually causes an immediate expiratory effort without a preliminary inspiration[3]. This has the advantage that any foreign body will not be first drawn into the lungs. However, when cough is elicited from the bronchial tree, a deep inspiration normally precedes the expulsive effort. This allows a more forceful expiratory effort, but may have a disadvantage if the cough is being induced by a chemical irritant, as more would be drawn into the lungs and might be absorbed. Cough cannot be induced from the small bronchi, bronchioles or alveoli[4,5]. In these regions it is likely that expiratory air velocities would be too low to produce enough turbulence and shearing forces to extrude material. The strength of the cough may also depend on the site activated. Chemical stimuli seem to be especially effective deep in the airways, and mechanical stimuli more effective at proximal sites[6]. The relative importance of the larynx as a tussigenic site is unclear, although one study suggests that in man it is rather insensitive[7]. In experimental animals, the bifurcations of the airways, such as the tracheal carina, are the most sensitive areas for eliciting cough.

Cough can be caused by a very wide variety of stimuli. In general there are four categories of stimulus: mechanical, chemical, inflammatory and other mediators, and various diseases[4,8] (Table 1.1). More than one stimulus may be present. For example, in asthma there will be the mechanical stimulus of mucus and the presence of many mediators that can cause cough.

MECHANISMS OF COUGH

The airway epithelium has long been known to contain sensory nerve fibres and these are thought to mediate cough[9,10] (Fig. 1.1). They can be seen under the electron microscope close and deep to the tight junctions that join epithelial cells. The nerves contain tachykinins such as substance P, neurokinin A (NKA) and calcitonin gene related peptide (CGRP), and connect with vagal nerve fibres running to the brain stem. Recording from these nerves shows that the receptors are sensitive to the various stimuli that cause cough[8,11] (Table 1.1).

There has been considerable discussion as to whether the "cough receptors" are C-fibre endings with non-myelinated vagal fibres, or rapidly adapting receptors

Table 1.1. Stimuli to C-fibre receptors and RARs

	C-fibre receptors	RARs
Mechanical	Inflation	Inflation
		Deflation
		Dust
		Mucus
		Foreign bodies
Chemical	Irritant gases	Irritant gases
	Cigarette smoke	Cigarette smoke
	Capsaicin	Capsaicin
	Volatile anaesthetics	Volatile anaesthetics
Mediators	Acetylcholine	Acetylcholine
	Histamine	Histamine
	Serotonin	Serotonin
	Prostaglandins	Prostaglandins
	Bradykinin	Bradykinin
	Substance P	Substance P
Diseases	Microembolism	Anaphylaxis
	Pulmonary oedema	Microembolism
	Pulmonary congestion	Atelectasis
	Pneumonia	Bronchoconstriction
		Pulmonary oedema

In general, both groups of receptor respond to the same stimuli. However, sensitivities vary greatly. The main differences in response relate to mechanical stimuli. The lists of chemical and mediator stimuli are incomplete, and not all agents have been tested on all groups of receptors.

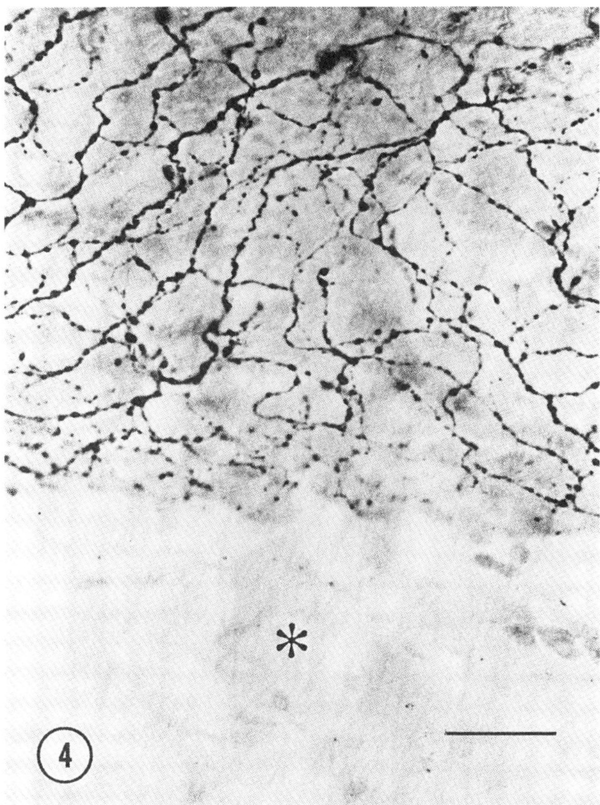

Figure 1.1. A region of the tracheal mucosa directly above a cartilaginous ring of a rat. Nerves are exhibited by immunofluorescence for substance P. The density and orientation of the intraepithelial plexus of substance P immunoreactive axons are similar to those found between the cartilaginous rings. The intraepithelial nerve plexus is absent in a region of the epithelium (*), which was accidentally removed during processing. Bar represents, 25 µm. Reproduced from Baluk *et al*[9] by permission

(RARs) with myelinated fibres[4,5,12]. The latter are certainly involved in cough caused by mechanical stimuli, to which they are extremely sensitive, and both may be active in cough caused by chemical irritation or mediators released in airway inflammation and disease. The interaction of the reflexes from the two types of receptor may explain in part the various patterns of cough that can occur. C-fibre receptors have been shown to inhibit cough centrally[13], but the tachykinins they release may excite RARs[4].

When cough is elicited, in addition to the reflex changes in the muscles of breathing, various other reflexes can be activated. These include closure of the glottis as a preliminary to the expulsive effort, bronchoconstriction, airway mucus secretion, airway vasodilatation and mucosal thickening, and various other cardiovascular events[8,11].

MECHANICS OF COUGH

Cough consists of three phases: inspiratory, compressive and expulsive[1-3] (Fig. 1.2). In the inspiratory phase, the glottis opens widely while the inspiratory muscles contract and the lungs inflate. The large lung volume allows a greater mechanical efficiency of the expiratory muscles plus a stronger elastic recoil of the lungs. In addition, it may enhance the expiratory phase of the cough by lung reflexes.

During the compressive phase of cough, the glottis usually closes and intrapleural pressure may increase to as much as 250 mm Hg. There has been much discussion as to whether the glottis always closes during the compressive phase of cough, and whether its closure is physiologically advantageous[14]. Certainly, cough can be effective without closure of the glottis, as can be seen in patients with a tracheostomy. Forced expiration with an open glottis can be effective in clearing material from the lower airways. The glottis only closes

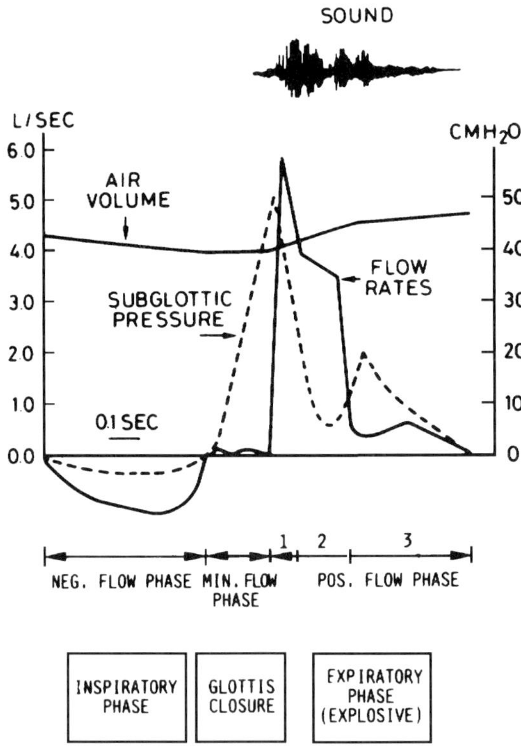

Figure 1.2. Diagrammatic representation of the changes in the following parameters during a representative cough: flow rate, volume, subglottic pressure, and sound level. During inspiration the flow rate is negative, at the glottic closure the flow rate is zero, and during the expiration phase the flow rate is positive. This last phase can be divided into three parts: growing, constant, and decreasing. Reproduced from Biancho *et al*[16] by permission

for about 200 ms, and then it opens in the expulsive phase of cough. Very rapid airflows occur in the larynx — often more than $10\,\text{m·s}^{-1}$. Vibration of the vocal cords during this phase causes the sound of cough, and there have been a number of studies on the diagnostic and prognostic value of the "tussiphonogram"[15]. The expulsive phase of cough may be long lasting, with a large expiratory tidal volume, or it may be interrupted into a series of short expiratory efforts, each having a compressive and an expulsive phase.

The maximum expiratory flow is limited by dynamic compression of the airways[1,2]. This occurs downstream from the equal pressure point at which pressures inside and outside the bronchial wall are equal. This equal pressure point shifts progressively towards the smaller airways as the lung empties. The effectiveness of cough depends on peak airflow, and dynamic compression of the airways will increase airflow velocity and the kinetic energy of the air, thus improving the clearing capacity of the cough.

The efficiency of cough depends on there being liquid in the airways of sufficient thickness, and airflow velocity and luminal area that cause turbulence of the expired gas[1,16]. Laminar flow, which would be ineffective in moving luminal

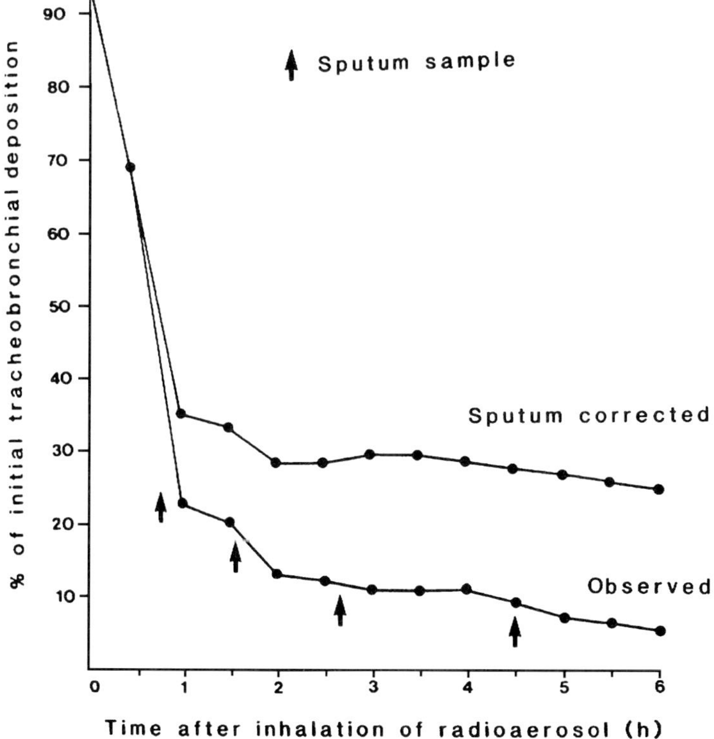

Figure 1.3. Observed and "sputum corrected" tracheobronchial clearance curves for a patient with chronic bronchitis. Cough occurred at the arrows and the volumes of sputum have been subtracted from the "observed" curve to give the "sputum corrected" curve. Reproduced from Hasani *et al*[19] by permission

debris, is more readily converted to turbulent flow when velocity is high and the airways are narrow. Under these conditions, the shearing forces on the luminal liquid or debris can be extremely high and will overcome any adhesiveness of the material to the mucosa, and thus the material will be expelled.

The influence of adhesiveness on the efficiency of cough has recently been studied and shown to be of considerable importance[17]. Phospholipids secreted onto the surface of the airway epithelium lessen adhesiveness[18], but if the epithelium is damaged and if the airway secretions are especially sticky as the result of plasma exudated into the lumen, adhesiveness may be considerably increased and limit the effectiveness of cough.

If clearance from the lungs is measured after inhalation of a radiolabel, it can be shown that coughing increases the rate of clearance by about 20% in patients with chronic bronchitis, but only by about 2.5% in healthy subjects[19] (Fig. 1.3).

AIRWAY MUCUS

A thin layer of airway surface liquid (ASL) is crucial for normal airway function. It allows the cilia to beat, and traps and absorbs inhaled material and irritants. ASL is usually divided into a sol phase, or periciliary liquid, about 5–10 µm deep, and a gel phase on the surface of the cilia[20] (Fig. 1.4). The thickness of the gel phase is uncertain, but most microscopic pictures give values of 2–20 µm. The gel is transported by mucociliary transport (MCT). The rate of flow of mucus in the human trachea is about 10 mm·min^{-1}, and that in the bronchioles probably about 10 times slower.

The composition of the sol phase of the ASL has not been determined, but presumably its ionic composition depends upon the various ionic pumps in the epithelial cell membranes. It has a much greater potassium concentration and a lower pH than interstitial liquid[22]. The composition of the gel phase has frequently been determined, in health and disease[23]. It consists of about 95% water, 1% salt, 1–3% proteins and mucoglycoproteins, and 1–3% proteoglycans and lipids.

The physical properties of mucus are provided mainly by mucins, which are high molecular mass (up to 15 MDa) mucoglycoproteins[24]. In addition, proteoglycans—of lower molecular mass but contributing much to mucus viscosity—are secreted from the surface of epithelial cells and from the glands.

Phospholipids are secreted by the epithelial cells and submucosal glands of the airways, and may be important in weakening adhesion of the mucus to the epithelium[18,25]. They may also change the physical properties of the mucus. Serum proteins, such as albumin, fibrinogen and immunoglobulins, exude from the blood vessels in the mucosa during airway inflammation[26]. The albumin can interact with mucins to make the mucus more viscous, and the exudate will also carry with it many active plasma components.

Serous cells in the epithelium and glands secrete lysozyme and lactoferrin; both have antibacterial properties[20,23]. Other important constituents of mucus are secretory IgA, antileukoproteases, various peroxidases, and proline-rich proteins. The actions of these components of secretion are described in later chapters.

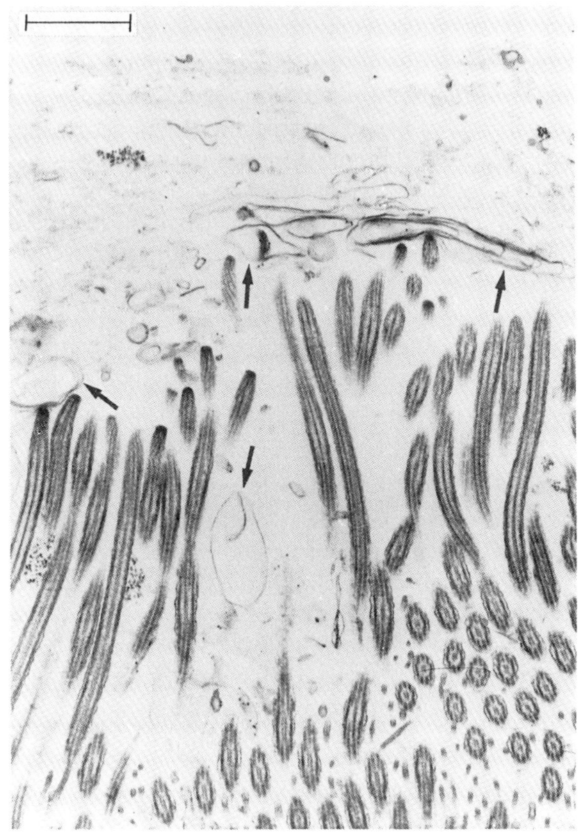

Figure 1.4. Arrangement of osmiophilic membranes (phospholipids) along the border between the sol and gel phases of mucus in a bronchus (arrows). Between the cilia a vesicular arrangement of the osmiophilic membranes can be seen. Transmission electron micrograph. Bar represents 1 μm. Reproduced from Morgenroth[21] by permission

MUCUS AND BACTERIA

The mucus gel acts as a barrier for bacteria, which adhere to it and can then subsequently multiply within it[25]. Mucins are polyanionic and also contain chemical receptors that can bind to the adhesins on many bacteria. The adhesins on common respiratory pathogens include the pilin proteins on fimbriae, mucoid exopolysaccharide, haemagglutinins, internal lectins, exoenzyme S and non-pilus protein components[27,28].

The respiratory pathogens that bind strongly to mucus include *Streptococcus pneumoniae, Haemophilus influenzae, Staphylococcus aureus* and *Pseudomonas aeruginosa*. The chemical receptors on the mucins may be of different types, but all seem to include carbohydrate. Sialic acid and *N*-acetylglucosamine are common in mucins, and are believed to bind *Ps. aeruginosa*. Binding can be blocked by addition of free sialic acid residues. Other mucus receptors that may be active in binding to bacterial adhesins are glycolipids, which are found in airway secretions.

Once the bacteria are bound to the mucus, two types of response will take place. The bacteria will multiply and in turn set up a range of tissue responses, and the other constituents of the airway secretions will act on the bacteria[25,27].

Colonized bacteria will also promote further mucus secretion which will add to the ASL[29,30]. This could be advantageous if it promotes greater clearance of mucus from the airway by cough. The disadvantage of the increased mucus secretion will be blockage of the smaller airways and a further chance to allow bacterial multiplication. The airway secretions would also bring to the ASL bactericidal products. Increased mucus secretion has been shown in response to *H. influenzae, Staph. aureus, Strep. pneumoniae* and *Ps. aeruginosa*, and the active secretory agents have been established as proteases and rhamnolipids[29,30].

SOURCES OF SECRETION

The mucus gel phase of secretion comes from several sources. These include goblet cells and serous cells in the airway epithelium[31]. At the bronchiolar level these are replaced by Clara cells, which are non-ciliated secretory cells. Epithelial ciliated cells have a glycocalyx on their luminal border, containing proteoglycans which may be released into the ASL[20,31].

The submucosal glands of the airways have two types of acini: serous ones which are distal and produce a thin secretion, and mucus acini that produce a more viscous secretion[20,32]. Presumably, the secretions mix before arrival in the airway lumen.

CONTROL OF SECRETION

In healthy lungs, control of secretion is probably mainly nervous[20,32]. Parasympathetic nerves promote secretion by cholinergic mechanisms, and sympathetic nerves can probably do the same by noradrenergic pathways. Other neurotransmitters such as vasoactive intestinal polypeptide (VIP) and nitric oxide (both in parasympathetic nerves), and neuropeptide Y (in sympathetic nerves) may have modulatory actions on secretion. The fact that atropine, an antiacetylcholine agent, seems to block glandular secretion almost completely, suggests that the dominant mechanism is parasympathetic and cholinergic. Secretion is also nervously induced during neurogenic inflammation of the airways, when sensory nerves are activated and release neuropeptides, such as substance P, that promote secretion.

The motor innervation of the submucosal glands can be activated by various reflexes, in particular those initiated by irritation and inflammation of the airways, the afferent pathways being the same as those that cause or modulate cough[8,11] (Table 1.2).

A very large range of inflammatory and other mediators have been shown to promote mucus secretion by local action[32]. These include histamine, bradykinin, archidonic acid, 5-hydroxytryptamine, several prostaglandins, leukotrienes, and platelet activating factor (PAF). Some bacterial products, such as rhamnolipids

Table 1.2. Reflex responses to receptor stimulation

C-fibre receptors	RARs
Apnoea	Cough
Tachypnoea	Tachypnoea
Cough inhibition	Augmented breaths
Bronchoconstriction	Bronchoconstriction
Mucus secretion	Mucus secretion
Laryngoconstriction	Laryngoconstriction
Vasodilatation	Vasodilatation
Somatic inhibition	

The main differences between the reflex responses are respiratory. The lists may be incomplete because not all reflexes have been studied for both groups of receptor.

and proteases, can also cause mucus secretion by a direct action on the glands[30]. Many of the inflammatory mediators also stimulate the airway sensory receptors that cause cough and reflex secretion of mucus. No mediator has yet been identified that inhibits secretion.

In airways disease, mucus secretion will be promoted by a complex interaction of local mediator release and central nervous reflexes. The pattern of response will presumably vary widely according to the nature of its initiation.

MUCOCILIARY CLEARANCE

CILIARY ACTIVITY

For most mammals including man, the ciliated cell predominates in the tracheo-bronchial epithelium, although there are reduced numbers at the bronchiolar level[32,33]. The cilia are 4–6 µm long, about 0.1–0.2 µm in diameter, and number about 200 per cell (Fig. 1.4). The tips of the cilia end in small claws that engage the overlying mucus gel, enabling it to be transported. In cross section, each cilium can be seen to contain a pair of central microtubules and nine pairs of peripheral microtubules, consisting mainly of the protein, tubulin. The microtubules in each peripheral pair are connected by strands of nexin, and each couplet has two dynein arms and a radial spoke that attaches it to the central microtubules. The bending of cilia depends on the active sliding of the peripheral microtubules relative to each other, based on the dynein bridges. ATP is the source of energy for this, dynein being an ATPase protein. The mechanisms of ciliary movement, the biochemical processes underlying it, and the ways in which it can go wrong have been studied extensively[33–35].

In most animals, ciliary beat frequency is slower in small airways (6 Hz) compared with the main bronchi (18 Hz)[33–35]. In man this difference has not been seen, and beat frequency appears uniform (15–18 Hz). The ciliary beat cycle has two components: movement towards the larynx, which is the effective stroke because the cilia are straight and attached to the mucus, followed by a recovery stroke in the opposite direction when the cilia disengage from the mucus and

     J. Widdicombe

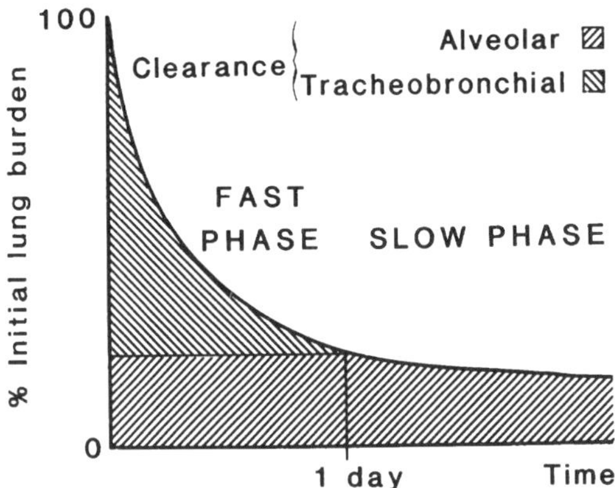

Figure 1.5. Schematic diagram of whole lung clearance of radioaerosol versus time showing two phases: a fast phase representing mucociliary clearance (with or without cough) and the slow phase representing "alveolar clearance." Reproduced from Clarke[37] by permission

bend while they travel backwards[36] (Fig. 1.5). There is no reason to believe that periciliary fluid is transported by the ciliary beat. The action of cilia both in a single cell and between adjacent cells is co-ordinated and appears as part of a metachronal wave, with adjacent cilia beating in succession[38].

There has been much research on the intracellular control of ciliary action. It depends on ATP cATP, cGMP, and protein kinase C, in addition to ionic calcium[34]. All these second messengers increase ciliary beat frequency except for protein kinase C, which decreases it. Baseline ciliary activity does not seem to be under nervous control, but acetylcholine and β_2-adrenoceptor agonists increase ciliary beat frequency, as also does adrenaline, although noradrenaline has little effect. Thus the potential for the nervous control of ciliary movement is present. Of the other neurotransmitters, VIP stimulates ciliary movement, and may coact with acetylcholine, as both are released from parasympathetic nerves. The sensory neuropeptides substance P, NKA and CGRP all stimulate ciliary activity, so this action may be a component of neurogenic inflammation when the sensory nerves are excited.

Most of the inflammatory mediators have been shown to affect ciliary activity[34]. It is increased by prostaglandins E_1 and E_2 and by leukotrienes C_4 and D_4. PAF is said to inhibit ciliary beating, possibly by release of a major basic protein which causes ciliary inhibition. Bradykinin also stimulates the cilia, possibly by acting on sensory nerves with release of tachykinins.

Some of the proteases active in airways disease inhibit the cilia[27,39]. This is true for human neutrophil elastase, and the elastases from *Ps. aeruginosa*. Other bacterial products such as rhamnolipid and pyocyanin inhibit cilia, as do oxygen radicals. Some of these effects seem to be due to activation of protein kinase C. Many of the ciliotoxic agents that act in inflammation also damage the airway epithelium when applied in higher concentrations.

Thus whereas mucus secretion is increased by virtually all mediators associated with inflammation, ciliary beating is increased by some and decreased by others[20,34,40]. Physical damage to the cilia and their cells may be more important than changes in ciliary beat frequency.

MUCOCILIARY TRANSPORT

The clearance of mucus together with any attached material or debris depends only in part on ciliary activity[19,41–43]. Other factors include cough (already mentioned), the amount of mucus present, the viscoelasticity of the mucus, and its adhesiveness to the airway epithelium.

MCT is usually measured by assessing the clearance rate of inhaled radiolabelled particles[19,43]. The clearance curve shows two phases: a fast phase, taking a few hours in healthy subjects, that is due to clearance by cilia and cough, and a slower phase, with a half life of weeks or months (Fig. 1.5), that represents alveolar clearance. The alveoli have no cilia and cough is not effective at this site, consequently removal of the labelled particles into the tissues and blood stream is slow.

Inflammatory mediators may have actions that are different for ciliary beat frequency and MCT[34]. Thus histamine increases MCT in dogs and man, but has little action on the ciliary beat. Leukotriene D_4 stimulates cilia but inhibits MCT.

In airway diseases, structural damage to the epithelium and secretion of mucus with increased adhesiveness may be more important factors in determining MCT than are changes in ciliary beat frequency[25,28]. MCT is impaired in asthma, chronic bronchitis and cystic fibrosis, when the ciliary beat frequency of individual epithelial cells may be normal. Antigen challenge in sensitive animals and man can increase both MCT and ciliary beat frequency[34]. An abnormal structure of the cilia has been observed in some airways diseases such as chronic bronchitis, but the most extreme example is the primary ciliary dyskinesia syndrome, in which there is ciliary immobility and interciliary discoordination, with virtually absent MCT[34]. As mentioned earlier, a number of bacterial products are ciliotoxic, which could contribute to decreased MCT in airway infections.

THE AIRWAY EPITHELIUM

If the layer of the mucus overlying the epithelium is inadequate to protect the mucosa, the airway epithelium presents the next important barrier[44,45]. In general terms, damage to the epithelium is often related to hyperresponsiveness to inhaled agents; this occurs in asthma and on inhalation of toxic agents such as ozone, sulphur dioxide and nitrogen dioxide.

There have been many experimental studies of the effects of epithelial removal on the response of underlying smooth muscle to contractile drugs[45,46]. Responses to luminal acetylcholine, histamine and 5-hydroxytryptamine are all enhanced by epithelial removal. This change may be due to more ready penetration of the agent to the smooth muscle, or to the absence of smooth muscle relaxant factors that arise from the epithelium itself. In general, the smooth muscle becomes about 3–5 times more responsive.

Damage to the epithelium, but without its destruction, can be caused by agents such as PAF and hydrogen peroxide[47,48]. Under these conditions, agents that contract the smooth muscle are far more effective, although again one cannot be sure whether this is the result of increased penetration of the agents through the damaged epithelium or the presence of epithelium derived mediators, or both.

Experiments with smooth muscle relaxants, such as β_2-adrenoceptor agonists, show that these are far more effective when applied to the serosal side of the airway wall than when presented at the mucosal side[45]. This difference in sensitivity disappears when the epithelium is removed, however, which suggests strongly that the epithelium is acting as a barrier to penetration of the drugs.

Measurements of the permeability of radiolabelled tracers through the epithelium or the airway mucosa support the view that the epithelium can be a major barrier[49,50]. This is certainly true for hydrophilic molecules such as diethylene triaminopentacetic acid (DTPA), which are believed to pass mainly through paracellular pathways. In isolated ferret trachea, epithelial damage with PAF, or its destruction by the surface active agent Triton X-100 or by epithelial rubbing, increases the permeability coefficient about eightfold[49,51]. This model involves penetration through the entire mucosa, but *in vivo*, when penetration has only to be through the epithelium to reach the copious vascular network just below, the coefficient of permeability to DTPA is increased 50-fold[48] by epithelial destruction. With a lipophilic agent such as antipyrine, damage to or destruction of the epithelium makes no difference to the permeability[49,51]. This is because the permeability of antipyrine is about 200 times greater than that of DTPA, and the agent is believed to pass mainly through cells because of its solubility in cell membranes.

The epithelium is also a strong barrier to macromolecules. In healthy airways, horseradish peroxidase penetrates the epithelium only up to the tight junctions between cells[52]. However, if the tight junctions are opened, for example by histamine or cigarette smoke, the peroxidase penetrates through the epithelium to the basement membrane[52,53].

BACTERIAL–EPITHELIAL INTERACTION

Many bacteria adhere more to mucus than to "clean" epithelium, provided the latter is healthy[25,27,28]. Most respiratory pathogens, apart from *Mycoplasma pneumoniae* and *Bordetella pertussis*, will not stick to epithelium until it has been damaged by toxins or proteases[54,55]. *Myco. pneumoniae* attaches to sialo-oligosaccharide receptors on cilia and microvilli on airway cells. The fact that such receptors may be scanty in secreted mucus may aid epithelial infection with this agent. *Bord. pertussis* also adheres to the proximal parts of cilia, but not to other cell bodies. The adhesion seems to be attributable to a filamentous haemagglutinin and to pertussis toxin. When these adhesins are added either to ciliated cells or to bacteria such as *Strep. pneumoniae* and *Staph. aureus*, which do not normally adhere to cells, adhesion is acquired both *in vivo* and *in vitro*. The receptors for adhesion by *Bord. pertussis* seem to be glycolipids containing galactose or glucose.

Airway pathogens such as *H. influenzae, Strep. pneumoniae* and *Staph. aureus* adhere powerfully to damaged cells, both ciliated and non-ciliated[27,56,57]. *Strep. pneumoniae* also adheres to differentiating cells in tracheal mucosa, presumably because these cells produce receptors during their proliferative phase. *Ps. aeruginosa* does not adhere to healthy human respiratory cells, but adheres to cilia of damaged or exfoliated cells, the adhesin being fimbriae. The membrane receptors for *Ps. aeruginosa* are believed to be glycolipids such as gangliotetraosylceramide (asialo GM1).

If damage to the mucosa is severe enough to denude it of epithelium, bacteria can adhere to the exposed extracellular matrix or basement membrane[58]. This process has been shown for *Strep. pneumoniae, H. influenzae* and *Ps. aeroginosa*.

REFERENCES

1. Leith D E, Butler J P, Sneddon S L, *et al.* Cough. In: Fisherman A P, Macklem P T, Mead J, *et al.*, eds. *Handbook of Physiology, Section 3, The Respiratory System.* Bethesda: American Physiological Society, 1986; 315–336.

2. Irwin R S, Widdicombe J G. Cough. In: Murray J F, Nadel J A, eds. *Textbook of Respiratory Medicine.* Philadelphia: W B Saunders Company, 1994; 529–544.

3. Korpas J, Tomori Z. *Cough and Other Respiratory Reflexes.* Basel: S Karger, 1979; 1–356.

4. Widdicombe J G. Relationship between the composition of mucus, epithelial lining liquid, and adhesion of micro-organisms. *Am J Crit Care Med* 1995; **151:** 2088–2093.

5. Karlsson J A, Sant'Ambrogio G, Widdicombe J G. Afferent neural pathways in cough and reflex bronchoconstriction. *J Appl Physiol* 1988; **65:** 1007–1023.

6. Widdicombe J G. Respiratory reflexes from the trachea and bronchi of the cat. *J Physiol* 1954; **123:** 55–70.

7. Stockwell M, Lang S, Yip R, *et al.* Lack of importance of the superior laryngeal nerves in citric acid cough in humans. *J Appl Physiol* 1993; **75:** 613–617.

8. Widdicombe J G. Physiology of cough. In: Braga P C, Allegra L, eds. *Cough.* New York: Raven Press Ltd, 1989; 3–25.

9. Baluk P, Nadel J A, McDonald D M. Substance P-immunoreactive sensory axons in the rat respiratory tract: a quantitative study of their distribution and role in neurogenic inflammation. *J Comp Neurol* 1992; **319:** 586–598.

10. Das R M, Jeffery P K, Widdicombe J G. The epithelial innervation of the lower respiratory tract of the cat. *J Anat* 1978; **126:** 123–131.

11. Coleridge H M, Coleridge J C G. Reflexes evoked from the tracheobronchial tree and lungs. In: Cherniack N S, Widdicombe J G, eds. *Handbook of Physiology, 3. The Respiratory System, Vol II, Control of Breathing.* Bethesda: American Physiological Society, 1986; 395–429.

12. Paintal A S. The visceral sensations — some basic mechanisms In: Cervero F, Morrisson J F B, eds. *Visceral Sensation.* Amsterdam: Elsevier, 1986; 3–19.

13. Tatar M, Webber S E, Widdicombe J G. Lung C-fibre receptor activation and defensive reflexes in anaesthetized cats. *J Physiol* 1988; **402:** 411–420.

14. Young S, Abdul-Sattar N, Caric D. Glottic closure and high flows are not essential for productive cough. In: Widdicombe J G, Korpas J, Salat D, eds. The cough reflex. Nerves and mediators in bronchial asthma. *Bull Europ Physiopath Resp* 1986; **23** (Suppl 10): 11–15.

15. Korpas J, Sadlonova J, Salat D, *et al.* The origin of cough sounds. In: Widdicombe J G, Korpas J, Salat D, eds. The cough reflex. Nerves and mediators in bronchial asthma. *Bull Europ Physiopath Resp* 1986; **23** (Suppl 10): 47–50.

16. Bianco S, Robuschi M. Mechanics of cough. In: Braga P C, Allegra L, eds. *Cough.* New York: Raven Press, 1989; 29–36.

17. Schurch S, Gehr P, Im Hof V, *et al.* Surfactant displaces particles toward the epithelium in airways and alveoli. *Respir Physiol* 1990; **80:** 17–32.

18. Rubin B K, Ramirez O, King M. The role of mucus rheology and transport in neonatal respiratory distress syndrome and the effect of surfactant therapy. *Chest* 1992; **101:** 1080–1085.
19. Hasani A, Pavia D. Cough as a clearance mechanism. In: Braga P C, Allegra L, eds. *Cough.* New York: Raven Press, 1989; 39–52.
20. Richardson P S, Somerville M, Sheehan J K. Airway mucus: What is it and how does it alter in disease? *Eur Resp Rev* 1992; **2:** 263–266.
21. Morgenroth K. Morphology of the bronchial lining layer and its alteration in IRDS, ARDS and COLD. In: van Golde L M G, Widdicombe J G, Vermeire P, eds. Endobronchial surface active phospholipids: Morphology, biochemistry, function and therapeutic aspects. *Eur J Respir Dis* 1984; **67** (Suppl 142): 7–18.
22. Widdicombe J G. Airway mucus. *Eur Respir J* 1989; **2:** 107–115.
23. Boat T F, Cheng P W, Leigh M W. Biochemistry of Mucus. In: Takishima T, Shimura S, eds. *Airway Secretion. Physiological Bases for the Control of Mucous Hypersecretion.* New York: Marcel Dekker, 1994; 217–282.
24. King M, Rubin B K. Rheology of airway mucus. Relationship with clearance function. In: Takishima T, Shimura S, eds. *Airway Secretion. Physiological Bases for the Control of Mucous Hypersecretion.* New York: Marcel Dekker, 1994; 283–314.
25. Puchelle E, Girod-de Bentzmann S, Jacquot J. Airway defence mechanisms in relation to biochemical and physical properties of mucus. *Eur Resp Rev* 1992; **2:** 259–263.
26. Persson C G. Plasma exudation from tracheobronchial microvessels in health and disease. In: Butler J, ed. *The Bronchial Circulation.* New York: Marcel Dekker, 1992; 443–473.
27. Widdicombe J G, Webber S E. Airway mucus secretion. *News Physiol Sci* 1990; **5:** 2–5.
28. Girod S, Zahm J -M, Plotkowski C, *et al.* Role of the physicochemical properties of mucus in the protection of the respiratory epithelium. *Eur Respir J* 1992; **5:** 477–487.
29. Adler K B, Hendley D D, Davis G S. Bacteria associated with obstructive pulmonary disease elaborate extracellular products that stimulate mucin secretion by explants of guinea pig airways. *Am J Pathol* 1986; **125:** 501–514.
30. Somerville M, Taylor G W, Watson D, *et al.* Release of mucus glycoconjugates by *Pseudomonas aeruginosa* rhamnolipids into feline trachea *in vivo* and human bronchus *in vitro*. *Am J Respir Cell Mol Biol* 1992; **6:** 116–122.
31. Kim K C. Epithelial goblet cell secretion. In: Takishima T, Shimura S, eds. *Airway Secretion. Physiological Bases for the Control of Mucous Hypersecretion.* New York: Marcel Dekker, 1994; 433–449.
32. Shimura S, Takishima T. Airway submucosal gland secretion. In: Takishima T, Shimura S, eds. *Airway Secretion. Physiological Bases for the Control of Mucous Hypersecretion.* New York: Marcel Dekker, 1994; 325–398.
33. Widdicombe J H, Widdicombe J G. Regulation of human airway surface liquid. *Respir Physiol* 1995; **99:** 3–12.
34. Wanner A. Possible control of airway hypersecretion. In: Takishima T, Shimura S, eds. *Airway Secretion. Physiological Bases for the Control of Mucous Hypersecretion.* New York: Marcel Dekker, 1994; 629–646.
35. Wanner A. Mucociliary clearance in the trachea. *Clin Chest Med* 1986; **7:** 247–258.
36. Sleigh M A, Blake J R, Liron N. The propulsion of mucus by cilia. *Am Rev Respir Dis* 1988; **137:** 726–741.
37. Clarke S W. Clearance of airway secretions. In: Petty T L, Cherniack R M, eds. *Seminars in Respiratory Medicine.* New York: Thieme-Stratton, 1984; 319–331.
38. Sanderson M J, Sleigh M A. Ciliary activity of cultured rabbit tracheal epithelium: beat pattern and metachrony. *J Cell Sci* 1981; **47:** 331–347.
39. Wilson R, Pitt T, Taylor G, *et al.* Pyocyanin and 1-hydroxyphenazine products by *Pseudomonas aeruginosa* inhibit the beating of human respiratory cilia *in vitro*. *J Clin Invest* 1987; **79:** 221–229.
40. Adler K B, Winn C Jr, Alberghinit T V, *et al.* Stimulatory effect of *Pseudomonas aeruginosa* on mucin secretion by the respiratory epithelium. *JAMA* 1983; **249:** 1615–1617.
41. Puchelle E, Zahm J M, Girard F. Mucociliary transport *in vivo* and *in vitro*. Relations to sputum properties in chronic bronchitis. *Eur J Respir Dis* 1980; **61:** 254–264.
42. Yeates D, Aspin N, Levison H, *et al.* Mucociliary tracheal transport rates in man. *J Appl Physiol* 1975; **39:** 487–495.

43. Pavia D. Lung mucociliary clearance. In: Clarke S W, Pavia D, eds. *Aerosols and the Lung.* Boston: Butterworths, 1984; 127–155.

44. Laitinen L A, Laitinen A, Heino M. Airway hyperresponsiveness, epithelial disruption, and epithelial inflammation. In: Farmer S G, Hay D W P, eds. *The Airway Epithelium.* New York: Marcel Dekker, 1991; 187–211.

45. Munakata M, Mitzner W. The protective role of the airway epithelium. In: Farmer S G, Hay D W P, eds. *The Airway Epithelium.* New York: Marcel Dekker, 1991; 545–564.

46. Barnes P J. Interaction between airway epithelium and peptides. In: Farmer S G, Hay D W P, eds. *The Airway Epithelium.* New York: Marcel Dekker, 1991; 527–544.

47. Webber S E, Morikawa T, Widdicombe J G. PAF-induced muscarinic cholinoceptor hyperresponsiveness of ferret tracheal smooth muscle and gland secretion in vitro. *Br J Pharmacol* 1992; **105:** 230–237.

48. Morikawa T, Webber S E, Widdicombe J G. The effect of hydrogen peroxide on smooth muscle tone, mucus secretion and epithelial albumin transport of the ferret trachea *in vitro. Pulm Pharmacol* 1991; **2:** 106–113.

49. Hanafi Z, Webber S E, Widdicombe J G. Permeability of the ferret trachea *in vitro* to ^{99m}Tc-DTPA and ^{14}C-antipyrine. *J Appl Physiol* 1994; **77:** 1263–1273.

50. Wells U M, Woods A J, Hanafi Z, *et al.* Tracheal epithelial damage alters tracer fluxes and the effects of tracheal osmolality in sheep *in vivo. J Appl Physiol* 1995; **78:** 1921–1930.

51. Hanafi Z, Wells U M, Widdicombe J G. Effects of epithelial damage on the permeability of the ferret trachea in vitro to ^{14}C-mannitol and ^{14}C-antipyrine. *J Appl Physiol* 1997; In Press.

52. Hogg J C. Mucosal permeability and smooth muscle function in asthma. *Med Clin N Am* 1990; **74:** 731–740.

53. Hulbert V M, Walker D C, Jackson A, *et al.* Airway permeability to horseradish peroxidase in guinea pigs; the repair phase after injury by cigarette smoke. *Am Rev Respir Dis* 1981; **123:** 320–326.

54. Tuomanen E, Hendley J O. Adherence of *Bordetella pertussis* to human respiratory epithelial cells. *J Infect Dis* 1983; **148:** 125–130.

55. Bredt W, Feldner J, Klauss B. Adherence of Mycoplasmas: phenomena and possible role in the pathogenesis of disease. *Infection* 1982; **10:** 199–202.

56. Plotkowski M C, Beck G, Tournier J M, *et al.* Adherence of *Pseudomonas aeruginosa* to respiratory epithelium and the effect of leucocyte elastase. *J Med Microbiol* 1989; **30:** 285–293.

57. Feldman C, Read R C, Rutman A, *et al.* Interaction of *Streptococcus pneumoniae* with human respiratory epithelium *in vitro. Am Rev Respir Dis* 1990; **141:** 335.

58. Ramphal R, Pyle M. Adherence of mucoid and nonmucoid *Pseudomonas aeruginosa* to acid-injured tracheal epithelium. *Infect Immun* 1983; **41:** 345–351.

2

Soluble Proteins in Lung Defence

ROBERT A. STOCKLEY

Queen Elizabeth Hospital, Birmingham, UK

INTRODUCTION

Proteins have been recognised as components of lung secretions for many years. Early studies using paper electrophoresis confirmed that several distinct protein bands were present in the secretions. Some were recognised as plasma proteins and some were unique to the lung. However, the factors that control the concentrations of these proteins in the lung secretions and their role in lung defence have been poorly studied. At present, in excess of 50 soluble proteins have been identified in lung secretions. Some, like albumin, are invariably present, whereas others may only be identified in the presence of established disease as they become "switched on" as part of the lung's response. Thus, at present, the study of the role of soluble proteins in lung defence is still going through the learning phase. Proteins are identified as absent or present only when they are specifically sought as part of the study of disease processes. More subtle changes, including modulation of protein concentrations and function, remain largely to be explored to determine the role of many of these proteins in the pathogenesis of lung disease.

With these reservations, however, it remains clear that many of the proteins identified within the lung secretions are relevant to its defence. This chapter summarises some of the factors that influence protein concentrations in the lung secretions and their potential roles.

THE SOURCE OF BRONCHIAL PROTEINS

Bronchial proteins have several potential sources. They may be derived solely from plasma as protein diffusing into the lung, or be entirely made locally within the lung tissue. In addition, some may come from both a lung and a plasma

Pulmonary Defences. Edited by Robert A. Stockley.
© 1997 John Wiley & Sons Ltd.

                                R. A. *Stockley*

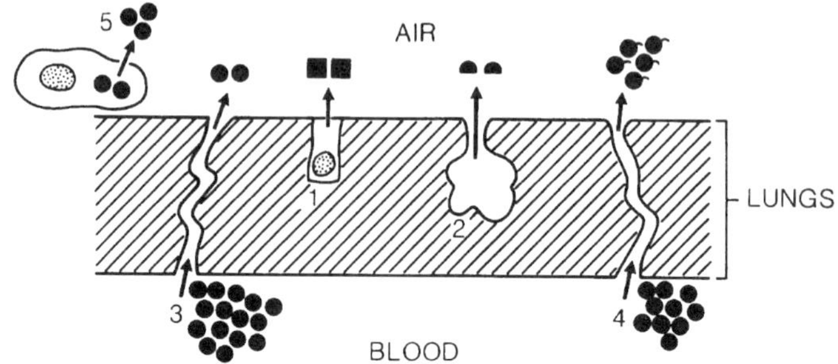

Figure 2.1. Potential sources of bronchial proteins. 1, 2 = Proteins made exclusively by bronchial epithelial cells or mucus glands, respectively; 3 = proteins derived from plasma by diffusion; 4 = selective transport mechanism for plasma proteins; 5 = local production of proteins also present in the plasma. Adapted from Stockley[5]

source, and there may be cells that normally circulate but may on occasions be recruited to the lung (neutrophils, monocytes, eosinophils, *etc.*). The factors which influence the concentrations of these various proteins will clearly depend upon their source and the pathological state of the lungs. Figure 2.1 summarises the potential source of bronchial proteins.

Plasma Derived

Many of the plasma proteins, including albumin, transferrin, haptoglobin and $\alpha_1$antitrypsin (α_1AT), are found within bronchial secretions[1]. These proteins are believed to diffuse from the pulmonary vasculature between both endothelial and epithelial cells. Although pinocytosis has been suggested as a mechanism, the concentration of many of these proteins is partly determined by their molecular size. Indeed, the larger plasma proteins such as $\alpha_2$macroglobulin (725 000 Da) are present (if at all) only at low concentrations in the healthy lung[2]. However, inflammatory conditions as diverse as adult respiratory distress syndrome (ARDS)[3] or sarcoid[4], in which size restriction is apparent, result in detectable levels. Thus the data would suggest that for some plasma proteins the lung seems to act as a filter, resulting in differential diffusion dependent upon their molecular size[1], whereas in the presence of inflammation the normal restriction of movement of larger proteins seems partially lost[1].

In addition to their size, the plasma concentration of the respective proteins will also influence the secretion levels. For instance, the increase in the concentrations of acute phase proteins during inflammation will also increase their respective concentrations in the lung. Thus, in summary, the concentration of plasma proteins in the lung is dependent upon the plasma concentration, molecular size and degree of lung inflammation[5].

"Local Lung Production"

Sometimes the concentration of a plasma protein is greater in the lung secretions than can be accounted for by simple diffusion from plasma (taking into account its size and plasma concentration). This suggests that "local mecha-nisms" exist to enhance the concentration in lung secretions. This may possibly reflect a local transport mechanism (as for secretory IgA) or that the protein is, at least in part, locally produced by lung cells. The source may include all cells found regularly or acutely in the lung (epithelial cells, type I and type II, pneu-mocytes, macrophages, lymphocytes and other inflammatory cells). For instance, the concentration of the plasma proteinase α_1 antichymotrypsin (α_1 ACh) is greater in lung secretions than would be predicted by diffusion from plasma[1]. Immuno-histochemistry has shown that macrophages contain the protein and do produce it[6], and hence are likely to be a source of local products.

Finally, some proteins may be virtually confined to the lung, other mucosal surfaces, or both. They may be constitutionally expressed (in addition to being subject to local modulation), as is the case for secretory leukoprotease inhibitor (SLPI) or produced only after appropriate stimulation (chemoattractants and cytokines).

PROBLEMS IN ASSESSING THE ROLE OF BRONCHIAL PROTEINS

Although it is possible to measure the concentration of proteins in bronchial secre-tions, the interpretation of the result is far from straightforward. The measurement itself may be influenced by antigenic alteration of the protein compared with the standard used for quantification. For instance, secretory IgA consists of two molecules joined by the J chain and bound to secretory component, and hence cannot be assessed accurately using a plasma IgA standard. Furthermore, there are also differences between the secretion and plasma proportions of the subclasses IgA1 and IgA2[7] that may also affect immunological measurement. In addition, some proteins may undergo major conformational change in the lung, as is seen for α_1 AT after interaction with enzymes[8] that will alter its antigenicity and hence may also alter its measurement immunologically.

Some proteins are likely to undergo active catabolism within the lung secre-tions, including uptake by inflammatory cells. Hence the balance between produc-tion and catabolism will also affect the concentration in the lung (although similar processes also affect plasma proteins). In addition, the proteins may be partitioned in the secretion. Some proteins may be cell associated (as for chemoattractants and other receptor ligands) and others may be partly localised to bronchial mucus. Thus the concentration in the soluble phase of the secretions may underestimate their actual quantity in the lung.

Finally, the concentration will depend upon the volume of secretion itself. Fluid and electrolyte shifts and mucus production will influence the volume of airways secretion, as will the harvesting technique[9]. Many techniques have been adopted to overcome this last problem of dilution during harvesting, although none is without its own drawbacks.

The simplest techniques involve comparison of protein measurements with an internal standard such as albumin or total protein[5]. However, although this may be useful for proteins such as α_1 AT when compared with albumin, it is inappropriate for proteins of different sizes, particularly when there is an element of local production or accumulation[5], unless these factors are also taken into account (Fig. 2.2).

 R. A. Stockley

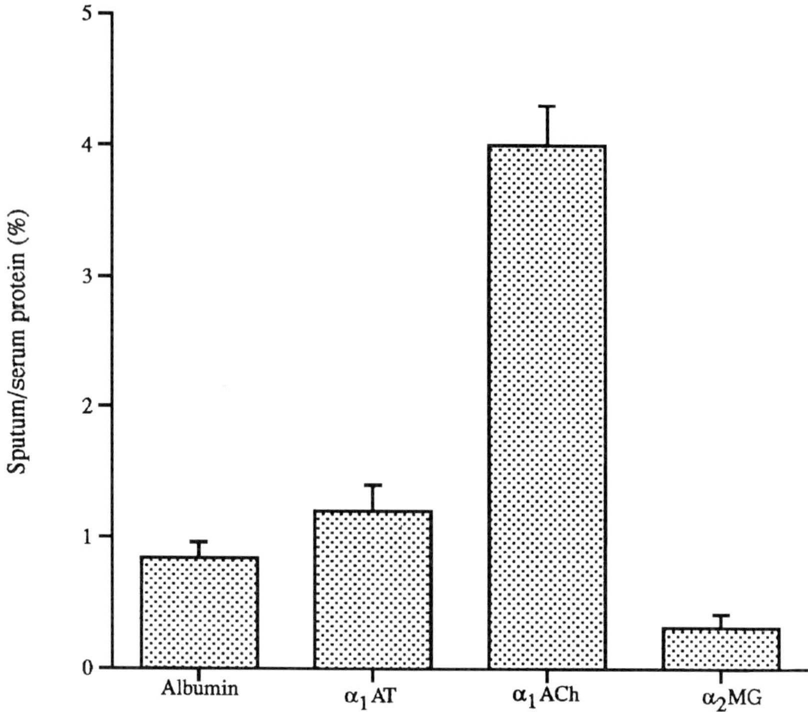

Figure 2.2. Secretion proteins expressed as a percentage of the plasma concentration. Representative value for α_1 antitrypsin (α_1AT), α_1 antichymotrypsin (α_1ACh) and α_2 macroglobulin (α_2MG) are shown in comparison with albumin. Data derived from Stockley *et al.*[1]

More recently, attempts have been made to determine the exact volume of the lung secretions harvested by measurement of the urea concentration[10]. It is argued that urea is freely diffusable and hence its secretion and plasma concentrations should be similar. Thus measurement of urea in the harvested sample (usually obtained by bronchoalveolar lavage) will determine the degree of secretion and hence protein dilution[10]. However, even this technique has been challenged, as urea can actively diffuse into the lavage fluid from plasma during harvesting[11].

It could be argued, however, that with all the drawbacks outlined above it may be just as valid to assess the concentrations in the harvested lavage sample alone, especially for proteins produced only in the lung or during inflammation. Alternatively, comparison with albumin may determine whether the concentration of a plasma protein is appropriate for the degree of inflammation alone or whether a significant degree of local production is present. Figure 2.3 shows some hypothetical results for four proteins. In Fig. 2.3A the secretion concentrations are shown in the presence and absence of lung inflammation and in Fig. 2.3B the secretion concentrations are corrected for the plasma concentrations where appropriate. In Fig. 2.3C the secretion/serum ratios of the plasma

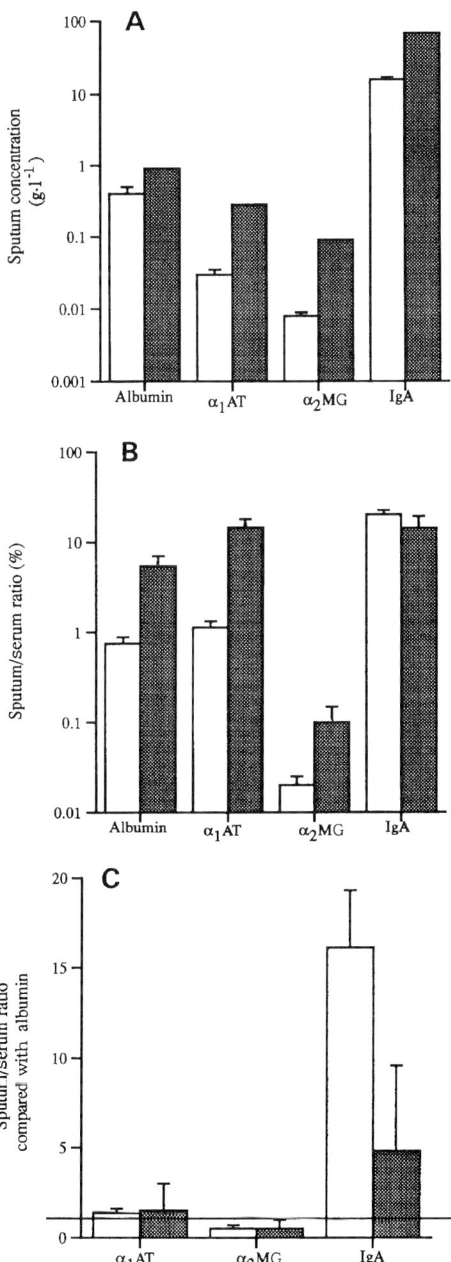

Figure 2.3. Representative results for secretion concentration of albumin, α_1 antitrypsin (α_1AT) α_2 macroglobulin (α_2MG) and IgA.   **A:** Sputum concentration.   **B:** Comparison with the relevant serum concentrations.   **C:** Ratio compared with the corresponding albumin values. The horizontal line equals unity (see text for further explanation). Shaded bars indicate presence of acute inflammation

proteins are compared with those of albumin to indicate those proteins that are locally produced (ratio >1). Note that when the lung is inflamed the protein transudation from plasma may overcome the amount of any protein produced locally. For proteins not present in plasma, comparison or correction for albumin may not be appropriate or necessary.

Once the method (or lack of it) for the measurement of bronchial proteins has been established, it is possible to derive a "normal" range for health. However, the effect of disease and the role of each protein are also difficult to interpret. Changes undoubtedly occur, including increased immunoglobulin production in sarcoid[12] and infections[13], but at present it is impossible to determine whether the changes reflect the disease itself, or are appropriate for the disease or are abnormal, thereby predisposing to the severity, pathogenesis or progression of the disease. Such information can only be determined in retrospect if the disease resolves completely with no lung damage (tissue destruction and fibrosis may represent an abnormal response), or progresses.

These problems of interpretation may currently appear insurmountable, but it is possible to obtain information about some of the protective proteins of the bronchial tree and hence determine factors that may have a role in their modulation to retain health.

PROTECTIVE PROTEINS

PROTEINASE INHIBITORS OF NEUTROPHIL ELASTASE

Proteolytic enzymes usually released from activated inflammatory cells possess the potential to damage and destroy many of the lung tissues. These enzymes have been implicated in the pathogenesis of diseases as diverse as bronchitis, emphysema, bronchiectasis and ARDS. However, several potent inhibitors of these enzymes have been identified in the lung secretions and are believed to play a major part in the protection of lung tissue from the destructive effects of the enzymes.

Studies of the form, function and regulation of the inhibitors have been concentrated on those perceived to be of major importance and this has been determined by those enzymes assumed to be the major mediators of destructive lung disease. In this respect, neutrophil elastase has been implicated in the pathogenesis of most of the diseases outlined above. Thus most research has concentrated on the role of inhibitors of neutrophil elastase.

α_1 Antitrypsin

α_1AT is a 54 000 Da glycoprotein coded for on chromosome 14. It is secreted by hepatocytes and cells of the monocytic lineage[14]. However, although alveolar macrophages are able to produce α_1AT[15], most of the lung protein is believed to derive from plasma by simple transudation.

The concentration of α_1AT in plasma is approximately $2\,\mathrm{g \cdot l^{-1}}$, but this increases during episodes of inflammation, to $4\,\mathrm{g \cdot l^{-1}}$ or more. The concentration in the normal lung is difficult to determine, but levels of $230\,\mathrm{\mu g \cdot l^{-1}}$ have been detected in epithelial lining fluid obtained by bronchoalveolar lavage[16] and $330\,\text{mg·l}^{-1}$ in expectorated bronchial secretions[17].

The protein is the major plasma inhibitor of neutrophil elastase and studies have suggested that this is also true in the secretions of the distal airways[18], although other studies have not confirmed this[19,20]. When the lung is inflamed (episodes in which increased release of elastase is likely to occur from recruited neutrophils), the lung concentration of α_1AT increases, partly as a result of the acute phase increase in plasma and partly as a result of increased protein transudation[17].

Studies of α_1AT function remain controversial. Some suggest that it is fully functional as an inhibitor in the healthy lung[21], which is surprising in view of its lability in the presence of the normal inflammatory cells in the lung. However, other studies have failed to confirm this in healthy subjects[19,20] and suggest that the physical nature of the lung protein differs from that in plasma[20]. Nevertheless, some of the protein remains capable of inhibiting neutrophil elastase[20], and evidence of this interaction is certainly present in the bronchial secretions during infective episodes, indicating that α_1AT does inactivate this potentially harmful enzyme.

The importance of α_1AT as a protective inhibitor is highlighted by the presence of neutrophil elastase related diseases (emphysema, bronchitis and bronchiectasis) in people with inherited α_1AT deficiency[22]. In these subjects the low plasma concentration of α_1AT is reflected in low secretion concentrations[23]. This is believed to reduce the protection of the lung from neutrophil elastase induced lung disease. Nevertheless, the observation that many subjects with α_1AT deficiency remain healthy suggests that alternative mechanisms of protection exist.

Secretory Leukoprotease Inhibitor

Studies in the 1970s identified a low molecular mass (12 kDa) inhibitor of neutrophil elastase in bronchial secretions. This protein was named antileukoprotease (ALP), although recently it has become more widely known as secretory leukoprotease inhibitor (SLPI). The protein is not glycoscylated, and is a potent inhibitor of neutrophil elastase. It is produced locally in the lung by epithelial cells[24] and is present in serous glands[25]. It is the major inhibitor of neutrophil elastase in bronchial secretions[26], accounting for up to 90% of all inhibition. Thus it is probably the most important protective inhibitor of neutrophil elastase, at least in the airways.

Regulation of the production of SLPI is uncertain. Early studies suggested that it was constitutionally expressed and that its production was constant[27]. However, more recent studies have shown that corticosteroids increase its concentration in the bronchial secretions *in vivo*[28] and its production by epithelial cells *in vitro*[29]. Furthermore, its secretion may actually decrease during infection (Fig. 2.4), suggesting negative control also, and recent studies have confirmed that neutrophil proteinases can reduce SLPI secretion by epithelial cells[30].

The role of this protein in the lower airways has been controversial. Early studies suggested that the only inhibitor of neutrophil elastase in the peripheral airways was α_1AT[18]. However, more recently the same group has confirmed that SLPI is present but non-functional[21]. This is at variance with other studies that

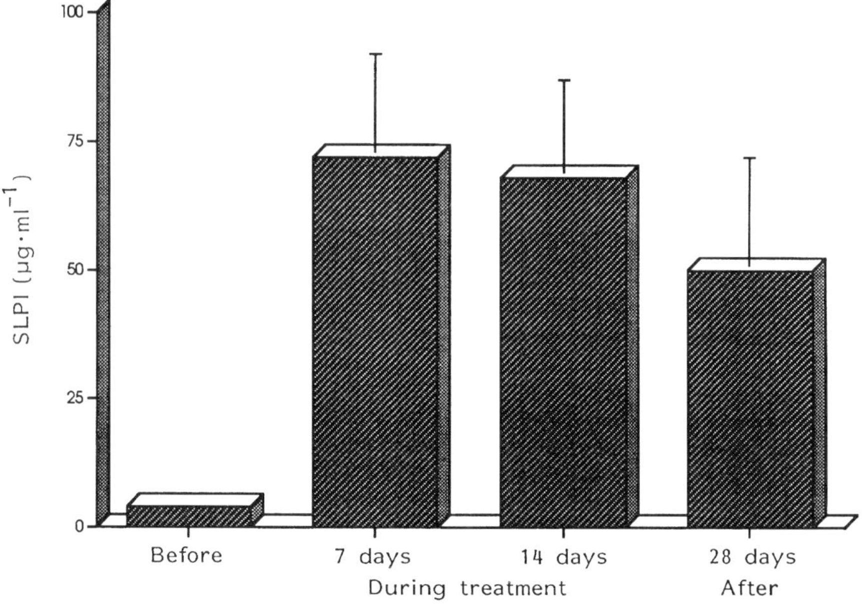

Figure 2.4. The average sputum concentration of secretory leukoprotease inhibitor (SLPI) before, during and after antibiotic treatment for an acute exacerbation of bronchitis. The bars are + 1 SE ($n = 8$)

have not only demonstrated the presence of SLPI in peripheral airways[19], but shown that it is functional[19,20] and can be produced by type II pneumocytes[30], suggesting a role at the alveolar level. Furthermore, SLPI may be secreted from the basolateral surface of epithelial cells[31] and can be identified in the lung interstitium[32], suggesting it may have a protective role there as well as in the airways.

Elafin

Early studies had suggested that at least one other inhibitor of neutrophil elastase was present in lung secretions[28]. Recently elafin, a 7 kDa inhibitor, has been purified and shown to inhibit neutrophil elastase[33]. This protein is also produced locally in the lung by type II pneumocytes[30] and has been identified in secretions[34]. Its role, however, has yet to be identified.

α_2 Macroglobulin

This serum protein is also an inhibitor of neutrophil elastase. However, its large mass (725 000 Da) largely prevents its diffusion into lung secretions unless the lung is inflamed[1]. In view of this restriction and its low serum concentration, it is rarely measurable in normal lung secretions[2], despite the ability of macrophages to produce the protein *in vitro*[35]. Even when present, α_2 macroglobulin contributes little to the lung antineutrophil elastase protection[36], and its role is far from clear.

OTHER ANTIPROTEINASES

α_1 Antichymotrypsin

This protein is a 68 kDa inhibitor of serine proteinases with chymotrypsin-like activity. The best characterised interaction is with neutrophil cathepsin G, which it rapidly inactivates. It has been suggested that the major role of this inhibitor is to protect tissues from cathepsin G activity released by the neutrophil[37].

α_1ACh is present in the plasma, is produced by liver cells and shows a rapid acute phase response, doubling in concentration within 8 h[38]. The protein is present in lung secretions but its concentration is greater than would be predicted by simple diffusion[39], suggesting an active transport system or local production. The protein can be produced by macrophages[6] and is present in bronchial epithelial cells (Stockley, unpublished observations), suggesting that they may be the source of a proportion of lung α_1ACh.

Local production or concentration of α_1ACh suggests it may have a significant role in the protection of the lung. However, little cathepsin G is released into the lung secretions, compared with elastase and, furthermore, lung α_1ACh does not appear to inhibit cathepsin G[40], whereas SLPI and α_1AT (which are present in greater concentrations) can inhibit cathepsin G.

These observations suggest that the form and function of lung α_1ACh may be different from those of the plasma protein[40]. Indeed, studies have suggested that α_1ACh may modulate neutrophil recruitment[41] and antibody dependent cell mediated cytotoxicity[42] — functions which may influence lung damage indirectly. Further studies will be required to clarify these possibilities.

Tissue Inhibitor of Metalloproteinases

Most of the studies of lung proteinase inhibitors have concentrated on the role of inhibitors of serine proteinases, as this class of enzyme has been considered to be the main mediator of tissue damage. However, metalloproteinases (those dependent upon metal ions for their activity) may have a potential role in tissue damage in the lung. The macrophage can secrete at least four metalloproteinases with the capability of degrading several collagen subtypes in addition to fibronectin and even elastin. Recent studies have shown that several subtypes of tissue inhibitor of metalloproteinases (TIMP) also exist, with varying inhibitory profiles; however, they have yet to be studied in the lung in detail.

One early study identified TIMP in lung secretions and its concentration reflected the collagenase inhibitory capacity[43]. This suggests that TIMP may have a role in the protection of lung tissues from damage by collagenolytic enzymes. However, the role of TIMP or its subtypes in the inhibition of other metalloproteinases has yet to be studied. For instance, many pathological bacteria release metalloproteinases that cleave IgA[44] and are believed to play a part in the survival of bacteria in the lung. Whether TIMP or other inhibitors of metalloproteinases can inhibit these enzymes and thereby protect important lung defences remains to be determined.

 R. A. Stockley

Cysteine Proteinase Inhibitors

Even less is known about inhibitors of cysteine proteinases. Bacteria can release them[45], and cathepsin B is present in lung secretions during infective episodes[46]. The source of this particular enzyme may be the macrophages or epithelial cells of the lung[47]. Cathepsin B can produce lesions similar to those of bronchitis[48] and emphysema[49], hence inhibitors of this enzyme would be expected to play a part in protection of tissues from these diseases, and several have indeed been identified in lung secretions[50]. Again, however, few studies have been carried out to date and the true role of cysteine proteinase inhibitors in the protection of the lung remains to be determined.

IMMUNOGLOBULINS

The large surface of the lungs is constantly exposed to inhaled antigens, including viable organisms. Health is maintained by the presence of a highly sophisticated local immune system that interacts constantly with the systemic system (see Chapter 4). Antigen presenting cells interact with localised T cells to generate specific cellular and humoral immunity. The immunoglobulins represent part of this immune response and are readily identified in the lung secretions. The nature and relative proportions of these immunoglobulins differ from those in plasma, confirming that much is made locally within the lung tissues. For instance, in plasma, IgG is the dominant immunoglobulin class, whereas IgA predominates in the upper respiratory tract[51].

Immunoglobulin A

In plasma, most of the IgA is monomeric and 90% is of the IgA1 subclass. However, in the lung most of the IgA is dimeric (as the secretory IgA molecule) and only 70% is of the IgA1 subclass (the remainder being the IgA2 subclass). This distribution is reflected in the type of B cells present. In the lamina propria, 26–33% of the IgA bearing cells stain positively for IgA2, compared with 10–20% in the bone marrow[52].

The immunoglobulins are relatively large molecules (compared with albumin) and transudation from plasma (particularly in health) is therefore limited. Thus most of the immunoglobulins detected in the lung secretions represent those made locally. In addition, there is a special transport system to facilitate passage of dimeric IgA into the lumen of the lung. "Secretory component" is the N-terminal sequence of a transmembrane Fc_α receptor[53]. This is expressed on the basal surface of bronchial epithelial cells and avidly binds dimeric IgA. The complex is internalised by endocytosis, sorted in an endosomal compartment and incorporated into transcytotic vesicles. These vesicles translocate to the apical surface, fuse with the membrane and the amino terminus, with the IgA attached, is cleaved, releasing the secretory IgA molecule (Fig. 2.5).

This complex process probably confers advantages to IgA in performing a protective role in the airway. First, it facilitates movement of the protein into the airway and second, it may stabilise the IgA, permitting it to retain its function. Most pathogenic bacteria secrete proteolytic enzymes with the ability to cleave

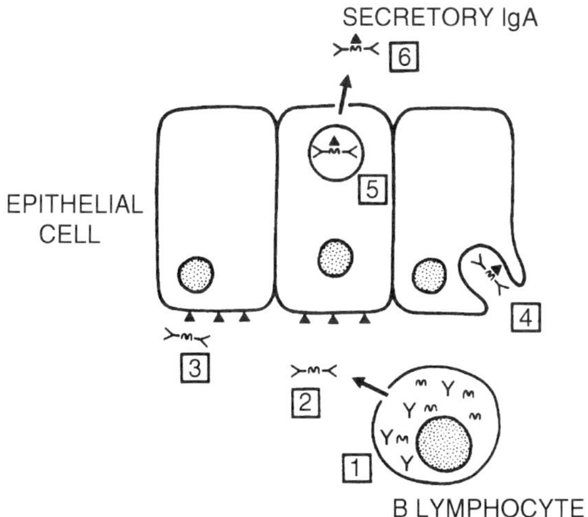

Figure 2.5. Mechanism of secretory IgA transport into secretions. 1 = Production by B lymphocytes in the lung interstitium; 2 = released IgA dimer linked by J chain; 3 = binding to polymeric IgA receptor; 4 = internalisation; 5 = transcellular transport; 6 = cleavage of receptor and release of secretory IgA molecule. Reproduced from Stockley RA (in *Respiratory Medicine*; Brevis RAL, ed. 1990), with permission of WB Saunders

specifically the heavy chain of IgA at a Pro–Thr bond in the hinge region. This would separate the IgA heavy chain from the Fab portion, inactivating it as an opsonin. Secretory component restricts the access of these proteinases to the heavy chain, thereby protecting the molecule. In addition, secretory component can stabilise the IgA2 antibody[54], which tends to dissociate spontaneously. This may also have an advantageous effect, as IgA2 is resistant to cleavage by these bacterial proteolytic enzymes.

The function of secretory IgA is only partly understood and has been the subject of some controversy. The dimeric form of the protein has four antigen binding sites that can prevent the epithelial adherence of bacteria and viruses. However, the joining of the two Fc regions by J chain and the presence of secretory component would be expected to interfere with the ability of the immunoglobulin to activate complement or act as an opsonin. Nevertheless, some studies have shown that secretory IgA can enhance macrophage phagocytosis[55] in addition to stimulating antibody dependent cell mediated cytotoxicity in synergism with IgG[56], indicating an ability to interact with other arms of the immune system.

Despite these studies, the role of IgA in the lung has to be inferred from indirect studies including animal experiments. IgA antibody levels increase after local administration of antigen, whereas this does not occur following systemic challenge[57]. However, some studies have indicated that antigens administered orally can afford protection to the lung[58], suggesting a close link between the gastrointestinal and lung immune systems (see Chapter 4). The response (when achieved) may last up to three years[59], suggesting long lived and specific protection to the airway.

The IgA system shows an adaptive response in the presence of chronic lung disease. First, the concentrations of IgA in secretions may increase, especially in the presence of an acute infection[60] when increased leakage of plasma IgA occurs. However, in addition, studies have shown an increase in the number of IgA-bearing plasma cells (both IgA1 and IgA2) in the presence of chronic bronchitis and chronic bronchial infection[52]. Whether this adaptive change is appropriate but ineffective, or insufficient, has yet to be determined.

Immunoglobulin G

Immunoglobulin G (subclasses 1–4) is regularly identified in the lung secretions of healthy subjects[61] in addition to those with lung disease[62]. Unlike lung IgA, the IgG seems to be quantitatively similar to plasma IgG. Plasma cells bearing IgG are present in the lung, suggesting that a proportion is locally synthesised in both health and disease although, again, some is derived from the plasma. In healthy lungs, IgG predominates in the lower airways[61] and the concentration of all subclasses is greater than that predicted for diffusion from plasma alone, supporting the concept that a small proportion is produced locally. Indeed, studies from normal subjects have confirmed active synthesis of immunoglobulins by interstitial lymphocytes, although not those free in the airways[63]. In contrast, in the upper airways IgA predominates, suggesting that IgG has a lesser role in the primary defence of the lung at this site.

Indeed, evidence would suggest that IgG plays a more important part in secondary defence in the lung. First, inflammation results in an increase in IgG transudation from the plasma. This may be important, as animal studies have shown that bacterial proliferation can be prevented in the lung by simultaneous administration of specific IgG systematically, and its subsequent movement into the lung secretions[64]. Second, the proportion of IgG subclasses produced locally in the lung is increased in patients with chronic lung disease and bacterial colonisation[62]. These subjects also show an increase in lung B cells[65], suggesting that chronic immune stimulation may result in a secondary expansion of these cells and hence their products.

Once IgG is present in the secretions, its ability to opsonise bacteria and activate complement appears to be crucial. The importance of these processes has been intimated indirectly by studies in patients with cystic fibrosis. The secretions of patients with cystic fibrosis are often colonised with *Pseudomonas aeruginosa*, even in the presence of a highly active immune system. It has been suggested that the organism survives because of two mechanisms. First, *Pseudomonas* releases proteases that can cleave IgG into its Fab and Fc portions[66], resulting in fragments which bind bacteria through the Fab fragment but do not link to complement or the Fc receptor on cells. Second, the IgG subclass in the secretions is predominantly IgG2[67]. It is believed that binding of this antibody to bacterial antigens blocks effective binding of the other subclasses such as IgG3 and IgG4, which are more effective opsonins.

These studies indicate that the production of ineffective IgG or the wrong subclass can prove detrimental in the defence of the lung. Nevertheless, IgG remains crucial to the maintenance of health. Subjects with

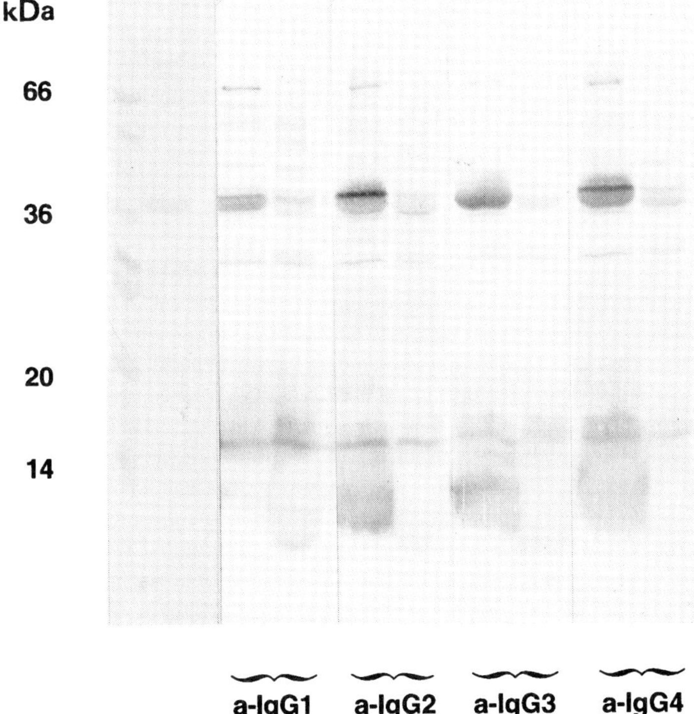

Figure 2.6. Outer membrane protein profiles from two strains of *Haemophilus influenzae* blotted onto nitrocellulose and incubated with secretions obtained from the respective patient. Immunoglobulin binding to antigen was identified with peroxidase labelled anti-human IgG (a-IgG) subclass antibodies as shown. The patients' antibodies of all four IgG subclasses bind to several bacterial antigens. (Gel kindly provided by JL Mitchell)

panhypogammaglobulinaemia suffer from recurrent respiratory tract infections. In addition, subjects with more subtle defects including IgG2 and IgG4 deficiency[68] or deficiency of IgG2 or IgG3 with IgA deficiency[69] also suffer from recurrent respiratory tract infections. Furthermore, some patients may have antigen specific deficiency even though the total immunoglobulin concentration may appear normal[70]. Bacteria express many potential antigens and these promote an antibody response (Fig. 2.6). However, it is not known which antigen or antigens are important in bacterial clearance by the immune system. As our understanding of the role of these bacterial antigens develops, the interaction with the immune system will become clarified. Thereafter, it should be possible to determine how the antibody response is critical in lung defence and whether subtle antigen specific defects account for recurrent respiratory tract infections.

Other Immunoglobulins

The roles of other immunoglobulins in lung defence are even less certain. IgM is regularly found in lung secretions despite its size, indicating significant local production. Its role, however, may be limited to the vascular space, although it has been suggested that IgM may replace IgA in the protection of the airways in subjects with IgA deficiency[71]. IgD is present in secretions at low concentrations, but its role in both the lung and plasma remains uncertain. Finally, IgE is also present in the lung secretions. Its role may be limited to activation of mast cells as a result of cross linking of antigens. This may have a crucial role in defence against metazoan parasites[72].

COMPLEMENT

Many proteins from the complement system have been identified in lung secretions. Factors C4 and C1q from the classic pathway are occasionally found, whereas factor B from the alternative pathway and C3 and C6 of the classic pathway are invariably present. Most of the complement components can be synthesised by alveolar macrophages. It is generally believed, however, that the majority of the complement factors in secretions are derived by diffusion from plasma during the secondary inflammatory response. Early activation of small amounts of C3 and C5 in the secretions may nevertheless have a crucial role in the establishment of the inflammatory process. Macrophages and bacteria possess the ability to split C3 and C5 into their active components, C3a, C3b and C5a. Of these, C3a and C5a are markedly chemotactic for neutrophils, monocytes and eosinophils and provide a major stimulus to the recruitment of those cells. The active components have been readily identified in the secretions of patients with a variety of inflammatory lung conditions. In addition, C3b is a non-specific stimulant of antibody formation, lymphokine production and antibody dependent cellular cytotoxicity, and C5a also possesses opsonic activity.

As inflammation develops, recruitment of other complement components from plasma results in activation of the complement cascade. C567 complexes may further enhance chemotaxis and as the later components, C8 and C9, bind they result in cell and bacterial lysis.

The importance of complement components is highlighted by the effect of deficiencies of the individual components. Mice with genetic deficiency of C5 are unable to clear bacteria efficiently from the lung unless this component is given exogenously[73]. Deficiency of C2 is the most common complement deficiency diagnosed in humans and is often associated with collagen vascular disease. Few patients have recurrent infections, although there is an increased susceptibility to septicaemia[74]. This suggests that the classic complement pathway is most important in removal of bacteria from the vascular space and is of less importance in the lung. Complement C3 has a key role in both the classic and alternative pathways. Activation of C3 results in the production of two active fragments: C3a which is a chemotactic factor and anaphyltoxin, and C3b which is an opsonin acting via specific receptors on phagocytes, but also binds factor B which activates the alternative pathway. Patients with deficiency of C3 have recurrent infections with many organisms, including *Streptococcus pneumoniae* and *Haemophilus influenzae*. These often affect the upper and lower respiratory tract. This suggests that the alternative pathway of complement activation is the most important one in the protection of the respiratory tract. Nevertheless, studies of complement components in the pathogenesis of acute and chronic lung infections remain in their infancy and their true role remains to be clarified.

BACTERIOSTATIC OR BACTERICIDAL PROTEINS

Lung secretions contain several proteins that may influence bacterial viability and proliferation by a non-immune mechanism. These include the iron binding proteins, lactoferrin and transferrin, that may reduce the availability of elemental iron which is a cofactor for bacterial replication. However, in addition, lactoferrin may also be bactericidal by binding to endotoxin[75], particularly in the presence of lysozyme.

Lysozyme is a muramidase that degrades a glycosidic linkage of bacterial membrane peptidoglycan[75]. It is regularly found in lung secretions and, when purified, it demonstrates bactericidal properties[76]. It may be derived from many sources, including epithelial cells, serous cells of submucosal glands, macrophages and neutrophils. Indeed, it is released from neutrophils at the same time as lactoferrin and this may be critical in view of their synergistic activity[75]. Their role in primary defence of the lung in the absence of inflammatory cell infiltration remains less certain.

CYTOKINES

Most metabolically active cells of the immune system possess the potential to secrete peptides with the ability to activate themselves or other cells. These activating peptides or cytokines include proteins such as the interleukins, interferons, tumour necrosis factor, colony stimulating factors and the chemotaxins. These are often thought of as the chemical mediators of inflammation and its resolution. Few of these agents are constitutively expressed, but can be rapidly manufactured as required. Consequently, they are rarely found in significant quantities in normal bronchial fluids. When they are required and are rapidly produced, their activity is carefully regulated at several levels. First, they are usually produced in response to a new signal that affects gene transcription. The resultant mRNA has a specific signal (multiple adenine uracil nucleotides) at the 3′ end which shortens its half life[77], and thus removal of the initiating signal results in rapid disappearance of the mRNA and hence the cytokine. Second, many cytokines are manufactured as precursor proteins which have to be cleaved to release the active form. Finally, the target cell receptor can also be regulated to influence its response.

Cytokines usually act over short distances and bind to target cells. Few are detected in the plasma unless highly sensitive assays are used and few have distant effects. They function in three ways:

(i)   Cell–cell communication: the cytokine remains on the surface of its cell of origin and results in close contact with a receptor bearing cell.

(ii) Autocrine: the cytokine activates its cell of origin.

(iii) Paracrine: the cytokine binds to and activates nearby cells.

Clearly, the detection of cytokines in bronchial secretion depends upon release of the cytokine and this largely reflects paracrine function.

The assessment of cytokines has taken two forms in respiratory disease: either the assessment of mRNA expression by respiratory cells, or the assay of the free cytokine. Each approach has its merits, but it should not be assumed that they are synonymous. The presence of mRNA does not necessarily indicate production of its product, and release of the product does not indicate its function. This latter statement is particularly apt, as cytokines can even demonstrate diametrically opposed function and may have their effects influenced by other cytokines. For instance, transforming growth factor β stimulates fibroblasts to grow in the presence of platelet derived growth factor, but inhibits this growth in the presence of epidermal growth factor[78].

With these reservations, it seems likely that tissue homeostatic mechanisms are controlled by cytokine cascades and networks[79]. Thus the cytokine content of the lung secretions will vary depending upon the disease process and its evaluation and resolution. There are several reviews on the role of cytokines and their receptors[80,81] and it would be inappropriate here to do more than touch upon this complex phenomenon. Their importance in the protection of the lung is poorly understood, but it is believed that chemoattractants are critical in the recruitment of secondary phagocytic cells in lung defence. In particular, the role of interleukin-8 (IL-8) has been the subject of recent study and is believed to be a major chemoattractant for lung neutrophils.

IL-8 is a 16 kDa protein that is a member of the C-X-C family of cytokines. It is made by bronchial epithelial cells[82], monocytes/macrophages[83] and even the

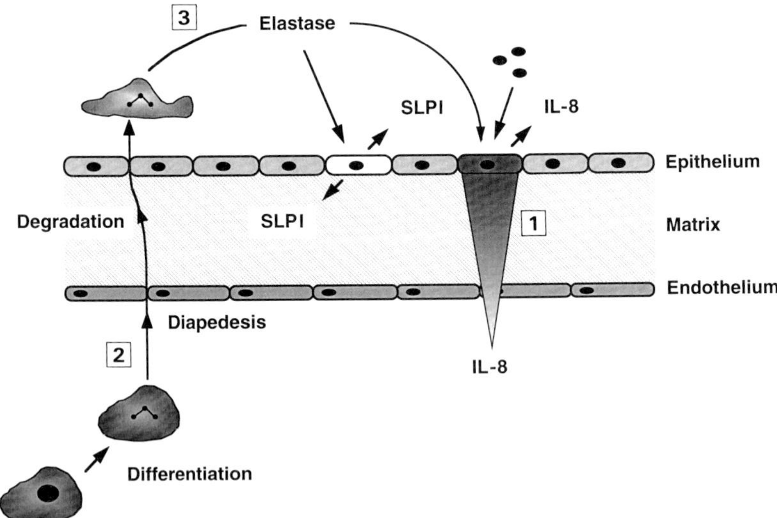

Figure 2.7. Putative potentiating circle of neutrophil recruitment. 1 = Release of interleukin-8 (IL-8) by epithelial cells in response to bacterial antigen; 2 = neutrophil recruitment; 3 = release of neutrophil elastase resulting in further IL-8 production. SLPI = Secretory leukoprotease inhibitor

neutrophils themselves[84]. IL-8 is identified within bronchoalveolar lavage fluids[85] and its concentration may be as high as $10\,\text{nmol·l}^{-1}$ in bronchial secretions from patients with major neutrophil influx[86]. The regulation of IL-8 is becoming clarified. It is known that tumour necrosis factor α can increase the expression of the IL-8 gene[87], but whether this is a major mechanism in the lung remains to be clarified. Perhaps of more relevance is the recent demonstration that bacteria can induce IL-8 expression by epithelial cells[87,88]. This would clearly represent a mechanism to "switch on" the secondary host defences. The presence of excessive numbers of bacteria would induce IL-8 production, which in turn would lead to neutrophil recruitment in order to phagocytose and kill the organism. Indeed, the process may become amplified by the neutrophils themselves, as they can also secrete IL-8, and as they become activated and release their proteolytic enzymes these can also induce epithelial cell IL-8 production[82]. This process can become

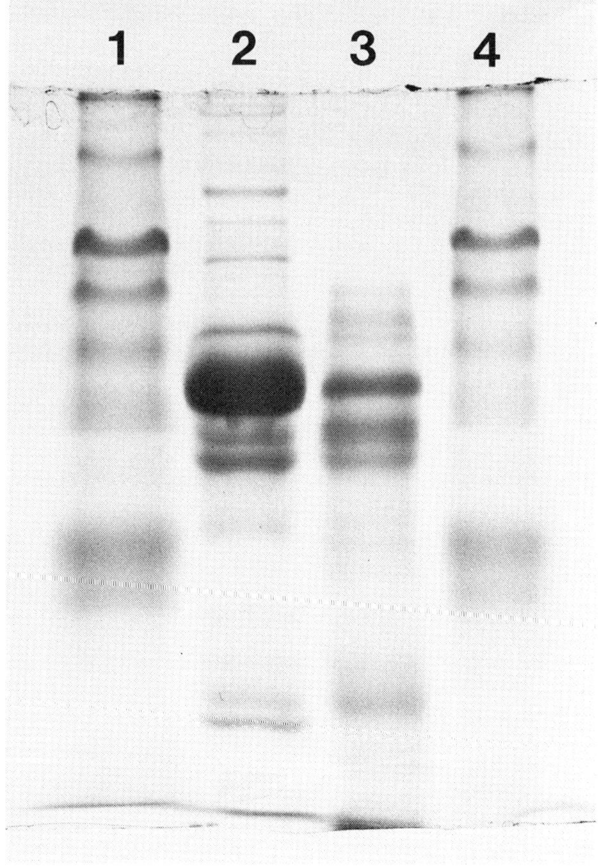

Figure 2.8. Sodium dodecyl sulphate polyacrylamide gel of major protein bands in sputum (lane 3) compared with serum (lane 2). Standard size markers are included in lanes 1 and 4

self-perpetuating, resulting in continued neutrophil influx and further IL-8 release (Fig. 2.7, p. 32). However, in most instances the process is short lived and hence there must also exist mechanisms to reverse the process, although these have yet to be identified.

The study of cytokines is in its infancy. The intermittent nature of their release, their low concentrations and their varied effects make their role difficult to pursue. However, because of their major effects on cell recruitment and activation they will be key factors in the defence of the lung.

In summary, the bronchial secretions contain many proteins, although perhaps fewer and in lower concentrations than in plasma (Fig. 2.8, p. 33). There are several that appear to be unique to the secretions and many that appear to be present intermittently. The role of those proteins in the protection of the lung is only partly understood, but deficiencies occur and are related to lung damage, suggesting a major role for some. Others may be intermittently expressed and further studies are necessary to define their role in the pathogenesis of lung disease.

REFERENCES

1. Stockley R A, Mistry M, Bradwell A R, *et al*. A study of plasma proteins in the sol phase of sputum from patients with chronic bronchitis. *Thorax* 1979; **34:** 777–782.
2. Warr G A, Russell Martin R, Sharp P M, *et al*. Normal human bronchial immunoglobulins and proteins: effects of cigarette smoking. *Am Rev Respir Dis* 1977; **116:** 25–30.
3. Holter J F, Weiland J E, Pacht E R, *et al*. Protein permeability in the adult respiratory distress syndrome. Loss of size selectivity of the alveolar epithelium. *J Clin Invest* 1986; **78:** 1513–1523.
4. Delacroix D L, Marchandise F X, Francis C, *et al*. Alpha-2-macroglobulin, monomeric and polymeric immunoglobulin A and immunoglobulin M in bronchoalveolar lavage. *Am Rev Respir Dis* 1985; **133:** 829–835.
5. Stockley R A. Measurement of soluble proteins in lung secretions. *Thorax* 1984; **39:** 241–247.
6. Burnett D, McGillivray D H, Stockley R A. Evidence that alveolar macrophages can synthesise and secrete α_1-antichymotrypsin. *Am Rev Respir Dis* 1984; **125:** 473–476.
7. Burnett D, Hill S L, Bradwell A R, Stockley R A. IgA subclasses in sputum from patients with bronchiectasis. *Respir Med* 1990; **84:** 123–127.
8. Stockley R A, Afford S C. Qualitative studies of lung lavage α_1-proteinase inhibitor. *Hoppe-Seylers Z Physiol Chem* 1984; **365:** 503–510.
9. Wiggins J, Hill S L, Stockley R A. Lung secretions sol phase proteins: comparison with secretions obtained by direct sampling. *Thorax* 1983; **38:** 102–107.
10. Rennard S, Basset G, Leossier D, *et al*. Estimation of the absolute volume of epithelial lining fluid recovered by bronchoalveolar lavage using urea as an endogenous marker of dilution. *J Appl Physiol* 1986; **60:** 532–538.
11. Marcy T W, Merrill W M, Rankin J A, *et al*. Limitations of using urea to quantify epithelial lining fluid recovered by bronchoalveolar lavage. *Am Rev Respir Dis* 1987; **135:** 1276–1280.
12. Rankin J A, Naegel G P, Schrader C E. Air-space immunoglobulin production and levels in bronchoalveolar lavage fluid of normal subjects and patients with sarcoidosis. *Am Rev Respir Dis* 1983; **127:** 442–448.
13. Stockley R A, Burnett D. Local IgA production in patients with chronic bronchitis: the effect of acute respiratory infection. *Thorax* 1980; **35:** 202–206.
14. Perlmutter D H, May L T, Sehgal P B. Interferon β_2/interleukin 6 modulates synthesis of α_1-antitrypsin in human mononuclear phagocytes and in human hepatoma cells. *J Clin Invest* 1989; **84:** 138–144.

15. Barbey-Morel C, Pierce J A, Campbell E J, *et al*. Lipopolysaccharide modulates the expression of α_1 proteinase inhibitor and other serine proteinase inhibitors in human monocytes and macrophages. *J Exp Med* 1987; **166:** 1041–1054.

16. Hubbard R C, Ogushi F, Fells G A, *et al*. Oxidants spontaneously released by alveolar macrophages of cigarette smokers can inactivate the active site of α_1-antitrypsin, rendering it ineffective as an inhibitor of neutrophil elastase. *J Clin Invest* 1987; **80:** 1289–1295.

17. Stockley R A, Burnett D. Alpha$_1$-antitrypsin and leukocyte elastase in infected and non-infected sputum. *Am Rev Respir Dis* 1979; **120:** 1081–1086.

18. Gadek J E, Fells G A, Zimmerman R L, *et al*. Antielastases of the human alveolar structures. Implications for the protease-antiprotease theory of emphysema. *J Clin Invest* 1981; **68:** 889–898.

19. Boudier C, Pelletier A, Pauli G, *et al*. The functional activity of α_1-proteinase inhibitor in bronchoalveolar lavage fluids from healthy human smokers and non smokers. *Clin Chim Acta* 1983; **132:** 309–315.

20. Afford S C, Burnett D, Campbell E J, *et al*. The assessment of α_1-proteinase inhibitor form and function in lung lavage fluid from healthy subjects. *Biol Chem Hoppe Seyler* 1988; **369:** 1065–1074.

21. Vogelmeier C, Hubbard R C, Fells G A, *et al*. Anti-neutrophil elastase defence of the normal human respiratory epithelial surface provided by the secretory leukoprotease inhibitor. *J Clin Invest* 1991; **87:** 482–488.

22. Stockley R A. The pathogenesis of chronic obstructive lung diseases: implications for therapy. *Q J Med* 1995; **88:** 141–146.

23. Morrison H M, Kramps J A, Burnett D, *et al*. Lung lavage fluid from patients with alpha-1-proteinase inhibitor deficiency or chronic obstructive bronchitis: antielastase function and cell profile. *Clin Sci* 1987; **72:** 373–381.

24. Maruyama M, Hay J G, Yoshimura K, *et al*. Modulation of secretory leukoprotease inhibitor gene expression in human bronchial epithelial cells by phorbol ester. *J Clin Invest* 1994; **94:** 368–375.

25. Mooren H W D, Kramps J A, Franken C, *et al*. Localisation of a low molecular weight bronchial protease inhibitor in the human peripheral lung. *Thorax* 1983; **38:** 180–183.

26. Morrison H M, Kramps J A, Afford S C, *et al*. Elastase inhibitors in sputum from bronchitic patients with and without alpha$_1$-proteinase inhibitor deficiency: partial characterization of a hitherto unquantified inhibitor of neutrophil elastase. *Clin Sci* 1987; **73:** 19–28.

27. Dijkman J H, Kramps J A, Franken C. Antileukoprotease in sputum during bronchial infections. *Chest* 1986; **89:** 731–736.

28. Stockley R A, Morrison H M, Kramps J A, *et al*. Elastase inhibitors of sputum sol phase: variability, relationship to neutrophil elastase and the effect of corticosteroids. *Thorax* 1986; **41:** 442–447.

29. Abbinante-Nissen J M, Simpson L G, Keikauf G D. Corticosteroids increase secretory leukocyte protease inhibitor transcript levels in airway epithelial cells. *Am J Respir Crit Care Med* 1994; **149:** A869.

30. Sallenave J-M, Shulmann J, Crossley J, *et al*. Regulation of secretory leukocyte proteinase inhibitor (SLPI) and elastase-specific inhibitor (ESI/Elafin) in human airway epithelial cells by cytokines and neutrophilic enzymes. *Am J Respir Cell Mol Biol* 1994; **11:** 733–741.

31. Dupuit F, Jacquot J, Spilmont C, *et al*. Vectorial delivery of newly-synthesised proteins by human tracheal gland cells in culture. *Epith Cell Biol* 1993; **2:** 91–99.

32. Willems L N A, Otto-Verberne C J M, Kramps J A, *et al*. Detection of anti-leukoprotease in connective tissue of the lung. *Histochemistry*, 1986; **86:** 165–168.

33. Sallenave J-M, Marsden M D, Ryle A P. Isolation of elafin and elastase-specific inhibitor (ESI) from bronchial secretions. *Biol Chem Hoppe Seyler* 1992; **373:** 27–33.

34. Sallenave J-M, Israel-Assayag E, Dakhama A, *et al*. Elafin and secretory leukocyte proteinase inhibitor in bronchoalveolar lavage fluid of farmer's lung. *Am Rev Respir Dis* 1994; **4:** A867.

35. White R, Habicht G S, Godfrey H P, *et al*. Secretion of elastase and alpha-2-macroglobulin by cultured murine peritoneal macrophages: studies on their interaction. *J Lab Clin Med* 1981; **97:** 718–728.

36. Stockley R A. Antielastases in lung lavage from patients with emphysema. In: Taylor J C, Mittman C, eds. *Pulmonary Emphysema and Proteolysis, 1986*. Orlando: Academic Press, 1987; 277–282.

37. Beatty K, Bieth J, Travis J. Kinetics of association of serine proteinases with native and oxidised alpha-1-proteinase inhibitor and alpha-1-antichymotrypsin. *J Biol Chem* 1980; **255:** 3931–3934.

38. Aronsen K F, Ekelund G, Kindmark C O, *et al*. Sequential changes of plasma proteins after surgical trauma. *Scand J Clin Lab Invest* 1972; **29** (suppl)**:** 127–136.

39. Stockley R A, Burnett D. Alpha$_1$-antichymotrypsin in infected and non-infected sputum. *Am Rev Respir Dis* 1980; **122:** 81–88.

40. Berman G, Afford S C, Burnett D, *et al*. α-1-Antichymotrypsin in lung secretions is *not* an effective proteinase inhibitor. *J Biol Chem* 1986; **261:** 14094–14099.

41. Stockley R A, Shaw J, Afford S C, *et al*. Effect of alpha-1-proteinase inhibitor on neutrophil chemotaxis. *Am J Respir Cell Mol Biol* 1990; **2:** 163–170.

42. Gravagna P, Gianazza E, Arnaud P, *et al*. Modulation of the immune response by plasma protease inhibitors. III. Alpha-1-antichymotrypsin inhibits human natural killing and antibody-dependent cell-mediated cytotoxicity. *J Reticuloendothel Soc* 1982; **32:** 125–130.

43. Burnett D, Reynolds J J, Ward R V, *et al*. Tissue inhibitor of metalloproteinase (TIMP) and collagenase inhibitory activity in sputum from patients with chronic obstructive bronchitis: the effect of corticosteroid therapy. *Thorax* 1986; **41:** 740–745.

44. Kilian M, Mestecky J, Kulhavy R, *et al*. IgA proteases from *Haemophilus influenzae, Streptococcus pneumoniae, Neisseriae meningitidis* and *Streptococcus sangus:* comparative immunochemical studies. *J Immunol* 1980; **124:** 2596–2600.

45. Potempa J, Dubin A, Korzus G, *et al*. Degradation of elastin by a cysteine proteinase from *Staphylococcus aureus*. *J Biol Chem* 1988; **263:** 2664–2667.

46. Burnett D, Stockley R A. Cathepsin B-like cysteine proteinase activity in sputum and bronchoalveolar lavage samples: relationship to inflammatory cells and effects of corticosteroids and antibiotic treatment. *Clin Sci* 1985; **68:** 469–474.

47. Burnett D, Crocker J, Stockley R A. Cathepsin B-like cysteine proteinase activity in sputum and immunohistological identification of cathepsin B in alveolar macrophages. *Am Rev Respir Dis* 1983; **128:** 915–919.

48. Stockley R A. The role of proteinases in the pathogenesis of chronic bronchitis. *Am Rev Respir Dis* 1994; **150:** S109–S113.

49. Lesser M, Padilla M L, Cardozo C. Induction of emphysema in hamsters by intratracheal instillation of cathepsin B. *Am Rev Respir Dis* 1992; **145:** 661–668.

50. Buttle D J, Burnett D, Abrahamson M. Levels of neutrophil elastase and cathepsin B activities, and cystatins in human sputum: relationship to inflammation. *Scand J Clin Lab Invest* 1990; **50:** 509–516.

51. Morgan K L, Hussein A M, Newby T J, *et al*., Quantification and origin of the immunoglobulins in porcine respiratory tract secretions. *Immunology* 1980; **41:** 729–736.

52. Andre C, Andre F, Fargier C. Distribution of IgA1 and IgA2 plasma cells in various normal human tissues and in the jejunum of plasma IgA-deficient patients. *Clin Exp Immunol* 1978; **33:** 327–331.

53. Mostov K E, Kraehenbuhl J-P, Blobel G. Receptor mediated transcellular transport of immunoglobulin: synthesis of secretory component as multiple and larger transmembrane forms. *Proc Natl Acad Sci USA* 1980; **77:** 7257–7261.

54. Jerry L M, Kunkel H G, Adams L. Stabilization of dissociable IgA2 proteins by secretory components. *J Immunol* 1972; **109:** 275–283.

55. Richards C D, Gauldie J. IgA-mediated phagocytosis by mouse alveolar macrophages. *Am Rev Respir Dis* 1985; **132:** 82–85.

56. Shen L, Fanger M W. IgA antibodies synergise with IgG in promoting ADCC by human polymorphonuclear cells, monocytes and lymphocytes. *Cell Immunol* 1981; **59:** 75–81.

57. Ogra P L, Karzou D T, Righthoud F, *et al*. Immunoglobulin responses in serum and secretions after immunisation with live and inactivated polio vaccine and natural infection. *N Engl J Med* 1968; **279:** 893–900.

58. Mestecky J, McGhee J R, Arnold R R, *et al*. Selective induction of an immune response in human external secretions by ingestion of bacterial antigen. *J Clin Invest* 1978; **61:** 731–737.

59. Ogra P L. Effect of tonsillectomy and adenoidectomy on nasopharyngeal antibody response to polio virus. *N Engl J Med* 1971; **284:** 59–64.

60. Stockley R A, Afford S C, Burnett D. Assessment of 7S and 11S immunoglobulin A in sputum. *Am Rev Respir Dis* 1980; **122:** 959–964.

61. Merrill W W, Naegel G P, Olchowski J J, *et al*. Immunoglobulin G subclass proteins in serum and lavage fluid of normal subjects: quantitation and comparison with immunoglobulins A and E. *Am Rev Respir Dis* 1985; **131:** 584–587.

62. Hill S L, Mitchell J L, Burnett D, *et al*. IgG subclasses in sputum from patients with chronic bronchial sepsis. *Thorax* 1990; **45:** 780–781.

63. Hances A J, Saltini C, Crystal R G. Does *de novo* immunoglobulin synthesis occur on the epithelial surface of the human lower respiratory tract? *Am Rev Respir Dis* 1988; **137:** 17–24.

64. Toews G B, Hart D A, Hansen E J. Effect of systemic immunisation on pulmonary clearance of *Haemophilus influenzae* type b. *Infect Immun* 1985; **48:** 343–349.

65. Lapa E, Silva J R, Jones J A H, *et al*. The immunological component of the cellular inflammatory infiltrate in bronchiectasis. *Thorax* 1989; **44:** 668–673.

66. Fick R B, Baltimore R S, Squier S U, *et al*. The immunoglobulin G proteolytic activity of *Pseudomonas aeruginosa* in cystic fibrosis. *J Infect Dis* 1985; **151:** 589–598.

67. Fick R B, Olchowski J, Squier S U, *et al*. Immunoglobulin-G subclasses in cystic fibrosis. IgG2 response to *Pseudomonas aeruginosa* lipopolysaccharide. *Am Rev Respir Dis* 1986; **133:** 418–422.

68. Oxelius V-A. Chronic infections in a family with hereditary deficiency of IgG2 and IgG4. *Clin Exp Immunol* 1974; **17:** 19–24.

69. Bjorkander J, Bake B, Oxelius V-A, *et al*. Impaired lung function in patients with IgA deficiency and low levels of IgG2 or IgG3. *N Engl J Med* 1985; **313:** 720–724.

70. Lane P J, MacLennan I C M. Impaired IgG2 anti-pneumococcal antibody responses in patients with recurrent infection and normal IgG2 levels but no IgA. *Clin Exp Immunol* 1986; **65:** 427–433.

71. Brandtzaeg P, Fellanger I, Bjeruldsen S T. Immunoglobulin M: local synthesis and selective secretion in patients with immunoglobulin A deficiency. *Science* 1968; **160:** 789–791.

72. Kay A B, Moqbel R, Durham S R, *et al*. Leucocyte activation initiated by IgE-dependent mechanisms in relation to helminthic parasitic disease and clinical models of asthma. *Int Arch Allergy Appl Immunol* 1985; **77:** 69–72.

73. Toews G B, Vial W C. The role of C5 in polymorphonuclear leukocyte recruitment in response to *Strepotococcus pneumoniae*. *Am Rev Respir Dis* 1984; **129:** 82–86.

74. Friend P, Repine J E, Kim Y, *et al*. Deficiency of the second component (C2) with chronic vasculitis. *Ann Intern Med* 1975; **83:** 813–816.

75. Ellison R T III, Giehl T J. Killing of gram-negative bacteria by lactoferrin and lysozyme. *J Clin Invest* 1991; **88:** 1080–1091.

76. Jacquot J, Puchelle E, Zahm J M, *et al*. Effect of human airway lysozyme on the *in vitro* growth of type 1 *Streptococcus pneumoniae*. *Eur J Respir Dis* 1987; **71:** 295–305.

77. Shaw G, Kamen R. A conserved AU sequence from the 3′ untranslated region of GM-CSF mRNA mediates selective mRNA degradation. *Cell* 1986; **46:** 659–667.

78. Roberts A B, Anzano M A, Wakefield L M, *et al*. Type-β transforming growth factor: a bifunctional regulator of cellular growth. *Proc Natl Acad Sci USA* 1985; **82:** 119–123.

79. Kelly J. Cytokines of the lung. *Am Rev Respir Dis* 1990; **141:** 765–788.

80. Kelly J, ed. *Cytokines of the lung*. (*Lung Biology in Health and Disease* Series). New York: Marcel Dekker, 1993.

81. Shepherd V L. Cytokine receptors of the lung. *Am J Respir Cell Mol Biol* 1991; **5:** 403–410.

82. Nakamura H, Yoshimura K, McElvaney N G, *et al*. Neutrophil elastase in respiratory epithelial lining fluid of individuals with cystic fibrosis induces interleukin-8 gene expression in a human bronchial epithelial cell line. *J Clin Invest* 1992; **89:** 1478–1484.

83. Standiford T J, Kunkel S L, Rolfe M W, *et al*. Regulation of human alveolar macrophage and blood monocyte-derived interleukin-8 by prostaglandin E2 and dexamethasone. *Am J Respir Cell Mol Biol* 1992; **6:** 75–81.

84. McCain R W, Holden E P, Blackwell T R, *et al*. Leukotriene B4 stimulates human polymorphonuclear leukocytes to synthesise and release IL-8 in vitro. *Am J Respir Cell Mol Biol* 1994; **10:** 651–657.

85. McCrea K A, Ensor J E, Nall K, *et al.* Altered cytokine regulation in the lungs of cigarette smokers. *Am J Respir Crit Care Med* 1994; **150**: 696–703.
86. Richman-Eisenstat J B Y, Jorens P G, Herbert C A, *et al.* Interleukin-8: an important chemoattractant in sputum of patients with chronic inflammatory airway diseases. *Am J Physiol* 1993; **264**: L413–L418.
87. Khair O A, Devalia J L, Abdelaziz M M, *et al.* Effect of *Haemophilus influenzae* endotoxin on the synthesis of IL-6, IL-8, TNF-α and expression of ICAM-1 in cultured human bronchial epithelial cells. *Eur Resp J* 1994; **7**: 2109–2116.
88. Inoue H, Massion P P, Ueki I F, *et al. Pseudomonas* stimulates interleukin-8 mRNA expression selectively in airway epithelium, in gland ducts, and in recruited neutrophils. *Am J Respir Cell Mol Biol* 1994; **11**: 651–663.

3

Immunoglobulins

R. JEFFERIS

University of Birmingham Medical School, Birmingham, UK

INTRODUCTION

The basic facts of antibody structure and function may be familiar to us and review articles and chapters in standard texts on this topic abound. However, these descriptions invariably refer to the biological activities of individual antibody isotypes in isolation and record profiles of effector function established in heterologous systems, for example using guineapig complement. These studies cannot easily be translated to an understanding of humoral immune responses *in vivo* in which multiple isotypes may participate and activate effector mechanisms mediated through human ligands. New and relevant knowledge and understanding has been gained in recent years through the development and application of human or humanised monoclonal antibodies. These studies are vital to the evolution of protocols for therapeutic use of monoclonal antibodies. Similarly, advances in vaccine development offer the potential to maximise the production of individual classes or subclasses of antibody that may be optimal for humoral protection. It is necessary, therefore, that the field of antibody function be kept under constant review to allow rational development. I shall attempt to give a background that reflects current understanding whilst indicating, where possible, fertile ground for future study. Several earlier reviews have been published[1-4].

SYSTEMIC AND MUCOSAL HUMORAL IMMUNE RESPONSES

Mucosal surfaces offer a first line of defence against invasion by micro-organisms. This is afforded as a physical barrier, through protection by non-specific biomolecules and specific local immunological responses. Any breakdown in the integrity of the individual may result in systemic infection and an accompanying systemic immune response. The interface between mucosal and systemic immune

Pulmonary Defences. Edited by Robert A. Stockley.

 R. Jefferis

responses is thus both intimate and vital. It may be summarised that systemic immune responses are characterised by the early appearance of immunoglobulin IgM antibodies, with a switch to a predominant IgG response after secondary stimulation. Antibodies of the humoral response are essentially confined to the circulation or interstitial fluids, and are not reflected in the antibody content of mucosal secretions. This includes IgA antibody secreted from plasma cells in the bone marrow, spleen or lymph nodes. Conversely, stimulation of local immune responses within the respiratory, gastrointestinal and urinary tracts results in the production of secretory IgA that is transported to mucosal surfaces and predominates in external secretions. This local production of IgA is not reflected in the antibody content of the blood or tissue fluids. Because of the ease of access to the circulatory (blood) system, systemic immune responses have been studied much more widely than mucosal ones.

BASIC STRUCTURAL FEATURES: THE Fab, HINGE AND Fc REGIONS

The fundamental structural features of antibody molecules are exhibited by the IgG isotype. The molecular mass of 150 kDa is determined by three globular regions, each of mass 50 kDa, linked together by a flexible hinge region (Fig. 3.1). There is an axis of symmetry and two of the globular regions recognise and bind antigen in identical manner. These regions can be released, by digestion with the enzyme papain, to yield the Fab (*f*ragment *a*ntigen *b*inding) fragments. The third region is released as the Fc fragment (*f*ragment *c*rystallisable; a property of the

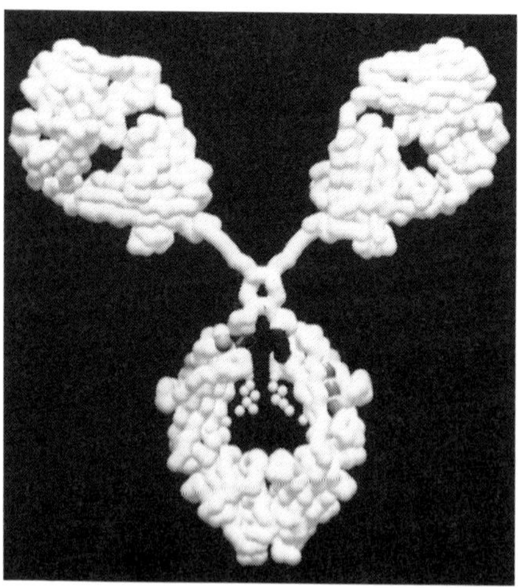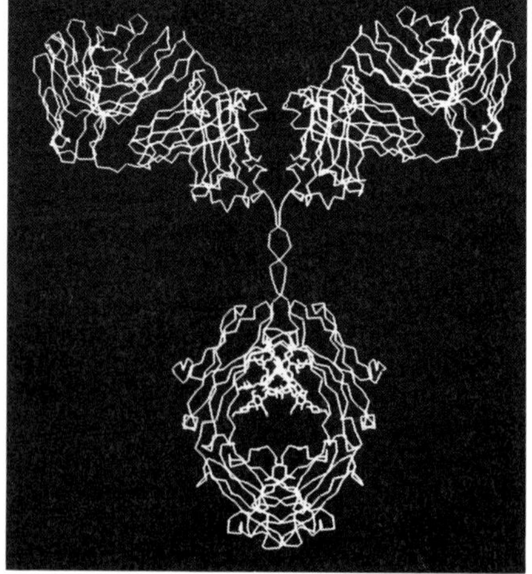

Figure 3.1. Cartoons of an intact human IgG1 molecule, based on X-ray crystal structures obtained for isolated Fab and Fc fragments. The left hand picture shows the molecule in a semi-spacefilling format with the Fab moieties in the upper half and the Fc in the lower. The right hand picture shows the α-carbon backbone of the molecule

fragment originally obtained from rabbit IgG by Rodney Porter[5]. In the intact antibody molecule, the steric disposition of the Fab and the Fc regions relative to each other is determined by the structure of the hinge region. The flexible nature of the hinge is illustrated by the lack of resolution of the Fc region in x ray crystallographic studies of intact antibody molecules, and is due to the distribution of the Fc among differing orientations within the crystal lattice[6]. The x ray crystallographic structure of isolated Fc fragments allows a composite structure for the intact IgG molecule to be generated and it is assumed that models for the other Ig isotypes can be derived, because of the high sequence homology.

The basic structural component of an immunoglobulin is the domain. This refers to the tertiary protein structure of a 110 amino acid residue polypeptide sequence which may be described as two surfaces of antiparallel β-pleated sheet linked through a disulphide bridge[7]. Additional stability is gained by the packing of hydrophobic side chains into the interior bounded by the β sheets, whilst hydrophilic side chains are exposed to the aqueous environment. The tertiary structure of a domain is referred to as the immunoglobulin fold. Proteins are identified as members of the immunoglobulin supergene family if they have primary sequences that are homologous with immunoglobulin domains[8]. The immunoglobulin fold is a basic structural feature that is retained in this large and growing family of proteins.

The first (variable) domain of both the heavy (V_H) and the light chain (V_L) is highly variable in amino acid sequence and determines the antigen binding specificity of an antibody molecule. The random (presumed!) pairing of V_H and V_L domains increases the antibody repertoire and is referred to as "combinatorial pairing". The other light and heavy chain domains are referred to as the "constant domains", as they have a conserved sequence that is characteristic for a light chain type or heavy chain isotype. In the IgG molecule and all Fab fragments analysed, pairing of domains is observed, with the exception of the second constant domains of the heavy chains (C_H2 domains). A complex oligosaccharide moiety attached to this domain has been shown to be integral to the quaternary structure and essential for the expression of effector functions (see below). This glycosylation site is conserved in all mammalian IgGs sequenced and in human IgM, IgD and IgE, but not in IgA. Each constant region domain is encoded by a separate exon, whereas the light and heavy chain variable domains are products of two and three V gene segments respectively (see later).

We are familiar with representations of the IgG molecule as Y- or T-shaped, reflecting variations in the angle between the Fab arms. Additionally, the Fabs may have rotational and lateral degrees of freedom — wagging and wobbling motions[1,9,10]. Given that the antigen binding sites have opposed orientations (they "point" in different directions), the mobility of the Fabs allows the potential divalency of the IgG molecule to be realised when the epitopes recognised have differing orientations and separations in space. Mobility of the Fc region is also necessary to the expression of ligand binding activities[10], for example, the engagement of membrane bound Fc receptors and the large multimeric C1 component of complement after the formation of antigen–antibody complexes. The primary interaction sites for each of these activities has been mapped to the N-proximal end of the C_H2 domain[2,11,12]. It can be appreciated, therefore, that

Fc mobility may be essential to allow differing spatial orientations, thus avoiding Fab arm obstruction of access to ligand binding sites.

Having emphasised the contribution of the hinge region to the expression of effector functions for IgG antibody, it is important to note that the IgM and IgE isotypes do not have an equivalent of the IgG hinge structure. However, there is evidence that a degree of flexibility may be possible within the Fc region. This facilitates the activation of complement by IgM–antigen complexes[13] and the binding of antigen by IgE bound to its high affinity receptor[14]. It is well documented that monomeric IgM is not agglutinating and is functionally monovalent for macromolecular antigens. This would appear to be, at least in part, the result of the lack of a functional hinge region resulting in the absence of Fab mobility. It is of interest to note that immunoglobulins first evolved to function as membrane bound receptors and that, in ontogeny, the earliest immune response (induction of anergy or tolerance) is mediated by immature B cells expressing monomeric IgM as an antigen receptor. It is possible that the monovalency of membrane bound IgM is essential to its function as a membrane bound receptor.

ANTIBODY ISOTYPES

There are nine human immunoglobulin isotypes that are defined by the structure and antigenicity of the constant regions of their heavy chains (Table 3.1). Each heavy chain type is encoded by a distinct gene within the heavy chain gene locus on chromosome 14. There are two types of light chain, κ and λ, encoded on chromosomes 2 and 22 respectively, that are expressed with each of the heavy chain types[15]. An individual plasma cell secretes antibody of a single specificity that is the product of one heavy chain and one light chain gene, consequently an antibody molecule has either κ or λ chains and never a mixture of the two. The proportion of molecules bearing κ and λ chains may vary between antibody isotypes, but there is little or no evidence to suggest that this has any influence on the effector functions activated. In the context of this volume, it is the IgA isotype that is central to the discussion, consequently a more comprehensive review of this isotype will be presented. Other reviews of IgA have been published elsewhere[4,16,17].

IMMUNOGLOBULIN
Serum IgA

The structure of the serum form of IgA is similar to the prototype IgG molecule. The source of serum IgA is plasma cells present in bone marrow, the spleen or lymph nodes. The predominant form is a monomer; however, IgA paraproteins in multiple myeloma may be comprised of many polymeric forms. There are two IgA isotypes or subclasses, IgA1 and IgA2, and the IgA1 subclass predominates (>90%) in the blood. While it is assumed that specific antibody responses may be generated for each isotype, it has been observed that responses to certain bacterial polysaccharide antigens may be predominantly those of the IgA2 subclass[18]. The constant regions of IgA1 and IgA2 are highly homologous (>90%), but there is

Table 3.1. Biochemical and biological properties of human immunoglobulins

	IgG1	IgG2	IgG3	IgG4	IgA1	IgA2	IgM	IgD	IgE
H chain class	γ_1	γ_2	γ_3	γ_4	α_1	α_2	μ	δ	ε
Number of heavy chain domains	4	4	4	4	4	4	5	4	5
Molecular weight	148 000	148 000	159 000	148 000	160 000	160 000	970 000	172 000	188 000
H chain molecular weight	50 000	50 000	55 000	50 000	56 000	57 000	71 000	60 000	71 000
Reference range concentration in adults ($g \cdot l^{-1}$)	3–10	1–7	0.02–2	<0.03–1.3	0.7–2.3	0.1–0.5	0.5–2.0	5–200 ($mg \cdot l^{-1}$)	<5–120 ($\kappa U \cdot l^{-1}$)
Complement activation:									
Classical pathway	++	−	++	−	−	−	+++	−	−
Alternative pathway	±	+	±	±	ND	+++	±	−	−
Interaction with									
$Fc_\gamma RI$	++	−	++	+	−	−	−	−	−
$Fc_\gamma RII$	++	+*	++	−	−	−	−	−	−
$Fc_\gamma RIII$	++	−	++	−	−	−	−	−	−
Mucosal transfer	−	−	−	−	+	+	+	−	−
Placental transfer	+	+	+	+	−	−	−	−	−

ND = Not determined. *Interacts with $Fc_\gamma RII$ LR only, see text a major structural difference in the hinge region, with an effective 13 amino acid deletion in IgA2 relative to IgA1.

The 13 amino acid residue sequence of the IgA1 hinge comprises seven proline, three serine and three threonine residues. Short oligosaccharide chains are attached (*O*-glycosidic linked) to five of the serine/threonine residues. This is a very unusual feature for a serum protein and it has been speculated that it may assist the "anchoring" of the secretory form to mucins present on epithelial tissues. A further consequence of this hinge structure is that it is extended, relative to the hinge of IgA2, is accessible, and may be cleaved by specific enzymes produced by micro-organisms — referred to as IgA proteases. The IgA2 isotype is not susceptible to these enzymes; however, there is emerging evidence that some micro-organisms also produce enzymes that specifically cleave, and hence inactivate, IgA2.

Two well defined allotypes of IgA2 are recognised: A2m(1) and A2m(2). Whilst there are only six differences in primary amino acid sequence between A2m(1) and A2m(2) proteins, there is a major consequence for chain assembly. The light chains of A2m(1) are disulphide linked, not to the α chains, but to each other; consequently light chain and heavy chain dimers can be obtained under dissociating but non-reducing conditions. This allows for chemical "typing" of IgA2 proteins as an alternative to use of antisera. Differences in the susceptibility of A2m(1) and A2m(2) molecules to enzymes produced by micro-organisms have been reported. As the frequency of the A2m alleles differs widely between populations — A2m(1) predominates in white and A2m(2) in black populations — these allelic differences could be factors in racial variations in disease resistance and susceptibility.

A receptor for IgA, $Fc_\alpha R$, is constitutively expressed on mono-cytes/macrophages, neutrophils and eosinophils[19,20]. The receptor binds both serum and secretory forms of IgA and can activate phagocytosis, degranulation and superoxide release by monocytes/macrophages and neutrophils. There is no evidence that IgA can activate complement through the classical pathway, but it can do so through the alternative pathway. Studies using chimeric mouse/human antibodies with specificity for the NIP (iodonitrophenyl) hapten, demonstrated IgA2 to be the most efficient of the human isotypes in activating the alternative pathway[21]; IgA1 was not available for study. The ability to activate was tolerant of both the epitope density on the target cell and the antigen/antibody ratio used.

Secretory IgA

The secretory form of IgA is produced locally in mucosal lymphoid tissue and is specifically transported across epithelial cells into the external milieu. Secretory IgA has been observed in all mammals investigated and in chickens[22]; however, it appears that in some other avian species IgM acts as the secretory form of antibody. Transportation of IgA required the emergence in evolution of new functional molecules. Both IgA and IgM heavy chains have an extended C-terminal 18 amino acid sequence referred to as the "tail piece". The penultimate amino acid residue is a cysteine, which may form disulphide bonds internally between heavy chains or with the glycosylated polypeptide J chain[23]. J chain is an evolutionarily conserved molecule exhibiting 70% homology between man, mouse and rabbit and a high degree of homology between that of the earthworm and man. There are eight cysteine residues that form three intra-J-chain disulphide bridges, while the two cysteines close to the N-terminus are available to form interchain disulphide bridges with α or μ heavy chains. The J chain gene is expressed early in B cell ontogeny and continues to be expressed in all plasma cells except those producing serum IgA. This explains why the predominant form of serum IgA is monomer. However, higher polymers can be generated through disulphide bond formation between the penultimate cysteines of different IgA molecules. Plasma cells in mucosal lymphoid tissue synthesise both IgA and J chain, resulting in the formation and secretion of IgA dimers[3,4,16,17].

The secretory form of IgA present in external secretions has a further polypeptide component, "secretory component", covalently attached. Secretory component has a mass of approximately 70 kDa and is comprised of five Ig-like domains with carbohydrate accounting for approximately 20% of the mass. This glycoprotein moiety is the extracellular region of a transmembrane transport receptor, the poly-Ig receptor (pIg), expressed on the basolateral membrane of mucosal epithelial cells. The binding of IgA dimers to the pIg receptor activates a transcytosis mechanism that results in transit of the IgA through the cell to be expressed on the apical membrane surface. The pIg receptor is then cleaved by a membrane localised enzyme to release the secretory form of IgA. This is an IgA dimer bound to the cleaved portion of the receptor, first identified as secretory component. The pIg receptor can also bind and transport IgM, and this mechanism may provide effective local immunity in individuals with selective IgA deficiency[3,4,16,17,23−25].

Biological Functions of Secretory IgA

The proportion of IgA1 and IgA2 in mucosal secretions varies with the site sampled. This reflects local synthesis and the observed frequency of IgA1 and IgA2 producing plasma cells present in the mucosal lymphoid tissue. While IgA1 cells predominate in most mucosal tissues, in the large intestine and the female genital tract IgA2 secreting cells are as numerous as or outnumber IgA1 cells. When bound to micro-organisms, specific IgA antibody may inhibit their motility, growth and ability to adhere to cellular receptors. Colonisation is thus frustrated and the organisms may be destroyed or voided from the body[24]. In the intact individual, few phagocytic cells or little complement will be present in mucosal secretions; however, local damage to epithelial tissue could result in both increasing. The specificity of the IgA antibodies present in mucosal secretion reflects the antigenic environment of the mucosal tissue. Intact antigens can be transported across the epithelium, with consequent stimulation of mucosal lymphoid tissue.

There is evidence of further mechanisms by which secretory IgA may afford local immune protection. In the event of an episode of mucosal infection, antigens or micro-organisms may pass into the tissue of the lamina propria and immune complexes may be formed with locally produced IgA. These complexes may then bind to the pIg receptor and be transported to the external surface

46 *R. Jefferis*

(excreted!). Alternatively, such complexes might activate clearance mechanisms after interaction with $Fc_\alpha R$ expressed on inflammatory cell activation or the alternative pathway of complement[19-21]. It is also possible that micro-organisms that penetrate into epithelial cells and reproduce intracellularly may encounter IgA antibody that is being transported through the same cell. Several model systems suggest that exocytotic and endocytotic pathways may interact so that the contents of each may be exposed to the other.

Selective IgA deficiency

The complexity of the secretory immune system argues for positive selection through evolution. It may appear paradoxical, therefore, that selective IgA deficiency is the most commonly encountered primary immune deficiency[16,17,25]. It occurs with a frequency of one in 500–700 in Europeans, but at a much lower frequency in Japanese and Afro-Americans. Many IgA deficient individuals are healthy, while others may exhibit one or more of a variety of clinical manifestations. These include recurrent upper respiratory infections and allergic, autoimmune, gastrointestinal and skin disorders. In a large proportion of healthy IgA deficient individuals, IgM functions as the secretory immunoglobulin. A significant proportion of IgA deficient individuals exhibiting clinical manifestations of immune dysfunction have an accompanying deficiency of one or more of the IgG subclasses. A combined IgA, IgG2 and IgG4 deficiency is particularly associated with the sequelae of humoral deficiency[26]. It is interesting to speculate that this may be evidence of a vital interface between secretory and systemic humoral immunity.

IMMUNOGLOBULIN G

An overview of structure of the IgG class of antibody has been presented above; however, in humans four subclasses of IgG are recognised. The constant domains exhibit >95% primary amino acid sequence homology, but each has a structurally distinct hinge region and expresses a unique profile of biological effector functions (Table 3.1)[1,2,27]. Total serum IgG levels vary between healthy adults, but the proportion of each subclass is maintained within a relatively narrow range: IgG1, 60–65%; IgG2, 20–25%; IgG3, 5–10%; IgG4, approximately 6%. However, the proportion of each subclass (profile) present within antigen specific IgG may differ substantially from the mean values for total IgG. The broad generalisation may be made that IgG responses to protein antigens are predominantly of the IgG1 and IgG3 subclass, while responses to bacterial polysaccharides may be predominantly or exclusively of the IgG2 subclass; individuals with selective IgG2 deficiency may be susceptible to recurrent infection. Thus polysaccharide antigens are frequently presented to the immune system to provoke a protective IgG2 response. Failure to produce this response may result in the individual suffering episodes of recurrent infection[2,28]. However, if such a polysaccharide antigen is coupled to a protein antigen, the conjugate may provoke an IgG1/IgG3 response to the polysaccharide that is protective. This strategy has been utilised successfully for *Haemophilus* b, with a conjugate vaccine composed of the polyribose phosphate carbohydrate moiety conjugated to tetanus toxoid protein[28].

Whilst the apparent requirement for an IgG2 response to polysaccharide antigens is well established, the mechanism(s) by which immune protection might be afforded has not been clear. It has usually been reported that IgG2 is poor at activating complement and is not recognised by Fc$_\gamma$ receptors (Fc$_\gamma$R). However, recent studies have shown that at high epitope density and at equivalence or antibody excess, IgG2 activates both the classical and alternative complement pathways[21]. It is now established that a polymorphic form of Fc$_\gamma$RII recognises IgG2, and that IgG2 complexes can trigger phagocytosis and superoxide release[29].

IMMUNOGLOBULIN M

The first antibody isotype expressed in human ontogeny is the monomeric transmembrane receptor form of IgM on B lymphocytes. This characterises the immature B cell, whereas the mature B cell expresses receptors of both the IgM and IgD isotypes, each having identical specificity[30]. These B cells may be stimulated by antigen to proliferate and differentiate to plasma cells secreting specific IgM antibody. This primary IgM response may be interpreted as evidence that IgM is the prototypic humoral antibody and that the membrane receptor role of immunoglobulin predates its function as a secreted product. Support for this proposal comes from the finding that the earliest humoral antibody response observed phylogenetically is constituted of the IgM isotype only. The secreted form of IgM is a pentamer of the basic four chain molecule[10,31]. This pentameric form is very efficient at agglutinating particulate antigens and activating complement through the classical pathway, as a result of its multivalency both for antigen and C1q binding. However, it should be appreciated that the uncomplexed IgM molecule is also, potentially, multivalent for C1 binding (see later). Hence it is posited that, when IgM binds to a multivalent antigen, the Fab arms may bend out of the plane of the Fc and become "fixed" in this steric from, which is made possible by an element of flexibility within a region between the second and third domains of the heavy chain. The IgM pentamer may be dissociated, on mild reduction, to monomer units that are functionally univalent with respect to binding of macromolecular antigens. This is thought to be attributable to the lack of a hinge region between the C$_\mu$1 and C$_\mu$2 domains and hence a lack of Fab mobility such that the binding of a large antigen to one Fab results in the binding site on the other Fab being sterically inaccessible. Plasma cells secreting IgM also synthesise J chain that functions to effect the ordered assembly of IgM to yield a pentamer. In the absence of J chain a mixture of pentamers and hexamers is formed[31].

IMMUNOGLOBULIN E

The IgE heavy chains are composed of four constant region domains. IgE is present in serum as a monomer, but normally only in trace amounts (Table 3.1). However, a substantial proportion of total IgE is bound to mast cells and basophils through the high affinity Fc$_\varepsilon$RI receptor[32]. IgE is believed to play an important part in protective immunity against helminth parasites such as schistosomulae. Antigens of these parasites provoke a vigorous IgE response, with the result that mast cells and basophils present in the underlying tissue become sensitised through Fc$_\varepsilon$RI; other inflammatory cells, especially eosinophils, may also be sensitised through the low affinity Fc$_\varepsilon$RII receptor (cluster of differentiation (CD) 23). Mast cell degranulation triggered by the binding of parasite antigens to cytophilic IgE causes a local inflammatory response and may contribute directly to expulsion of parasites from the gut. *In vivo* studies in rats suggest that a more important role for IgE mediated mast cell degranulation may be the attraction of eosinophils to the site of infection by eosinophil chemotactic factors[33]. Eosinophils are very effective in killing large parasites sensitised with IgE antibodies. Macrophages and platelets are also capable of IgE dependent cytotoxicity and may have an additional role in protective responses to helminth infestations. The demonstration of Fc$_\varepsilon$RII mediated cytotoxic responses of human eosinophils, macrophages and platelets[34] to IgE sensitised helminths *in vitro* would be consistent with such a role in man. IgE also plays an immunoregulatory role through Fc$_\varepsilon$RII expressed on B lymphocytes[35]. The membrane bound receptor may be enzymatically cleaved to release soluble receptor proteins that regulate B cell function, and IgE production in particular[36].

The debilitating and potentially life-threatening nature of allergic diseases has attracted basic and clinical scientists in efforts to understand the underlying mechanisms. A crucial element of the allergic reaction is the binding of antigen to mast cells and basophils sensitised with specific IgE bound to the high affinity Fc$_\varepsilon$R receptor. Attempts have been made, therefore, to isolate a small univalent peptide fragment of the IgE Fc that could be used to inhibit IgE binding *in vivo*. This has proven to be a controversial field of investigation and several claims for success have failed to be substantiated. Modern experimental approaches, using genetic engineering techniques, have allowed the Fc$_\varepsilon$RI interaction site to be localised to a 76 amino acid peptide that spans the C-terminal portion of the second domain and the N-terminal portion of the third domain in the native molecule[37−39]. These studies provide a basis for the production of a recombinant or synthetic peptide that could, potentially, inhibit IgE binding to Fc$_\varepsilon$RI and hence the allergic response. However, any such treatment must be approached with extreme caution, because if such a peptide aggregated or bound to host protein it could effect Fc$_\varepsilon$RI cross linking and trigger an anaphylactic reaction.

The interaction site on the IgE molecule for Fc$_\varepsilon$RII has been localised to the C$_\varepsilon$3 domain, but it is apparent that the C$_\varepsilon$4 domain is also required, possibly in order to stabilise the Fc$_\varepsilon$RII binding site. The Fc$_\varepsilon$RI and Fc$_\varepsilon$RII binding sites on IgE appear to be close to each other[40]. It is essential, therefore, that any treatment aimed at inhibiting IgE–Fc$_\varepsilon$RI interactions should be carefully evaluated to ensure that it does not also inhibit IgE–Fc$_\varepsilon$RII binding and perturb immunoregulatory pathways.

IMMUNOGLOBULIN D

The production of antibodies of the IgD isotype is thought to be a normal, but quantitatively minor characteristic of a humoral immune response. It has not been possible to demonstrate effector functions for this isotype that would suggest a role for IgD in the clearance or destruction of IgD complexed antigens. As coexpression of membrane IgM and IgD characterises the mature B lymphocyte[30], it is assumed, though not proven, that membrane IgD contributes to B cell responsiveness. A subpopulation of T cells has been shown to express receptors that bind IgD; however, it has been shown that it is not Fc_δ specific but is a lectin that binds IgD and IgA1 associated *O*-linked carbohydrates[41−43], and studies in mice suggest that IgD–antigen complexes may mediate an immunoregulatory function[44]. It is of interest to note that murine IgD lacks the equivalent of the second constant domain of the human molecule[45], therefore the functions of this isotype could differ substantially between the species.

INTERACTION OF IMMUNOGLOBULINS WITH CELLULAR Fc RECEPTORS

Cellular receptors that specifically recognise the Fc regions of each of the immunoglobulin classes have been reported, but only those for IgG, IgE (see above) and IgA are well characterised. $Fc_\alpha R$ has only recently been identified. It is constitutively expressed on monocytes and granulocytes and its engagement by IgA antibody–antigen complexes can trigger metabolic activation, with resultant phagocytosis, degranulation and superoxide production[9,20,46,47]. $Fc_\alpha R$ also has a role in IgA catabolism and the clearance of immune complexes from the circulation. Receptors for the IgG isotypes ($Fc_\gamma R$) play a major part in the processes of removal and destruction of antigen–IgG antibody complexes — for example phagocytosis, antibody dependent cell-mediated cytotoxicity and superoxide production[48,49]. Three types of human Fc_γ receptors have been defined physicochemically and with monoclonal antibodies; the genes have been cloned. Each has a characteristic profile of cellular expression.

$Fc_\gamma RI$ is a high affinity receptor that binds monomeric IgG1, IgG3 and IgG4 and is expressed constitutively only on mononuclear phagocytes. $Fc_\gamma RII$ is a family of highly homologous receptors, encoded by three genes, that all bind monomeric IgG1 and IgG3 with low affinity. Alternative splicing of the primary transcripts results in the expression of multiple forms differing in the structure and function of the cytoplasmic domains. There are two polymorphic variants of the $Fc_\gamma RIIa$ gene, the products of which have different IgG subclass recognition profiles. Initially, the two forms were defined functionally as high (HR) and low responder (LR) forms; it was subsequently shown that the LR form recognises IgG2 in addition to IgG1 and IgG3; the HR form recognises IgG1 and IgG3 only. There is evidence that the HR/LR status of an individual may be of clinical significance. As mentioned above, protective antibody responses to bacterial polysaccharides may be exclusively of the IgG2 isotype; however, IgG2–antigen complexes will not activate clearance mechanisms in individuals homozygous for the HR form of $Fc_\gamma RII$[50].

There are two forms of $Fc_\gamma RIII$, encoded by distinct genes, that have low affinity recognition specificity for monomeric IgG1 and IgG3. Alternate RNA splicing results in the biosynthesis of transmembrane and phosphatidyl linked $Fc_\gamma RIII$ receptors, the latter being expressed on neutrophils. $Fc_\gamma RII$ and $Fc_\gamma RIII$ are believed to fulfil their biological roles by interaction with complexed IgG;

the normal blood levels of IgG suggest that all high affinity $Fc_\gamma RI$ receptors will be saturated with monomeric IgG. The nature of the $Fc_\gamma R$ that transports monomeric IgG across the placenta is unclear at present, but may be related to the $Fc_\gamma R$ that transports IgG across the gut in the newborn rat. This receptor is a heterodimer homologous to the major histocompatibility class I molecules and utilises β_2 microglobulin[51]. A unique $Fc_\gamma R$ has been reported to occur on human intestinal epithelium[52]; its role in the lung has yet to be delineated.

COMPLEMENT ACTIVATION

THE CLASSICAL PATHWAY

Only IgM, IgG1 and IgG3 have been consistently reported to activate complement efficiently through the classical pathway; numerous reports have suggested that IgG2 has a weak ability to activate the classical pathway and the evidence, at present, is that it is at best a poor activator of human C1. IgM is generally the most effective isotype, as a single molecule of IgM bound to cell surface antigen can activate complement mediated lysis, whereas at least two closely spaced IgG molecules are required[53,54]. This is because there is a requirement for two C1q heads to engage the Fc binding sites of antibody. This requirement is met by a single molecule of multimeric IgM. It must be emphasised that epitope density, distribution and the relative proportion of antigen and antibody reacting have a critical influence on the size and nature of immune complexes formed and consequently their ability to activate complement[21].

THE ALTERNATIVE PATHWAY

The physicochemical structure and nature of the immune complex formed also determine the efficacy with which the Ig isotypes activate the alternative complement pathway. In a study using a wide range of immune complexes[21], only IgA2 and IgG2 were consistently active (but note that IgA1 antibodies of the same specificity were not available for study). IgA2 was the most effective isotype and its activity was relatively tolerant to epitope density and antigen/antibody ratio. Alternative pathway activation by IgG2 was dependent on high epitope density and immune complexes formed at equivalence or in antibody excess. It is not yet known whether the mechanism of alternative pathway activation by immunoglobulins differs from that of other activators such as bacterial polysaccharides.

The clinical relevance of epitope density may be illustrated by a comparison of DNA antibodies in systemic lupus erythematosus and thyroglobulin antibodies in autoimmune thyroiditis. The high epitope density of DNA results in the formation of complexes that activate complement very efficiently, while the restricted specificity of the autoantibody response to thyroglobulin results in few epitopes being recognised and the formation of complexes that do not fix complement. A very important role for complement *in vivo*, after fixation to immune complexes, is attachment to erythrocytes via complement receptor 1(CR1) to facilitate transport to the liver for clearance by the Kupffer cells[55].

ISOTYPE CONCENTRATIONS AND SPECIFIC ANTIBODY RESPONSES

Systemic immunity is provided by antibody secreted from plasma cells within the bone marrow, whereas antibody present at mucosal surfaces and in external secretions is produced by plasma cells in lymphoid tissue underlying the epithelium. A primary systemic immune response is characterised by the production of IgM antibody, whilst a secondary response results in a predominant IgG response, although all isotypes are usually present. Some antigens are processed and presented to evoke a sustained IgM response. Mechanisms determining isotype expression and regulation within immune responses have only recently begun to be elucidated[56]. The nature of the antigen can determine the antigen processing cells activated and hence the profile of cytokines released. This in turn determines patterns of lymphocyte activation, isotype switching, *etc.* For many years, evaluation of the status of systemic antibody production has been determined by quantitation of the total levels of the individual classes, subclasses, or both. However, there are an increasing number of situations in which it is the isotype profile of specific antibody responses that is most relevant to diagnosis[2,27].

The IgG subclass profile of some specific antibodies is shown in Table 3.2. As each antibody isotype expresses an individual profile of effector functions, the isotype composition of a given antibody response may significantly affect the clearance mechanisms activated. It also suggests that selective immunoglobulin deficiencies may compromise an individual's ability to generate a fully protective humoral response[2,27]. Thus antibody responses to bacterial polysaccharides may be predominantly or exclusively of the IgG2 subclass. Selective IgG2 subclass deficiency is associated with recurrent respiratory tract and chest infections. Some individuals with a similar history of recurrent infection may have normal levels of total IgG2; however, this may mask a deficiency in the individual's ability to produce antibodies of the required specificity within this subclass. It is likely that the observed IgG2 deficiency in these groups of patients is indicative of multiple deficits within their immune systems, as there are individuals within the normal healthy population having an apparent IgG2 deficiency. Indeed, healthy individuals have been identified who lack the genes encoding one or more of the IgG subclasses[57].

The antibody response to the rhesus D antigen is another clear example of isotype restriction. This response, which results from sensitisation of rhesus

Table 3.2. Subclass profile of specific antibody responses

Antigen	IgG1	IgG2	IgG3	IgG4
Tetanus toxoid	+++	+	+	++
Polysaccharides	+	+++	+	(+)
Rhesus-D	+++	−	+++	−
Factor VIII	−	−	−	+++
Phospholipase A2	+++	+	+	+
Phospholipase A2[†]	+	+	+	+++

[†]Following long term (chronic) antigenic stimulation in bee keepers who are constantly stung

52   R. Jefferis

negative mothers by fetal red cells bearing the paternally inherited antigen, comprises predominantly IgG1 and IgG3 antibodies[58]. Secondary stimulation (a subsequent pregnancy) results in the production of IgG antibodies that cross the placenta and cause red cell destruction, by a non-complement-dependent process[59], leading to haemolytic disease of the newborn. Early attempts to correlate the severity of haemolytic disease of the newborn with a predominance of IgG1 or IgG3 anti-Rh(D) in maternal serum yielded conflicting results, as has been reviewed elsewhere[60]. Recent evidence, however, suggests that the important factor in predicting severity of the disease is the presence of both of the isotypes[61].

Fc: STRUCTURAL AND FUNCTIONAL HETEROGENEITY

Multiple alleles of human constant region genes are present within the human population. They have been documented for each of the IgG subclasses and the IgA2 subclass. The close linkage between the genes encoding the heavy chain constant regions results in their inheritance as a haplotype. Certain haplotypes are characteristic for a population group, and the observation of linkage disequilibrium suggests positive selection and thus survival value for certain haplotypes, within the context of the antigenic environment experienced over evolutionary time. Recent studies have revealed disease associations for certain haplotypes and it is possible that allotype may be one genetic parameter that contributes to disease susceptibility. Thus individuals homozygous for the G2m(n) allotype of IgG2 have greater serum concentrations of IgG2 than those homozygous for the G2m(n$^-$) allele, with heterozygotes having intermediate levels[62]. As protective immune responses to certain bacteria are restricted to the IgG2 isotype, these findings may have implications for disease susceptibility. Such an effect has been reported for postimmunisation levels of IgG2 antibody to *Haemophilus influenzae* type b polyribose phosphate and *Meningococcus* C capsular polysaccharides: individuals lacking the G2m(n) allele had an increased risk of vaccine failure[63]. Because allotypic differences result in structural differences within the Fc region, this could result in functional differences. Whilst this aspect has not been adequately investigated, differences in complement activation have been reported for allotypic forms of human chimeric IgG3[64].

Immunoglobulins are glycoproteins that may bear simple, complex or high mannose oligosaccharide moieties. As in other glycoproteins, the simple sugars are *O*-linked through the hydroxyl groups of serine or threonine, whereas the complex and high mannose varieties are linked through an asparagine, within an acceptor site with an asparagine–X–threonine/serine motif. Whereas the heavy chain constant regions of IgM, IgA, IgD and IgE bear several *N*-linked oligosaccharide moieties, the IgG heavy chain bears a single oligosaccharide of the complex type[2,11,65], covalently linked through a conserved glycosylation site (297 Asn) within the $C_\gamma2$ domain[11,65,66] (Fig. 3.2). Approximately 20% of the mass of this domain is contributed by the carbohydrate. It has been demonstrated that glycosylation of IgG antibody is essential for recognition and activation of Fc$_\gamma$RI, Fc$_\gamma$RII, Fc$_\gamma$RIII and the classical pathway of complement

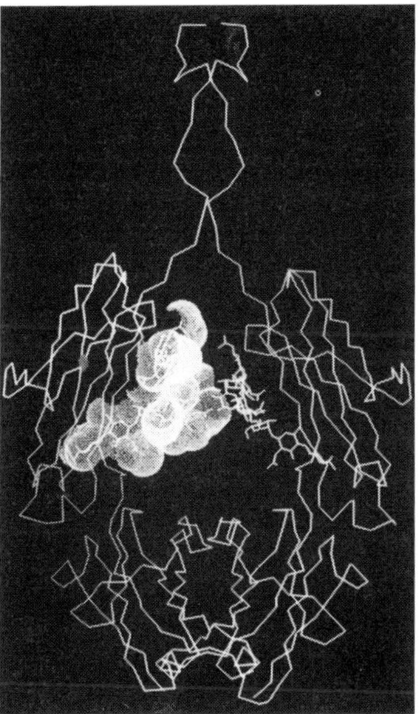

Gal (β 1-4) GlcNac (β 1-2) Man (α 1-6)

Gal (β 1-4) GlcNac (β 1-2) Man (α 1-3)

Fuc (α 1 -6)

Man (β 1-4) GlcNac (β 1-4) GlcNac

Figure 3.2. An α-carbon backbone cartoon of the Fc region of human IgG1 with the solvent accessible surface of one of the carbohydrates highlighted. The structure of a fully galactosylated biantennary, *N*-linked oligosaccharide is given in the lower hand section

activation[11,12,65,66]. Changes in the pattern of IgG glycosylation have been shown to be associated with disease states. For example, an increased proportion of IgG lacking galactose has been observed in the serum of patients with certain chronic inflammatory diseases, notably rheumatoid arthritis[67] and Crohn's disease[68]. The significance of this finding is not clear, but it is believed to be indicative, at least,

 R. Jefferis

of a significant underlying defect. Heavy chains of the IgA1[69] and IgD[70] isotypes also bear simple *O*-linked sugars covalently linked at multiple sites within the hinge region.

RHEUMATOID FACTORS

A diagnostic feature of rheumatoid arthritis is the presence in the serum of an autoantibody, rheumatoid factor (RF) which, by definition, has specificity for the Fc region of IgG[71,72]. In rheumatoid arthritis, the synovium is infiltrated with lymphocytes and essentially becomes a secondary lymphoid organ. Within this tissue, both the autoantibody and the autoantigen are produced[73,74] and secreted into the joint space. This results in the formation of immune complexes *in situ* that are assumed to initiate self perpetuating inflammatory reactions. Most studies of the antigen specificity of RF have used IgM RF, which may also occur in the serum of patients with mixed essential cryoglobulinaemia, primary Sjögren's syndrome and several chronic infections. However, IgG and IgA RF also occur in rheumatoid sera[71,74,75]. Thus the proportions of both the autoantibody isotype and the autoantigen present in the synovium will influence the composition of the immune complexes formed and, consequently, the inflammatory mechanisms activated.

IMMUNOGLOBULIN GENES

While a detailed account of our knowledge of the organisation and expression of immunoglobulin genes is not appropriate to this volume, some consideration is warranted. Examples have been given of particular antigens that provoke antibody responses with restricted isotype profiles that in turn, determine the range of effector functions activated. The isotype profile is determined by the antigen processing pathway and the cytokines released that influence isotype switching of the activated B cells. An alternative possibility could be selective expression of certain Ig V gene segments with the genes encoding Ig heavy chains.

The specificity of an antibody molecule is determined by the sequence of the variable regions of the heavy and light chains. Each variable region is composed of about 110 amino acid residues that generate a domain structure and an immunoglobulin fold that is characteristic for a variable region and distinct from, but related to, that formed by the constant regions. Amino acid sequence differences between antibody molecules of differing specificity are maximal at three distinct sites, the hypervariable regions, within the linear sequence of the variable region[1,7,76]. However, the immunoglobulin fold brings them into close proximity with each other in such a way that they can each contribute to the formation of an antigen binding site[7,76]. The pairing of light and heavy chain variable regions (combinatorial association) brings all six hypervariable regions together to form a continuous protein "surface" that, in charge distribution and shape, is complementary to the surface of the epitope recognised and bound. The antibody residues contributing to antigen binding are referred to as the complementary determining regions and, in essence, they correspond to the hypervariable regions. During B cell ontogeny, the first immunoglobulin gene product is a functional μ heavy chain[30]. This signals rearrangement at the κ light chain locus to occur, and the production of the monomeric membrane form of IgM that is the antigen receptor on the B cell. Rearrangement at the κ locus does not always occur with appropriate fidelity (unproductive rearrangement), in which case rearrangement is initiated at the λ locus. These events result in the generation of a primary B cell repertoire of $>10^8-10^{10}$ different specificities. This repertoire is expanded in a secondary immune response when the process of somatic mutation is activated.

The initial heavy chain transcript of a B cell has the information sufficient for the production of both μ and δ heavy chains. However, this transcript is processed so that only a μ chain is synthesised and IgM is expressed as a membrane bound receptor on the surface of the immature B cell. At the next stage in ontogeny, the primary RNA transcript is processed to allow synthesis of both a μ and a δ chain, and subsequent expression of both isotypes on the surface of the B cell[30]. Both isotypes have identical V regions and, hence, antigen recognition specificity. Thus the antigen recognition repertoire is represented by the virgin B cell pool. Antigen specific stimulation can result in a primary immune response with the generation, after proliferation and differentiation, of IgM secreting plasma cells and memory B cells. The site at which the initial contact with antigen occurs may determine the profile and concentration of cytokines that will influence its further development and the isotype commitment of the memory cells produced. The lymphoid tissue first encountering an antigen will be determined by the site of infection or entry. In addition, antigen processing and presentation may also vary from tissue to tissue. It is likely that these influences determine the isotype of the response, rather than the genes used to generate the V region or epitope specificity, *per se*.

CONCLUDING REMARKS

Significant advances in our understanding of the structure and effector functions of antibody molecules have been achieved in the past decade. These advances are of practical significance, as monoclonal antibodies are increasingly being applied to human therapy[77-79]. Although originating in mice or rats, these antibodies are converted to chimerics or humanised to overcome the problem of recipient responses to these foreign proteins and to utilise human effector mechanisms. The understanding contained in this review allows for a rational choice of antibody isotype to be made, depending on what one wishes to achieve *in vivo*. The application of protein engineering techniques has allowed the generation of new antibody constructs with profiles of effector function not found in nature. This approach increases the armoury of potential therapeutic agents available.

REFERENCES

1. Burton D R, Woof J M. Human antibody effector functions. *Adv Immunol* 1992; **51**: 1–48.
2. Jefferis R, Pound J, Lund J, *et al*. Effector mechanisms of human IgG subclass antibodies: clinical and molecular aspects. *Ann Biol Clin* 1994; **52**: 57–65.

3. Kerr M A. The structure and function of IgA. *Biochem J* 1990; **271**: 285–296.

4. Underdown B J, Mestecky J. Mucosal immunoglobulins. In: Mestecky J, ed. *Handbook of Mucosal Immunology*. New York: Academic Press, 1994; 79–97.

5. Porter R R. Separation and isolation of fractions of rabbit gamma globulin containing the antibody and antigenic combining sites. *Nature* 1958; **182**: 670–671.

6. Ely K R, Colman P M, Abola E E, *et al*. Mobile Fc region in the ZieIgG2 cryoglobulin: comparison of crystals of the F(ab′)₂ fragment and the intact immunoglobulin. *Biochemistry* 1978; **17**: 820–823.

7. Alzari P M, Lascombe M-B, Poljak R J. Three-dimensional structure of antibodies. *Ann Rev Immunol* 1988; **6**: 555–580.

8. Williams A F, Barclay A N. The immunoglobulin superfamily: domains for cell surface recognition. *Ann Rev Immunol* 1988; **6**: 381–405.

9. Hanson D C, Yguerabide J, Schumaker V N. Segmental flexibility of immunoglobulin G antibody molecules in solution: a new interpretation. *Biochemistry* 1981; **20**: 6842–6852.

10. Burton D R. Is IgM-like dislocation a common feature of antibody function? *Immunol Today* 1986; **7**: 165–167.

11. Lund J, Takahashi N, Pound J D, *et al*. Oligosaccharide–protein interactions in IgG can modulate recognition by Fc receptors. *FASEB J* 1995; **9**: 115–119.

12. Duncan A R, Winter G. The binding site for C1q on IgG. *Nature* 1988; **332**: 738–741.

13. Feinstein A, Richardson N, Taussig M J. Immunoglobulin flexibility in complement activation. *Immunol Today* 1986; **7**: 169–174.

14. Zheng Y, Shopes B, Holowka D, *et al*. Dynamic conformations compared for IgE and IgG1 in solution and bound to receptors. *Biochemistry* 1992; **31**: 7446–7456.

15. McBride O W, Hieter P A, Hollis G F, *et al*. Chromosomal location of human kappa and lambda immunoglobulin light chain constant region genes. *J Exp Med* 1982; **155**: 1480–1486.

16. Underdown B J, Schiff J M. Immunoglobulin A: strategic defense at the mucosal surface. *Ann Rev Immunol* 1986; **4**: 389–417.

17. Mestecky J, McGhee J R. Immunoglobulin A: molecular and cellular interactions involved in IgA biosynthesis and immune response. *Adv Immunol* 1987; **40**: 404–412.

18. Leu C, Tarkovski A, Mestecky J. Systemic immunisation with pneumococcal polysaccharide vaccine induces predominant IgA2 reponse of peripheral blood lymphocytes and increases of both serum and secretory anti-pneumococcal antibodies. *J Immunol* 1988; **140**: 3793–3800.

19. Maliszweski C R, March C J, Scheonborn M A, *et al*. Expression cloning of a human receptor for IgA. *J Exp Med* 1990; **172**: 1665–1672.

20. Shen L, Collins J E, Scheonborn M A, *et al*. Lipopolysaccharide and cytokine augmentation of human monocyte IgA receptor expression and function. *J Immunol* 1994; **152**: 4080–4086.

21. Lucisano Valim Y M, Lachmann P J. The effect of antibody isotype and antigenic density on the complement-fixing activity of immune complexes: a systematic study using chimeric anti-NP antibodies with human Fc regions. *Clin Exp Immunol* 1991; **84**: 1–8.

22. Vaerman J-P. Phylogenetic aspects of mucosal immunoglobulins. In: Mestecky J, ed. *Handbook of Mucosal Immunology*. New York: Academic Press, 1994; 99–104.

23. Brandtzaeg P. The role of J chain and secretory component in receptor mediated glandular and hepatic transport of immunoglobulins in man. *Scand J Immunol* 1985; **22**: 111–146.

24. Kilain M, Russell M W. Function of mucosal immunoglobulins. In: Mestecky J, ed. *Handbook of Mucosal Immunology*. New York: Academic Press, 1994; 127–137.

25. Schaffer F M, Monteiro R C, Volanakis J E, *et al*. IgA deficiency. In: Rosen F S, Seligmann M, eds. *Immunodeficiency*. Switzerland: Harwood Academic Press, 1993; 77–88.

26. French M A, Denis K A, Dawkins R, *et al*. Severity of infection in IgA deficiency: correlation with decreased serum antibodies to pneumococcal polysaccharides and decreased serum IgG2 and/or IgG4. *Clin Exp Immunol* 1995; **100**: 47–53.

27. Jefferis R, Kumararatne D S. Selective IgG subclass deficiency: quantification and clinical significance. *Clin Exp Immunol* 1990; **81**: 357–368.

28. Statement on *Haemophilus influenzae* type B conjugate vaccines for use in infants and children. *Can Med Assoc J* 1993; **148**: 199–204.

29. Bredius R G M, de Vries C E E, Troelstra A, *et al*. Phagocytosis of *Staphylococcus aureus* and *Haemophilus influenzae* type b opsonised with polyclonal human IgG1 and IgG2 antibodies. Functional hFcγRII a polymorphism to IgG2. *J Immunol* 1993; **151**: 1271–1280.

30. Reth M. Antigen receptors on lymphocytes. *Ann Rev Immunol* 1992; **10**: 97–121.
31. Davis A C, Shulman M J. IgM—molecular requirements for its assembly and function. *Immunol Today* 1989; **10**: 118–120.
32. Metzger H. Receptors of high affinity for IgE. *Immunol Rev* 1992; **125**: 37–48.
33. Capron A, Dessaint J P. Immunological aspects of schistosomiasis. *Ann Rev Med* 1992; **43**: 209–218.
34. Capron M, Capron A. IgE and effector cells in schistosomiasis. *Science* 1994; **264**: 1876–1877.
35. Gordon J, Flores-Romo L, Cairns J A, *et al*. CD23: a multi-functional receptor/lymphokine? *Immunol Today* 1989; **10**: 153–157.
36. Delespesse G, Sarfati M, Hofstetter H. Human IgE-binding factors. *Immunol Today* 1989; **10**: 159–164.
37. Helm B, Marsh P, Vercelli D, *et al*. The mast cell binding site on human immunoglobulin E. *Nature* 1988; **331**: 180–183.
38. Weetal M, Shopes B, Holowka D, *et al*. Mapping the site of interaction between murine IgE and its high affinity receptor with chimeric Ig. *J Immunol* 1990; **145**: 3849–3854.
39. Padlan E A, Helm B A. Modelling of the lectin-homology domains of the human and murine low-affinity Fc-epsilon receptor. *Receptor* 1993; **3**: 325–341.
40. Padlan E A, Helm B A. Modelling study of IgE/receptor interactions. *Biochem Soc Trans* 1993; **21**: 963–967.
41. Tamma S M L, Coico R F. IgD positive human T lymphocytes. Identification and partial characterisation of a human IgD binding factor. *J Immunol* 1992; **148**: 2050–2057.
42. Coico R F, Xue B, Wallace D, *et al*. T cell receptors for IgD. *Nature* 1985; **316**: 744–776.
43. Swenson C D, Amin A R, Edington J, *et al*. The role of IgD-receptors on T cells in young and aged mice. *FASEB J* 1994; **8**: A749.
44. Amin A R, Swenson C D, Wei C F, *et al*. The IgD receptor on human T cells is a lectin that binds carbohydrate sequences common to IgD and IgA. *FASEB J* 1994; **8**: A749.
45. Cheng H L, Blattner F R, Fitzmaurice L, *et al*. Structure of genes for membrane and secreted murine IgD heavy chains. *Nature* 1982; **296**: 410–415.
46. Weisbart R H, Kacena A, Schuh A, *et al*. GM-CSF induces human neutrophil IgA-mediated phagocytosis by an IgA Fc receptor activation mechanism. *Nature* 1988; **332**: 647–648.
47. Stewart W W, Mazengera R L, Shen L, *et al*. Unaggregated IgA binds to neutrophil Fc$_\alpha$R at physiological concentrations and is endocytosed but cross-linking is necessary to elicit a respiratory burst. *J Luekoc Biol* 1994; **56**: 481–487.
48. van de Winkel J G J, Anderson C L. Biology of human immunoglobulin G Fc receptors. *J Leukoc Biol* 1991; **49**: 511–524.
49. van de Winkel J G J, Capel P J A. Human IgG fc receptor heterogeneity: Molecular aspects and clinical relevance. *Immunol Today* 1993; **14**: 215–221.
50. Sanders L A M, Feldman R G, Voorhorstogink M M, *et al*. Human immunoglobulin G (IgG) Fc-receptor IIA (CD32) polymorphism and IgG2-mediated bacterial phagocytosis by neutrophils. *Infect Immun* 1995; **63**: 73–81.
51. Burmeister W P, Gastinel L N, Simister N E, *et al*. Crystal structure at 2.2A° of the MHC related neonatal Fc receptor. *Nature* 1994; **372**: 336–343.
52. Kobayashi K, Brown W R. Study of a colonic IgG-Fc binding site on cultured epithelial cells. *Dig Dis Sci* 1994; **39**: 526–533.
53. Borsos T, Rapp H J. Complement fixation on cell surfaces by 19S and 7S antibodies. *Science* 1965; **150**: 505–506.
54. Humphrey J H, Dourmashkin R R. The lesions in cell membranes caused by complement. *Adv Immunol* 1969; **11**: 75–115.
55. Schifferli J A, Ng Y C, Peters D K. The role of complement and its receptor in the elimination of immune complexes. *N Engl J Med* 1986; **315**: 488–495.
56. Banchereau J, Rousset F. Human B lymphocytes: phenotype, proliferation and differentiation. *Adv Immunol* 1992; **52**: 125–261.
57. Lefranc M, Lefranc G P, Rabbitts T H. Inherited deletion of immunoglobulin heavy chain constant region genes in normal human individuals. *Nature* 1982; **300**: 760–762.
58. Michaelson T E, Kornstad L. IgG subclass distribution of anti-Rh, anti-Kell and anti-Duffy antibodies measured by sensitive haemagglutination assays. *Clin Exp Immunol* 1987; **67**: 637–645.

59. Urbaniak S J, Greiss M A. ADCC (K-cell) lysis of human erythrocytes sensitised with rhesus alloantibodies. III. Comparison of IgG anti-D agglutination and lytic (ADCC) activity and the role of IgG subclasses. *Br J Haematol* 1980; **46:** 447–453.

60. Wiener, E. The ability of IgG subclasses to cause the elimination of targets *in vivo* and to mediate their destruction by phagocytosis/cytolysis *in vitro*. In: Shakib F, ed. *The Human IgG Subclasses. Molecular Analysis of Structure, Function and Regulation.* Oxford:Pergamon, 1990; 135–160.

61. Zupanska B M, Brojer E, Richards Y, *et al.* Serological and immunological characteristics of maternal anti-Rh(D) antibodies in predicting the severity of haemolytic disease of the newborn. *Vox Sang* 1989; **56:** 247–253.

62. Ambrosino D M, Schiffman G, Gotsschlich E C, *et al.* Correlation between G2m(n) immunoglobulin allotype and human antibody response and susceptibility to polysaccharide encapsulated bacteria. *J Clin Invest* 1985; **75:** 1935–1942.

63. Granoff D M, Munson R S. Prospects for prevention of *Haemophilus influenzae* type b disease by immunisation. *J Infect Dis* 1986; **153:** 448–461.

64. Brüggemann M, Williams G T, Bindon C I, *et al.* Comparison of the effector functions of human immunoglobulins using a matched set of chimeric antibodies. *J Exp Med* 1987; **166:** 1351–1361.

65. Jefferis R. Glycosylation of antibody molecules: functional significance. *Glycoconjugate J* 1993; **10:** 357–361.

66. Lund J, Winter G, Jones P T, *et al.* Human Fc$_\gamma$RI and Fc$_\gamma$RII interact with distinct but overlapping sites on human IgG. *J Immunol* 1991; **147:** 2657–2662.

67. Parekh R B, Dwek R A, Sutton B J, *et al.* Association of rheumatoid arthritis and primary osteoarthritis with changes in the glycosylation pattern of total serum IgG. *Nature* 1985; **316:** 452–457.

68. Tomana M, Schrohenloher R E, Koopman W J, *et al.* Abnormal glycosylation of serum IgG from patients with chronic inflammatory diseases. *Arthritis Rheum* 1988; **31:** 333–338.

69. Baenziger J, Kornfeld S. Structure of the carbohydrate units of IgA1 immunoglobulin. II. Structure of the *O*-glycosydically linked oligosaccharide units. *J Biol Chem* 1974; **249:** 7270–7281.

70. Mellis S J, Baenziger J U. Structures of the *O*-glycosidically linked oligosaccharides of human IgD. *J Biol Chem* 1983; **258:** 11557–11563.

71. Carson D A. Rheumatoid factor. In: Kelley W J, Harris E D, Ruddy S, *et al.*, eds. *Textbook of Rheumatology.* Philadelphia: Saunders, 1985; 664–676.

72. Jefferis R. Rheumatoid factors, B cells and immunoglobulin genes. *Br Med Bull* 1995; **51:** 312–331.

73. Smiley J D, Sachs C, Ziff M. *In vitro* synthesis of immunoglobulins by rheumatoid synovial membranes. *J Clin Invest* 1968; **47:** 624–632.

74. Munthe E, Natvig J B. Complement fixing intracellular complexes of IgG rheumatoid factor in rheumatoid plasma cells. *Scand J Immunol* 1972; **1:** 217–229.

75. Deftos M, Olee T, Carson D A. Defining the genetic origin of three rheumatoid synovium-derived IgG rheumatoid factors. *J Clin Invest* 1994; **93:** 2545–2553.

76. Padlan E A. Anatomy of the antibody molecule. *Mol Immunol* 1994; **31:** 169–217.

77. Adair J R. Engineering antibodies for therapy. *Immunol Rev* 1992; **130:** 5–40.

78. Wright A, Shin S U, Morrison S L. Genetically engineered antibodies—progress and prospects. *Crit Rev Immunol* 1992; **12:** 125–168.

79. Smith R I F, Morrison S L. Recombinant polymeric IgG—an approach to engineering more potent antibodies. *Bio-Technology* 1994; **12:** 683–688.

4

Localisation and Dynamics of Lymphoid Cells in the Different Compartments of the Lung

R. PABST

Medical School of Hannover, Germany

INTRODUCTION

The large volume of air we inhale each day ($>10\,000\,l$) contains variable amounts of foreign material, ranging from particulate matter of different sizes to minute microbial constituents, which are all potentially harmful. Each part of the respiratory tract has its own unspecific barrier system: for example, the air conducting parts are lined by a mucous layer, whereas the gas exchange parts contain numerous macrophages for unspecific clearance functions. In addition to such unspecific lines of defence, each organ needs an antigen specific defence system.

For a long time, lymphocytes were scarcely mentioned in detailed reviews on cells of the lung[1,2] but, more recently, interest has steadily increased[3-6]. Specific immune reactions are based on the presence and function of different lymphocyte subsets. Initiation of an immune response (afferent limb of immunity) requires the interaction of lymphoid cells with each other and with accessory cells such as antigen presenting cells. The effector side of immune reactions, such as cellular or humoral responses, also depends on the interaction of different cells of the immune system. Therefore, the localisation of the different lymphocyte subsets and accessory cells in the lung will be described, to facilitate understanding of pulmonary immune responses.

Antigens normally reach the lung in inhaled air, and encounter the air-conducting bronchial epithelium, the underlying mucosa, and specialised aggregations of lymphoid cells—the bronchus associated lymphoid tissue (BALT). In addition, there is a pool of pulmonary lymphocytes situated in the bronchoalveolar space and, finally, the intravascular pulmonary lymphocyte

                              R. Pabst

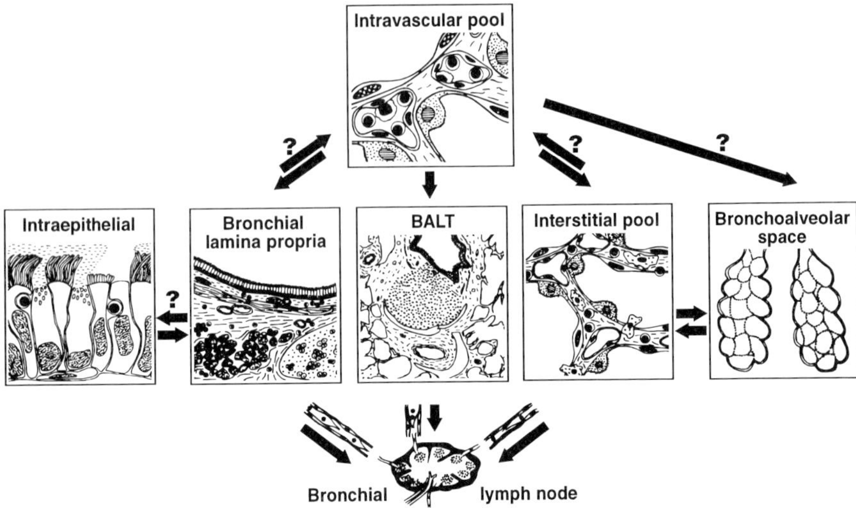

Figure 4.1. Schematic diagram of the different compartments of the lung containing lymphocytes. Their migratory routes are indicated by arrows. The question marks indicate lack of experimental data for that route. BALT = Bronchus associated lymphoid tissue. (Modified from Pabst[6])

pool, from which lymphocytes can leave the blood and migrate into the interstitium.

Phenotypic studies of lung lymphocytes have been difficult to interpret. For instance, there are several reports of unique markers on lymphocytes from the lung, including a predominance of $\gamma\delta$ T lymphocytes in the early postnatal period in mice and a specific pattern of V_γ gene usage, indicating that maturation takes place within the lung[7]. However, these data have been obtained from minced lung tissue and thus the lymphocytes cannot be attributed to specific compartments. Furthermore, these lymphocytes have been called "resident"—a designation which is not valid, in view of the absence of kinetic data. Therefore, in order to understand the role of lung lymphoid tissue, it is critical to understand the localisation of lymphocytes in different parts of the lung and the migratory routes of lymphocytes through the lung. These two aspects will be considered in detail in this chapter. Figure 4.1 summarises the general relationships.

LYMPHOCYTES IN THE BRONCHIAL EPITHELIUM

In the normal epithelium of the bronchi, lymphocytes are found interspersed with the many other cell types and are therefore called intraepithelial lymphocytes (IELs). In healthy control subjects, the numbers of the lymphocyte cluster of differentiation (CD) subsets per 100 epithelial nuclei were approximately 18 CD3+, 5 CD4+ and 11 CD8+ indicating a preponderance of CD8+ cells compared with CD4+[8]. As in the gut epithelium, there are few B lymphocytes in this compartment, and in man only about 1% of all T lymphocytes express the $\gamma\delta$ T cell receptor[9]. In the gut, an interesting heterodimeric cell surface glycoprotein of the integrin family is expressed on IELs, which seems to be critical for cell to cell adhesion and adhesion to matrix proteins. Initially, this adhesion molecule was identified by the HML-1 antibody, but it has now been identified as the $\alpha_E\beta_7$ integrin[10]. Immunohistology showed that IELs in mouse and rat tracheal and bronchial epithelium were positive for this integrin[11–13]. Two independent groups described large numbers of $\alpha_E\beta_7+$ lymphocytes in bronchoalveolar lavage (BAL) samples from human volunteers and patients with lung disease[10,14], which is compatible with the hypothesis that some IELs are released into the BAL fluid.

The turnover of cells, their rate of immigration from the mucosa, their fate and the role of local proliferation in determining the nature of this population have not been studied, either in experimental animals or in man. Very little is known about the function of the IELs in the bronchial tract. There are surprisingly high numbers of dendritic cells in the human bronchial epithelium[15] and their numbers increase rapidly in immune reactions[16], therefore it could be argued that these dendritic cells present antigen to the lymphocytes. The recent findings of Holt *et al*[17] on the short life span of dendritic cells, and that the increase in dendritic cell numbers in the epithelium lasts only 2 days, followed by a dramatic increase of dendritic cells in the draining nodes, might indicate that the antigen is taken up by dendritic cells in the epithelium but then transported to the bronchial lymph node, and that only there is an immune reaction initiated.

LYMPHOCYTES IN THE BRONCHIAL MUCOSA

The T lymphocyte subset composition in the mucosa is different from that in the epithelium (Table 4.1). The proportion of lymphoid cells in the mucosa is about 12% of the total, consisting of approximately 10% B and 70% T lymphocytes[19]. No differences have been found between central and subsegmental bronchial mucosa[20]. The number of lymphoid cells calculated either per area of lamina propria or per length of basement membrane[20] differed from that of the IELs, with CD4+ cells predominating (approximately 18 CD3+, 10 CD4+ and 5 CD8+). The vast majority of the T cells stained with the marker CD45RO, which is normally believed to identify so called "memory" lymphocytes[21]. Recently, small clusters of T lymphocytes around dendritic cells have been described in human bronchial mucosa, indicating the cell–cell contact required to initiate an immune response[22]. Furthermore, B lymphocytes and plasma cells, many of which secrete IgA, are preferentially concentrated around bronchial glands[23]. Despite an increasing wealth of detail about autonomous nerves[24,25] and neuropeptides in the bronchial wall[26], little is known about a possible regulatory function of neurotransmitters affecting lymphocyte function in the bronchial wall.

 R. Pabst

Table 4.1. Lymphocyte subsets (per mm^2) in the bronchial wall of
never smokers and ex-smokers (data derived from Richmond *et al.*[18])

	CD3+	CD4+	CD8+	CD25+ (IL-2R)
Epithelium	297	82	219	0
Submucosa	306	162	132	2
Glands	153	72	109	3

IL-2R = Interleukin-2 receptor.

BRONCHUS ASSOCIATED LYMPHOID TISSUE — A VARIABLY INDUCIBLE STRUCTURE

BALT is the most fascinating compartment of lymphocytes in the lung. Interest in this structure, and the variability between species with respect to histotopographical details and, particularly, function—which was often extrapolated from one experimental species to others including humans—have led to some confusion over the past 20 years.

In 1973, Bienenstock *et al*[27,28] introduced the term bronchial associated lymphoid tissue (BALT) to describe aggregations of lymphoid cells in the bronchial wall, often near to bronchial bifurcations, with an infiltration of the covering epithelium by lymphocytes. These structures were compared to the well known aggregated lymphoid follicles in the gut, the Peyer's patches. A further typical feature of the epithelium of BALT comprises specialised epithelial cells that show non-ciliated microvilli or short cytoplasmic projections and have therefore also been termed M cells, in analogy with the M cells in the Peyer's patches epithelium. As has been described in two reviews[29,30], the latter are well characterised in respect of their function of taking up and transporting both soluble and particulate antigens, such as viruses, bacteria and yeast, in addition to inorganic particles. In electron microscope (EM) studies, the uptake of large molecules and virus particles by M cells has been documented in rabbit and mouse BALT[31−34]. However, a critical review on the light and EM features of these cells summarised many differences compared with M cells in Peyer's patches[35].

Most experiments on BALT had initially been performed in rabbits and rats, and the results were assumed to be relevant for other mammals, including man[36]. However, the frequency of BALT in different species is very variable[37,38] and it would seem also that particular stimuli are responsible for the development of BALT. For instance, in germfree pigs no BALT is found, whereas it is present in variable amounts in conventional pigs, and after infection with the lung pathogenic bacterium *Actinobacillus pleuropneumoniae*, all animals are found to have large amounts of BALT[37,39]. A further difference between Peyer's patches and BALT is that a clear compartmentalisation of BALT is obvious in rabbits but not in rats[35,40]. As in several other peripheral lymphoid organs, well developed BALT contains high endothelial venules (HEV), the entry sites for lymphocytes[41], and lymphocytes leave BALT via lymphatics[42]. As with all lymphoid organs,

BALT is supplied by sensory and adrenergic nerves, and thus may serve as an important link between the nervous and immune systems[43].

For clinicians, however, the most important aspect is whether BALT has a significant role in the human lung. Several years ago BALT was described in the lungs of patients with sudden infant death syndrome[44], recurrent pneumonia[45] and several other diseases affecting the immune system[46-49]. However, a study of several samples from each lung of 34 patients who had died of acute diseases but had no history of respiratory diseases (ages ranging from 3 months to 99 years) failed to identity the presence of BALT[37]. It was therefore concluded that under everyday conditions of exposure to antigen, BALT is not a constitutive structure in the human lung, and is thus unlikely to have an important role in the uptake of reoviruses[34] or in lung transplantation[50-52], as had been suggested on the basis of data from experimental animals. The confirmation of the absence of BALT in the healthy lung of adults initiated new discussions on the role of BALT in lung immunology[53,54].

BALT has often been identified in specimens of human lungs. Sato *et al*[55] studied open lung biopsy specimens from 70 patients with diffuse shadows on chest radiographs and found BALT in 12 of 17 patients diagnosed as suffering from diffuse panbronchiolitis. This BALT fulfilled most of the criteria for its identification in experimental animals, in that it was localised mostly at bifurcations, the covering epithelium was infiltrated by lymphocytes which were mostly CD4+ T helper cells and there was a distinct area of T cells with some HEVs at the border of follicles, which consisted partially of germinal centres; M cells, however, could not be identified in the lymphoepithelium by electron microscopy. Diffuse panbronchiolitis is characterised by a chronic exposure to pathogens, and bacteria were cultured from the sputum of 11 of the 12 patients: *Pseudomonas aeruginosa* in six, *Klebsiella pneumoniae* in two, *Haemophilus influenzae* in two and *Streptococcus pneumoniae* in one[55]. These findings are thus consistent with the concept that microbial stimulation may lead to the development of BALT in the human lung.

In support of this concept, Gould and Isaacson[56] studied postmortem examination specimens of 102 fetal and 17 infant lungs retrospectively. BALT was found in 47% and was almost invariably associated with choriomeningitis or intrauterine pneumonia. Among 51 fetuses without obvious infection, BALT was seen in only 10%, while in infant lungs (sudden infant death, meningitis and bronchopneumonia) BALT was seen in 77%. When T and B cells were assessed, no clear cut compartmentalisation was found and the intraepithelial lymphocytes were B cells, which is in contrast with data from adults. The high frequency of BALT in fetuses and infants with infection is also consistent with the idea that the presence of BALT appears to be dependent on extensive antigenic stimulation.

Two groups have looked for BALT-like structures in the lungs of smokers. The 20 lungs studied by Bosken *et al*[57] were all from patients who underwent lung resection for a peripheral carcinoma. Most lymphoid aggregates were not associated with bronchi, but located more peripherally. Richmond *et al*[58] used 31 whole lung specimens obtained after pneumonectomy for lung carcinoma or from organ donors. Interestingly, lymphoid aggregates were seen beneath the muscularis mucosae close to bronchial glands, but these structures do not fulfil the criteria for BALT. Other follicular structures consisted of germinal centres, infiltrated epithelium and HEV.

Thirteen of 14 examples of "true BALT" were found in the lungs of smokers. Further interesting aspects were the lack of M cells and the increasing distribution of BALT from the main stem bronchus to the periphery of the lung, which is different from the proximal localisation in rabbits. As no data on bacterial infections were available in either of these studies, it cannot be determined whether BALT developed in the patients as a result of smoking alone, or whether bacterial stimulation was also involved.

Holt[59] has suggested that BALT developed in the presence of human lung disease, and might be utilised for therapeutic purposes, as a site of antigen uptake as part of immunisation protocols. This hypothesis awaits further data to determine appropriate stimulatory agents for the development of BALT in humans.

In a recent investigation, the frequency of BALT was studied in the lungs of children who had died of sudden infant death syndrome and of other causes such as congenital heart malformations or lethal trauma[60]. The results indicated that the probability of finding BALT increased with age (with a higher frequency in cases of sudden infant death syndrome in all age groups). The following concept for BALT in humans has therefore been proposed. There is no BALT present at birth, in contrast with other lymphoid organs such as lymph nodes, spleen, tonsils or Peyer's patches. During the first year of life, in particular when the child becomes mobile, many different inhaled antigens, mostly of microbial origin, stimulate the development of BALT. In healthy adults BALT is not present, as other structures of the bronchial tract may fulfil its role. Chronic microbial stimuli may subsequently induce the reappearance of BALT in adults, and further unknown factors may even result in malignant transformation, leading to the development of tumours of BALT[61].

Future studies are required to focus on the structure and function of BALT in humans, as these topics are not only of general immunological significance, but also of major clinical relevance. There remain many unanswered questions. What is the best animal model, and which age range should be studied? Can the development of BALT be induced and the specialised epithelium used as an entry site for microbial or other antigens, as an immunisation technique? Is it important to suppress the development of BALT in some instances because it may have a pathological role in the human lung?

LYMPHOCYTES IN THE LUNG INTERSTITIUM

In routine histological sections of the normal lung, lymphocytes are seen in the narrow interstitium only rarely[62], which is probably why this compartment has been neglected for study. Holt *et al*[63] recovered surprisingly large numbers of lymphocytes from human lung samples and this was not the result of contamination by lymphocytes from the blood compartment or the bronchoalveolar space[64]. On the basis of the number of lymphocytes per gram of lung tissue and the weight of the lung, the total number of lymphocytes in the interstitial space of the human lung was calculated as roughly equivalent to the total circulating blood pool (about 10×10^9 in a healthy adult). In many studies in experimental animals and humans, the number, phenotype and function of "lung lymphocytes" were assessed and taken as representative of lymphocytes of the lung interstitium. However, this did not exclude an admixture of lymphocytes from the vascular and bronchoalveolar pool, BALT or bronchial mucosa and hence the results must be interpreted with caution.

An interesting observation has been that sections of the lung contained more natural killer (NK) cells that were CD16+ than were found in the blood[65]. The lung contains approximately 10×10^9 NK cells, which is a high proportion of all NK cells in the human body[66]. Marathias *et al.*[67] studied lymphocyte subsets in human lung samples from patients with lung cancer and compared them with blood lymphocytes of the same patients. The vast majority of T lymphocytes from the lung expressed the $\alpha\beta$ T cell receptor and more than 90% were CD45RO+, indicating the phenotype of "memory" lymphocytes, which is in contrast to the subset distribution in the blood. The interstitial pool is thus large and seems to be more than just a transit pool for lymphocytes on their way from the blood to the alveolar space. As macrophages and dendritic cells which can act as antigen presenting cells are also present in the lung interstitium[22], immune reactions might be initiated by the interstitial lymphocytes.

LYMPHOCYTES IN THE BRONCHOALVEOLAR SPACE

Since bronchoalveolar lavage (BAL) became a routine procedure in the clinics and recommendations for a standardised technique were published[68,69], the number of reports on lymphocytes in BAL samples from patients with different diseases has increased. Results suggested that the total number of lymphocytes in the bronchoalveolar space is approximately 5×10^8, which is equivalent to about 5% of the whole circulating lymphocyte pool in humans, or 5% of that of the interstitial lung pool[63]. In healthy adults only about 10% of all cells recovered by bronchoalveolar lavage are lymphocytes; of these the majority are T cells, and the CD4+ lymphocytes outnumber the CD8+ cells with a CD4/CD8 ratio of 1.7[5,70−72]; there are only 5–10% of B lymphocytes. The memory T cells (86%) are much more numerous than "naive" T cells. The expression of adhesion molecules of the integrin family show a preference for $\alpha_E\beta_7$ (42% of CD3+ T cells) and more CD8+ than CD4+ cells are also positive for $\alpha_E\beta_7$[10]. Lymphocytes expressing the interleukin-2 (IL-2) receptor or human leucocyte antigen HLA-DR are found in greater numbers in BAL samples than in the blood[73]. While blood lymphocytes do not express the activation marker very late activating antigen-1 (VLA-1), about 20% of lymphocytes in BAL samples are VLA-1 positive[74]. Thus lymphocytes recovered by bronchoalveolar lavage show major differences from blood lymphocytes or lymphocytes obtained from other lung compartments. Comparison is difficult, as most studies considered only one or two compartments of the lung or compared them with the blood. Table 4.2 shows the lymphocyte subsets, NK cells and monocytes obtained from the same animals: the lungs were perfused, lavaged and then mechanically disrupted to

Table 4.2. Relative numbers (%) of lymphocyte subsets, natural killer (NK) cells and monocytes in different compartments of the lung and blood obtained from the same rats ($n = 6$)[75]

	Blood	Perfusate	Lung parenchyma	BAL fluid
B cells	19.1 (3.9)	20.2 (5.1)	16.8 (4.3)	7.0 (1.6)
T cells	69.9 (5.2)	56.8 (7.2)	57.4 (8.0)	77.3 (7.7)
CD8	17.2 (2.1)	13.5 (3.3)	10.4 (2.5)	10.8 (1.8)
CD4	49.9 (3.7)	41.3 (5.1)	40.5 (4.6)	58.5 (6.5)
"Naive"	70.9 (2.4)	67.9 (3.4)	19.3 (5.6)	1.2 (0.3)
"Memory"	29.1 (2.4)	32.1 (3.4)	80.7 (5.6)	98.8 (0.3)
NK cells	2.3 (0.7)	5.1 (2.0)	5.0 (1.5)	5.0 (3.8)
Monocytes	8.3 (2.5)	12.8 (5.6)	12.1 (3.5)	3.2 (1.1)*

Values are mean (SE). BAL = Bronchoalveolar lavage.
*Excluding macrophages.

obtain interstitial lymphocytes. These data agree with most of the available data on individual compartments.

LYMPHOCYTES IN THE PULMONARY VASCULAR BED

It is generally accepted that a large proportion of all granulocytes are found in the pulmonary vascular bed, where they "roll" along the endothelium or marginate[76]. This pool is therefore often called the "marginating pool", in contrast to the "circulating pool", and contains approximately 28×10^9 granulocytes in a normal healthy person[77]. The interaction of adhesion molecules on granulocytes and endothelial cells in the lung capillary bed depends on a variety of stimuli[78]. A similar phenomenon observed with lymphocytes in the lung vasculature has long been taken as an artefact[79,80]. In perfusion studies this intracapillary lymphocyte pool was characterised in the rat[9], rabbit[81,82] and pig[80]. In carefully controlled, perfusion-fixed rabbit lungs, 1.7×10^7 lymphocytes per 1 ml of parenchyma were found, equivalent to an approximately 50-fold enrichment compared with the capillary blood volume[81]. In further experiments, the washout kinetics of intravascular lymphocytes in the rabbit lung were studied by computer assisted measurements of digitalised EM images, revealing a pool much larger than the circulating pool[82]. Lymphocytes released from the isolated lungs of young pigs totalled approximately 1.5×10^9 over a period of at least $4\,h$[80]. The size of this pool is unique to the lung, as the marginal pool of lymphocytes in other non-lymphoid organs, including the kidney and liver, is several times smaller[83]. When the lymphoid cells of the pulmonary vascular pool were labelled *in vitro*, transferred to recipients and their migration pattern compared with that of blood lymphocytes or splenic emigrants, the lymphocytes and lymphoblasts from the intravascular pulmonary pool showed a typical migration pattern, with many lymphoid cells returning to the lung[84]. It is only possible to speculate on the function of this pool: it could be a depot to be mobilised quickly on demand, or it might only be the first step of emigration into the pulmonary interstitium, which might start when locally produced chemokines from the lung parenchyma activate adhesion molecules on pulmonary endothelial cells.

In addition to intravascular granulocytes and lymphocytes, monocytes also adhere to the vessel wall[82]. These might partially be identical to the pulmonary intravascular macrophages, which show major species variations in number and function. This aspect has been reviewed by Staub[85].

ADHESION MOLECULES AND LYMPHOCYTES IN THE LUNG

Growing numbers of adhesion molecules have been characterised at a molecular level. There are three major families: the integrins, the immunoglobulin super-family and the selectins[86–88]. Adhesion molecules are essential for cell–cell contacts, for example leucocyte–endothelium, but also for cell contacts with extracellular matrix proteins. The probable role of adhesion molecules in immune reactions in diseases of the lung has recently been reviewed[89,90]. Adhesion molecules can be upregulated by cytokines[91] or during inflammation, as has been documented for intercellular adhesion molecule-1 (ICAM-1) on lung endothelial cells in experimental Goodpasture syndrome[92] and pneumonia[93]. The adhesion molecule ICAM-1 is essential for leucocyte adhesion via CD18, as shown for monocyte retention in the lung[94] and in CD18 dependent emigration in rabbits[78]. Much less is known about soluble adhesion molecules such as sICAM-1, which is increased in BAL fluid in allergic subjects following segmental antigen challenge[95]. Antibodies against adhesion molecules affect granulocyte and eosinophil accumulation in the lung, making it possible to prevent pathological reactions[89,90].

Despite all the existing data on the role of adhesion molecules in lymphocyte migration[96], little is known about the role of the same adhesion molecules in lymphocyte function in the lung. When the effect of an antibody against the integrin $\alpha_4\beta_7$ or anti-L-selectin was tested on lymphocyte migration in the mouse, major differences were seen in the homing capacity to Peyer's patches or peripheral lymph nodes, but the number of lymphocytes recovered from the lung was not affected[97]. Thus other adhesion molecules are probably effective in the lung. When endotoxin or tumour necrosis factor α was infused intravenously in sheep, the number of lymphocytes in the lung increased and blood lymphocytes decreased[98]. Furthermore, lymphocyte output in lung lymph decreased, indicating an arrest of lymphocytes within the lung[99]. The molecular mechanisms behind this phenomenon are not known. In a recent study, an antibody against VLA-4 suppressed the antigen induced infiltration of the bronchial wall by CD4+ and CD8+ lymphocytes and prevented bronchial hyperactivity in guineapigs[100]. A comparable antibody to VLA-4 partially blocked the *in vitro* adherence of T lymphocytes to human airway smooth muscle cells[101], suggesting that VLA-4 has a major role in lymphocyte migration. These are a few examples of how it may be possible therapeutically to influence lymphocyte migration into the lung or from one compartment to another. However, there is a suggestion that allergen challenge in asthma patients tends to decrease localisation specificity expressed by typical homing receptors on lymphocytes in the bronchoalveolar space[102].

MIGRATION OF LYMPHOCYTES FROM ONE LUNG COMPARTMENT TO ANOTHER

Only for didactic purposes has the lung been divided into different compartments; these are not separated from each other in reality. In Fig. 4.1, the arrows indicate the flux of lymphocytes from compartment to compartment as discussed in detail previously[6]. The question marks indicate areas of uncertainty. The turnover, local proliferation, transit time of the different lymphocyte subsets and regulatory factors in this dynamic system are largely unknown. Without such data, a meaningful interpretation of an increase in a certain lymphocyte subset in one compartment is difficult.

INTEGRATION OF LUNG LYMPHOCYTES INTO THE IMMUNE SYSTEM

Lymphocytes enter the lung via the blood; from most compartments, they leave via lymphatics into regional lymph nodes. For a long time, lymphocytes in the bronchoalveolar space were considered to be endstage effete cells to be eliminated by the mucociliary escalator. Recently, it was demonstrated that lymphocytes return from the bronchoalveolar space to regional lymph nodes, with differences between the kinetics of the various lymphocyte subsets[103]. Thus lymphocytes from the lung can also emigrate to other organs, and hence the lung is part of the general route of trafficking lymphocytes (Fig. 4.2).

One aspect of the role of the lung as part of the general mucosal immune system is of major clinical relevance for preventing or even treating infections of the lung[104–107]. Until recently, only the migration of precursor cells of IgA-producing plasma cells from the gut to the bronchial mucosa had been studied (Fig. 4.3)[108,109]. However, T lymphocytes migrating from the gut to the bronchial tract also have an important role[110]. In a rat model, T lymphocytes protected the lung against colonisation with *H. influenzae*[111,112] and CD4+ lymphocytes enhanced the clearance of *Ps. aeruginosa*[113]. The clinical importance of this is shown by the effectiveness of oral immunisation protocols against lung viral and bacterial antigens[114,115]. In addition to influencing the bronchial mucosa, other immunisation protocols can modify the lymphocyte number and subset composition in the bronchoalveolar space. For example, the infection of pigs by the lung pathogenic bacterium *Actinobacillus pleuropneumoniae* is a major veterinary problem. Immunisation with viable or inactivated bacteria, applied as an aerosol or orally, has been shown to result in an increase in T lymphocytes (including CD4+ and CD8+ lymphocytes) and B lymphocytes, and in the appearance of lymphoblasts and plasma cells in the bronchoalveolar space[39]. The animals also become protected against a subsequent infection and develop

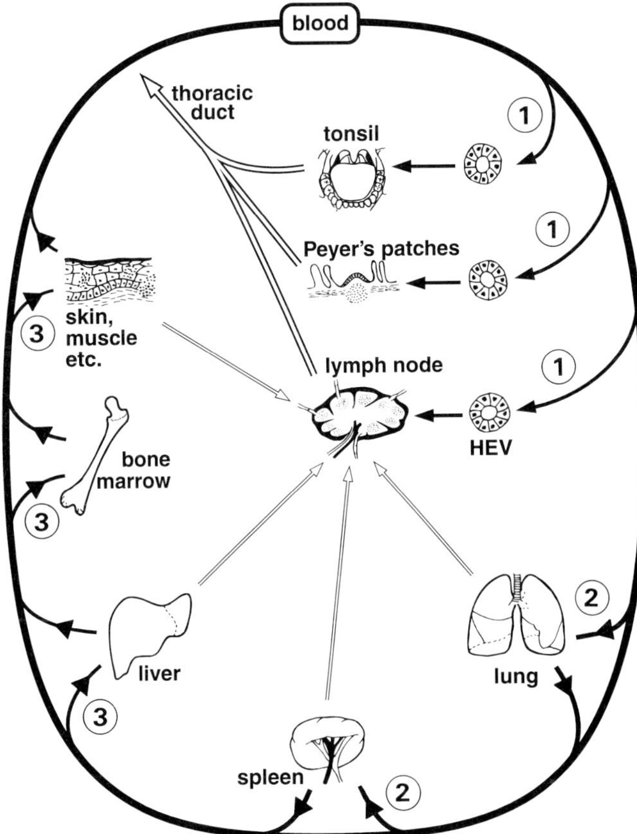

Figure 4.2. Different migratory routes of lymphocytes through the body. 1 = Exit from the blood via high endothelial venules (HEV) into typical lymphoid organs such as tonsil, Peyer's patches and lymph node. 2 = Exit into organs without specialised venules (e.g. lung, spleen) at high rates (indicated by the size of the arrows). 3 = Exit into other non-lymphoid organs, such as liver, bone marrow, skin and muscle. The lymphocytes return to the circulating blood pool either via lymphatics and finally the thoracic duct (open arrows), or directly into the blood (black arrows)

increased specific antibody titres in the lavage fluid[116]. Furthermore, after the pigs were exposed to viable bacteria in an aerosol, no further increase in lymphocytes in the bronchoalveolar space was observed[117]. These data confirm the successful exploitation of the migratory route from the gut to the bronchoalveolar space to obtain effective lung immunisation.

Such observations confirm that understanding the function of lymphocytes in the lung requires not only more detailed study of the organotypic compartmentalisation of these cells, but also of their migratory route between the compartments and from other organs to the lung. This will then provide a basis on which to develop effective immunisation and therapeutic strategies.

                                    R. Pabst

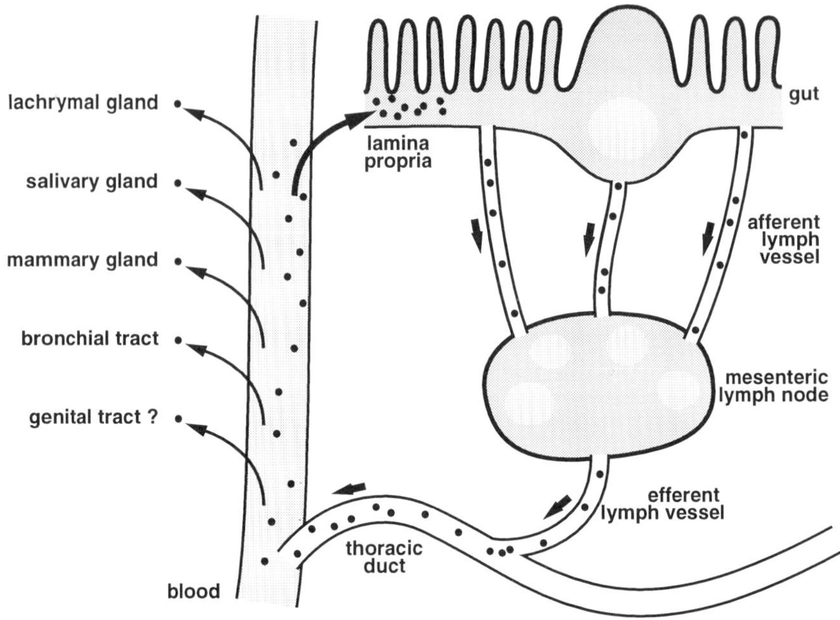

Figure 4.3. Migratory route of lymphocytes primed in the gut wall (Peyer's patches and lamina propria) to other mucosa lined organs. This route had initially been documented for precursors of IgA-producing cells, but there is increasing evidence that T lymphocytes also use this preferential migration route

ACKNOWLEDGEMENTS

The author's studies were supported by a grant from the German Federal Ministry of Research and Technology (01KE88141) and the German Research Foundation (Pa 240/7-1). The technical assistance of K. Westermann and the correction of the English by S. Fryk are gratefully acknowledged.

REFERENCES

1. Crapo J D, Barry B E, Gehr P, *et al*. Cell number and cell characteristics of the normal human lung. *Am Rev Respir Dis* 1982; **125:** 332–337.
2. Gail D B, Lenfant C J M. Cells of the lung: biology and clinical implications. *Am Rev Respir Dis* 1983; **127:** 366–387.
3. Daniele R P, ed. *Immunology and Immunologic Diseases of the Lung*. Boston: Blackwell, 1988.
4. Berman J S, Beer D J, Theodore A C, *et al*. Lymphocyte recruitment to the lung. *Am Rev Respir Dis* 1990; **142:** 238–257.
5. Saltini C, Richeldi L, Holroyd K J, *et al*. Lymphocytes. In: Crystal R G, West J B, eds. *The Lung: Scientific Foundations*. New York: Raven, 1991; 459–482.
6. Pabst R. Mucosa-associated lymphoid tissue. Only one part of the dynamic lung lymphoid system. In: Holgate S T, Busse W W, eds. *Asthma and Rhinitis*. Cambridge, MA: Blackwell, 1995; 415–425.

7. Sim G K, Rajaserkar R, Dessing M, *et al*. Homing and *in situ* differentiation of resident pulmonary lymphocytes. *Int Immunol* 1994; **6**: 1287–1295.

8. Bradley P A, Bourne F J, Brown P J. The respiratory tract immune system in the pig. I. Distribution of immunoglobulin-containing cells in the respiratory tract mucosa. *Vet Pathol* 1976; **13**: 81–89.

9. Scheuermann D W. Proliferation and transformation of lymphocytes in the lung capillaries of the rat: ultrastructure, acid phosphatase and peroxidase cytochemistry. *Acta Anat* 1982; **113**: 264–280.

10. Erle D J, Brown T, Christian D, *et al*. Lung epithelial lining fluid T cell subsets defined by distinct patterns of β7 and β1 integrin expression. *Am J Respir Cell Mol Biol* 1994; **10**: 237–244.

11. Cerf-Bensussan N, Jarry A, Brousse N, *et al*. A monoclonal antibody (HML-1) defining a novel membrane molecule present on human intestinal lymphocytes. *Eur J Immunol* 1987; **17**: 1279–1285.

12. Kilshaw P J, Baker K C. A unique surface antigen on intraepithelial lymphocytes in the mouse. *Immunol Lett* 1988; **18**: 149–154.

13. Cerf-Bensussan N, Guy-Grand D, Lisowska-Grospierre B, *et al*. A monoclonal antibody specific for rat intestinal lymphocytes. *J Immunol* 1986; **136**: 76–82.

14. Rosseau S, Friedrich J, Ziegler S, *et al*. Expression of alpha-IEL β7 integrin on bronchoalveolar lavage derived T-cells in interstitial lung disease. *Am J Respir Crit Care Med* 1994; **149**: A267.

15. Holt P G, Schon-Hegrad M A, Phillips M J, *et al*. Ia-positive dendritic cells form a tightly meshed network within the human airway epithelium. *Clin Exp Allergy* 1989; **19**: 597–601.

16. McWilliam A S, Nelson D, Thomas J A, *et al*. Rapid dendritic cell recruitment is a hallmark of the acute inflammatory response at mucosal surfaces. *J Exp Med* 1994; **179**: 1331–1336.

17. Holt P G, Haining S, Nelson D J, *et al*. Origin and steady-state turnover of class II MHC-bearing dendritic cells in the epithelium of the conducting airways. *J Immunol* 1994; **153**: 256–261.

18. Richmond I, Pritchard G E, Walters E H. Airway inflammation in the segmented bronchi of smokers and non-smokers. *Eur Respir J* 1994; **7** (suppl 18): 388S.

19. Hunninghake G W, Kawanami O, Ferrans V J, *et al*. Characterization of the inflammatory and immune effector cells in the lung parenchyma of patients with interstitial lung disease. *Am Rev Respir Dis* 1981; **123**: 407–412.

20. Azzawi M, Bradley B, Jeffery P K, *et al*. Identification of activated T lymphocytes and eosinophils in bronchial biopsies in stable atopic asthma. *Am Rev Respir Dis* 1990; **142**: 1407–1413.

21. Upham J W, McMenamin C, Schon-Hegrad M A, *et al*. Functional analysis of human bronchial mucosal T cells extracted with interleukin-2. *Am J Respir Crit Care Med* 1994; **149**: 1608–1613.

22. van Haarst J M W, de Wit H J, Drexhage H A, *et al*. Distribution and immunophenotype of mononuclear phagocytes and dendritic cells in the human lung. *Am J Respir Cell Mol Biol* 1994; **10**: 487–492.

23. Soutar C A. Distribution of plasma cells and other cells containing immunoglobulin in the respiratory tract of normal man and class of immunoglobulin therein. *Thorax* 1976; **31**: 158–166.

24. Barnes P J, Baraniuk J N, Belvisi M G. Neuropeptides in the respiratory tract. Part I. *Am Rev Respir Dis* 1991; **144**: 1187–1198.

25. Barnes P J, Baraniuk J N, Belvisi M G. Neuropeptides in the respiratory tract. Part II. *Am Rev Respir Dis* 1991; **144**: 1391–1399.

26. Barnes P J. Airway neuropeptides. In: Busse W W, Holgate S T, eds. *Asthma and Rhinitis*. Cambridge, MA: Blackwell, 1995; 667–685.

27. Bienenstock J, Johnston N, Perey D Y E. Bronchial lymphoid tissue. I. Morphologic characteristics. *Lab Invest* 1973; **28**: 686–692.

28. Bienenstock J, Johnston N, Perey D Y E. Bronchial lymphoid tissue. II. Functional characteristics. *Lab Invest* 1973; **28**: 693–698.

29. Kraehenbuhl J P, Neutra M R. Molecular and cellular basis of immune protection of mucosal surfaces. *Physiol Rev* 1992; **72**: 853–879.

30. Gebert A, Rothkötter H J, Pabst R. M cells in Peyer's patches of the intestine. *Int Rev Cytol* 1996; **167:** 91–159.

31. Tenner-Racz K, Racz P, Myrvik Q N, *et al.* Uptake and transport of horseradish peroxidase by lymphoepithelium of the bronchus-associated lymphoid tissue in normal and Bacillus Calmette-Guerin-immunized and challenged rabbits. *Lab Invest* 1979; **41:** 106–115.

32. Fournier M, Vai F, Derenne J P, *et al.* Bronchial lymphoepithelial nodules in the rat. Morphologic features and uptake and transport of exogenous proteins. *Am Rev Respir Dis* 1977; **116:** 685–694.

33. Pankow W, Wichert P. M cell in the immune system of the lung. *Respiration* 1988; **54:** 209–219.

34. Morin M J, Warner A, Fields B N. A pathway for entry of reoviruses into the host through M cells of the respiratory tract. *J Exp Med* 1994; **180:** 1523–1527.

35. Sminia T, Brugge-Gamelkoorn G J, Jeurissen S H M. Structure and function of bronchus-associated lymphoid tissue (BALT). *Crit Rev Immunol* 1989; **9:** 119–150.

36. Bienenstock J. Bronchus-associated lymphoid tissue. In: Bienenstock J, ed. *Immunology of the Lung and Upper Respiratory Tract*. New York: McGraw Hill, 1984; 96–118.

37. Pabst R, Gehrke I. Is the bronchus-associated lymphoid tissue (BALT) an integral structure of the lung in normal mammals including man? *Am J Respir Cell Mol Biol* 1990; **3:** 131–135.

38. Pabst R. Is BALT a major component of the human lung immune system? *Immunol Today* 1992; **13:** 119–122.

39. Delventhal S, Hensel A, Petzoldt K, *et al.* Effects of microbial stimulation on the number, size and activity of bronchus-associated lymphoid tissue (BALT) structures in the pig. *Int J Exp Pathol* 1992; **73:** 351–357.

40. Racz P, Tenner-Racz K, Myrvik Q N, *et al.* Functional architecture of bronchial associated lymphoid tissue and lymphoepithelium in pulmonary cell-mediated reactions in the rabbit. *J Reticuloendothel Soc* 1977; **22:** 59–83.

41. Brugge-Gamelkoorn G J, Kraal G. The specificity of the high endothelial venule in bronchus-associated lymphoid tissue (BALT). *J Immunol* 1985; **134:** 3746–3750.

42. Otsuki Y, Ito Y, Magari S. Lymphocyte subpopulations in high endothelial venules and lymphatic capillaries of bronchus-associated lymphoid tissue (BALT) in the rat. *Am J Anat* 1989; **184:** 139–146.

43. Nohr D, Weihe E. The neuroimmune link in the bronchus-associated lymphoid tissue (BALT) of cat and rat: peptides and neural markers. *Brain Behav Immun* 1991; **5:** 84–101.

44. Emery J L, Dinsdale F. Increased incidence of lymphoreticular aggregates in lungs of children found unexpectedly dead. *Arch Dis Child* 1974; **49:** 107–111.

45. Meuwissen H J, Hussain M. Bronchus-associated lymphoid tissue in human lung: correlation of hyperplasia with chronic pulmonary disease. *Clin Immunol Immunopathol* 1982; **23:** 548–561.

46. Rogers J, Langston C, Guerra I C. Pulmonary follicular lymphoid hyperplasia in a child with HTLV-III-related immunodeficiency. *Pediatr Pulmonol* 1986; **2:** 175–178.

47. Church J A, Isaacs H, Saxon A, *et al.* Lymphoid interstitial pneumonitis and hypogammaglobulinemia in children. *Am Rev Respir Dis* 1981; **124:** 491–496.

48. Yousem S A, Colby T V, Carrington C B. Follicular bronchitis/bronchiolitis. *Human Pathol* 1985; **16:** 700–706.

49. Yousem S A, Colby T V, Carrington C B. Lung biopsy in rheumatoid arthritis. *Am Rev Respir Dis* 1985; **131:** 770–777.

50. Prop J, Wildevuur C R H, Nieuwenhuis P. Lung allograft rejection in the rat. II. Specific immunological properties of lung grafts. *Transplantation* 1985; **40:** 126–131.

51. Prop J, Nieuwenhuis P, Wildevuur C R H. Lung allograft rejection in the rat. I. Accelerated rejection caused by graft lymphocytes. *Transplantation* 1985; **40:** 25–30.

52. Prop J, Wildevuur C R H, Nieuwenhuis P. Lung allograft rejection in the rat. III. Corresponding morphological rejection phases in various rat strain combinations. *Transplantation* 1985; **40:** 132–136.

53. McGhee J R, Kiyono H. New perspectives in vaccine development: mucosal immunity to infections. *Infect Agent Dis* 1993; **2:** 55–73.

54. Bienenstock J, Clancy R. Bronchial mucosal lymphoid tissue. In: Ogra P L, Strober W, Mestecky J, *et al*. eds *Handbook of Mucosal Immunology*. San Diego: Academic Press, 1994; 529–538.

55. Sato A, Chida K, Iwata M, *et al*. Study of bronchus-associated lymphoid tissue in patients with diffuse panbronchiolitis. *Am Rev Respir Dis* 1992; **146:** 473–478.

56. Gould S J, Isaacson P G. Bronchus-associated lymphoid tissue (BALT) in human fetal and infant lung. *J Pathol* 1993; **169:** 229–234.

57. Bosken C H, Hards J, Gatter K, *et al*. Characterization of the inflammatory reaction in the peripheral airways of cigarette smokers using immunocytochemistry. *Am Rev Respir Dis* 1992; **145:** 911–917.

58. Richmond I, Pritchard G E, Ashcroft T, *et al*. Bronchus associated lymphoid tissue (BALT) in human lung: its distribution in smokers and non-smokers. *Thorax* 1993; **48:** 1130–1134.

59. Holt P G. Development of bronchus associated lymphoid tissue (BALT) in human lung disease: a normal host defence mechanism awaiting therapeutic exploitation. *Thorax* 1993; **48:** 1097–1098.

60. Tschernig T, Kleemann W J, Pabst R. Frequency of bronchus-associated lymphoid tissue (BALT) in the lungs of children with sudden infant death syndrome and children who had died of other causes. *Thorax* 1995; **50:** 658–660.

61. Li G, Hansmann M L, Zwingers T, *et al*. Primary lymphomas of the lung: morphological, immunohistochemical and clinical features. *Histopathology* 1990; **16:** 519–531.

62. Weibel E R, Crystal R G. Structural organization of the pulmonary interstitium. In: Crystal R G, West J B, eds. *The Lung: Scientific Foundations*. New York: Raven, 1991; 369–380.

63. Holt P G, Robinson B W S, Reid M, *et al*. Extraction of immune and inflammatory cells from human lung parenchyma: evaluation of an enzymatic digestion procedure. *Clin Exp Immunol* 1986; **66:** 188–200.

64. Holt P G, Degebrodt A, Venaille T, *et al*. Preparation of interstitial lung cells by enzymatic digestion of tissue slices: preliminary characterization by morphology and performance in functional assays. *Immunology* 1985; **54:** 139–147.

65. Weissler J C, Nicod L P, Lipscomb M F, *et al*. Natural killer cell function in human lung is compartmentalized. *Am Rev Respir Dis* 1987; **135:** 941–949.

66. Westermann J, Pabst R. Distribution of lymphocyte subsets and natural killer cells in the human body. *Clin Invest* 1992; **70:** 539–544.

67. Marathias K P, Preffer F I, Pinto C, *et al*. Most human pulmonary infiltrating lymphocytes display the surface immune phenotype and functional responses of sensitized T cells. *Am J Respir Cell Mol Biol* 1991; **5:** 470–476.

68. Klech H, Pohl W, eds. Technical recommendations and guidelines for bronchoalveolar lavage (BAL). *Eur Respir J* 1989; **2:** 561–585.

69. Cherniack R M. Bronchoalveolar lavage constituents in healthy individuals, idiopathic pulmonary fibrosis, and selected comparison groups. *Am Rev Respir Dis* 1990; **141:** S169–202.

70. Reynolds H Y. Immunologic system in the respiratory tract. *Physiol Rev* 1991; **71:** 1117–1133.

71. Reynolds H Y. Integrated host defense against infections. In: Crystal R G, West J B, eds. *The Lung: Scientific Foundations*. New York: Raven, 1991; 1899–1911.

72. Saltini C, Kirby M, Trapnell B C, *et al*. Biased accumulation of T lymphocytes with "memory"-type CD45 leukocyte common antigen gene expression on the epithelial surface of the human lung. *J Exp Med* 1990; **171:** 1123–1140.

73. Walker C, Bode E, Boer L, *et al*. Allergic and nonallergic asthmatics have distinct patterns of T-cell activation and cytokine production in peripheral blood and bronchoalveolar lavage. *Am Rev Respir Dis* 1992; **146:** 109–115.

74. Saltini C, Hemler M E, Crystal R G. T lymphocytes compartmentalized on the epithelial surface of the lower respiratory tract express the very late activation antigen complex VLA-1. *Clin Immunol Immunopathol* 1988; **46:** 221–233.

75. Fliegert F G, Tschernig T, Pabst R. Comparison of lymphocyte subsets, monocytes and NK cells in three different lung compartments and peripheral blood in the rat. *Exp Lung Res* 1996; **22:** 677–690.

76. O'Byrne P M. Neutrophil dynamics in airway disease. In: Busse W W, Holgate S T, eds. *Asthma and Rhinitis.* Cambridge, MA: Blackwell, 1995; 389–396.

77. Hogg J C. Neutrophil traffic. In: Crystal R G, West J B, eds. *The Lung: Scientific Foundations.* New York: Raven, 1991; 565–579.

78. Burns A R, Doerschuk C M. Quantitation of L-selectin and CD18 expression on rabbit neutrophils during CD18-independent and CD18-dependent emigration in the lung. *J Immunol* 1994; **153:** 3177–3188.

79. Hall J. The study of circulating lymphocytes *in vivo:* a personal view of artifice and artifact. *Immunol Today* 1985; **6:** 149–152.

80. Pabst R, Binns R M, Licence S T, *et al.* Evidence of a selective major vascular marginal pool of lymphocytes in the lung. *Am Rev Respir Dis* 1987; **136:** 1213–1218.

81. Ermert L, Seeger W, Duncker H R. Computer-assisted morphometry of the intracapillary leukocyte pool in the rabbit lung. *Cell Tissue Res* 1993; **271:** 469–476.

82. Ermert L, Duncker H R, Rosseau S, *et al.* Morphometric analysis of pulmonary intracapillary leukocyte pools in *ex-vivo* perfused rabbit lungs. *Am J Physiol* 1994; **267:** L64–L70.

83. Pabst R. Compartmentalization and kinetics of lymphoid cells in the lung. *Reg Immunol* 1990; **3:** 62–71.

84. Binns R M, Licence S T, Pabst R. Homing of blood, splenic and lung emigrant lymphoblasts: comparison with the behaviour of lymphocytes from these sources. *Int Immunol* 1992; **4:** 1011–1019.

85. Staub N C. Pulmonary intravascular macrophages. *Annu Rev Physiol* 1994; **56:** 47–67.

86. Adams D H, Shaw S. Leucocyte-endothelial interactions and regulation of leucocyte migration. *Lancet* 1994; **343:** 831–836.

87. Picker J L. Control of lymphocyte homing. *Curr Opin Immunol* 1994; **6:** 394–406.

88. Springer T A. Traffic signals for lymphocyte recirculation and leukocyte emigration: the multi-step paradigm. *Cell* 1994; **76:** 301–314.

89. Hamacher J, Schaberg T. Adhesion molecules in lung diseases. *Lung* 1994; **172:** 189–213.

90. Wegner C D, Gundel R H, Rothlein R, *et al.* Expression and probable roles of cell adhesion molecules in lung inflammation. *Chest* 1992; **101:** 34S–39S.

91. Pilewski J M, Panettieri R A, Kaiser L R, *et al.* Expression of endothelial cell adhesion molecules in human bronchial xenografts. *Am J Respir Crit Care Med* 1994; **150:** 795–801.

92. Hill P A, Lan H Y, Nikolic-Paterson D J, *et al.* Pulmonary expression of ICAM-1 and LFA-1 in experimental Goodpasture's syndrome. *Am J Pathol* 1994; **145:** 220–227.

93. Burns A R, Takei F, Doerschuk C M. Quantitation of ICAM-1 expression in mouse lung during pneumonia. *J Immunol* 1994; **153:** 3189–3198.

94. Doherty D E, Downey G P, Schwab B, *et al.* Lipopolysaccharide-induced monocyte retention in the lung. Role of monocyte stiffness, actin assembly, and CD18-dependent adherence. *J Immunol* 1994; **153:** 241–255.

95. Takahashi N, Liu M C, Proud D, *et al.* Soluble intracellular adhesion molecule 1 in bronchoalveolar lavage fluid of allergic subjects following segmental antigen challenge. *Am J Respir Crit Care Med* 1994; **150:** 704–709.

96. Granger D N, Kubes P. The microcirculation and inflammation: modulation of leukocyte-endothelial cell adhesion. *J Leuk Biol* 1994; **55:** 662–675.

97. Hamann A, Andrew D P, Jablonski-Westrich D, *et al.* Role of alpha4-integrins in lymphocyte homing to mucosal tissues *in vivo. J Immunol* 1994; **152:** 3282–3293.

98. Duke S S, Guerry-Force M L, Forbes J T, *et al.* Acute endotoxin-induced lymphocyte subset sequestration in sheep lungs. *Lab Invest* 1990; **62:** 355–362.

99. Johnson J, Brigham K L, Jesmok G, *et al.* Morphologic changes in lungs of anesthetized sheep following intravenous infusion of recombinant tumor necrosis factor alpha. *Am Rev Respir Dis* 1991; **144:** 179–186.

100. Pretolani M, Ruffié C, Lapa e Silva J R, *et al.* Antibody to very late activation antigen 4 prevents antigen-induced bronchial hyperreactivity and cellular infiltration in the guinea pig airways. *J Exp Med* 1994; **180:** 795–805.

101. Lazaar A L, Albelda S M, Pilewski J M, *et al.* T lymphocytes adhere to airway smooth muscle cells via integrins and CD44 and induce smooth muscle cell DNA synthesis. *J Exp Med* 1994; **180:** 807–816.

102. Picker L J, Martin R J, Trumble A, *et al*. Differential expression of lymphocyte homing receptors by human memory/effector T cells in pulmonary versus cutaneous immune effector sites. *Eur J Immunol* 1994; **24:** 1269–1277.

103. Pabst R, Binns R M. Lymphocytes migrate from the bronchoalveolar space to regional bronchial lymph nodes. *Am J Respir Crit Care Med* 1995; **151:** 495–499.

104. Bienenstock J, Befus A D. Mucosal immunology. *Immunology* 1980; **41:** 249–270.

105. Merchant R K, Schwartz D A, Helmers R A, *et al*. Bronchoalveolar lavage cellularity. The distribution in normal volunteers. *Am Rev Respir Dis* 1992; **146:** 448–453.

106. Brandtzaeg P. Human immune response patterns of human mucosae: induction and relation to bacterial respiratory tract infections. *J Infect Dis* 1992; **165** (suppl 1): 167–176.

107. Husband A J. Mucosal immune interactions in intestine, respiratory tract and mammary gland. *Prog Vet Microbiol Immunol* 1985; **1:** 25–57.

108. Weisz-Carrington P, Roux M E, McWilliams M, *et al*. Organ and isotype distribution of plasma cells producing specific antibody after oral immunization: evidence for a generalized secretory immune system. *J Immunol* 1979; **123:** 1705–1708.

109. McDermott M R, Bienenstock J. Evidence for a common mucosal immunologic system. I. Migration of B immunoblasts into intestinal, respiratory, and genital tissues. *J Immunol* 1979; **122:** 1892–1898.

110. Dunkley M, Pabst R, Cripps A. An important role for intestinally-derived T cells in respiratory defence against gram-negative bacteria. *Immunol Today* 1995; **16:** 231–236.

111. Wallace F J, Cripps A W, Clancy R L, *et al*. A role for intestinal T lymphocytes in bronchus mucosal immunity. *Immunology* 1991; **74:** 68–73.

112. Cripps A W, Dunkley M L, Clancy R L. Mucosal and systemic immunizations with killed *Pseudomonas aeruginosa* protect against acute respiratory infection in rats. *Infect Immun* 1994; **62:** 1427–1436.

113. Dunkley M L, Clancy R L, Cripps A W. A role for CD4+ T cells from orally immunized rats in enhanced clearance of *Pseudomonas aeruginosa* from the lung. *Immunology* 1994; **83:** 362–369.

114. Clancy R, Murree-Allen K, Cripps A, *et al*. Oral immunisation with killed *Haemophilus influenzae* for protection against acute bronchitis in chronic obstructive lung disease. *Lancet* 1985; **II:** 1395–1397.

115. Bergmann K C, Waldman R H. Oral immunization with influenza virus: experimental and clinical studies. *Curr Top Microbiol Immunol* 1989; **146:** 83–89.

116. Hensel A, Pabst R, Bunka S, *et al*. Oral and aerosol immunization with viable or inactivated *Actinobacillus pleuropneumoniae* bacteria: antibody response to capsular polysaccharides in bronchoalveolar lavage fluids (BALF) and sera of pigs. *Clin Exp Immunol* 1994; **96:** 91–97.

117. Pabst R, Delventhal S, Gebert A, *et al*. Lymphocyte subsets in bronchoalveolar lavage after exposure to *Actinobacillus pleuropneumoniae* in pigs previously immunized orally or by aerosol. *Lung* 1995; **173:** 233–241.

5

Pulmonary Macrophages

L. W. POULTER

Royal Free Hospital School of Medicine, London, UK

INTRODUCTION

It is now approaching 100 years since Eli Metchnikoff first observed macrophages and introduced us to a population of cells that were seen for many years as garbage collectors! Even when it was revealed that macrophages constituted part of a systemic network, the reticuloendothelial system, and later the mononuclear phagocyte system[1], it was not realised just how diverse and complex the role of these cells might be. Over the past 20 years such a remarkable heterogeneity in terms of morphology, physiology and function has been discovered to reside in these populations that the term "macrophage" now needs to be constantly qualified when describing one specific cell.

We are now aware that, in addition to acting as phagocytes, these cells can stimulate or suppress lymphocyte function; act as cytotoxic cells against neoplasms; exhibit microbicidal activity; and secrete a multitude of soluble factors that can orchestrate not only the macrophage populations themselves but also most, if not all, other cells within the tissue milieu. Given this, and the fact that these functions can be modified repeatedly in response to local stimuli and vary from one tissue site to another, one begins to realise just how versatile these cells are.

Despite their diversity, it is clear that these cells are designed for defence. Macrophages in all their forms should be seen in the context of protection. Whether this be simple protection from the debris generated by the host (removal of effete cells) or protection from infectious agents (microbicidal capacity), promotion of specific acquired immunity (antigen presentation), or regulation of effector mechanisms and inflammation (promotion and suppression via secretion of soluble mediators), macrophages are central to the policing and preservation of tissue integrity.

The lung represents a unique challenge to any population of cells designed for host protection. Like the skin, it is constantly exposed to the environment and thus to any toxins, organic and inorganic particulate matter or microbes naturally present in that environment. As the physiological function of the lungs is vital to survival, it needs to be well protected. This chapter concentrates on the macrophage populations, although their function and distribution should be viewed in the context of a much broader defensive plan involving many other cells and mechanisms, which are considered comprehensively elsewhere in this book.

ORIGINS AND DISTRIBUTIONS

Pulmonary macrophages are bone marrow derived cells that differentiate from blood monocytes after they have emigrated into the tissues. Under steady state conditions there is constant recruitment of monocytes from the capillaries occurring in response to chemotactic factors. These cells then populate the various compartments of the lung, differentiating into mature macrophages. The possibility that pulmonary macrophages proliferate has been raised by several authors who have speculated on the contribution that division might make in sustaining the overall pulmonary macrophage pool. It seems likely that, although macrophages are known to have the capacity to divide, under normal conditions fewer than 0.5% of the pulmonary population would be dividing. (It is suggested, however, that this figure can increase significantly in inflammatory processes.) Thus, in health, local division of macrophages in the lung is not considered to make a significant contribution to their renewal[2].

The mature lung macrophage pool is conventionally divided into five types, distinguished by their anatomical location (Fig. 5.1): pleural macrophages, interstitial macrophages, alveolar macrophages (sometimes distinguished from "airway" cells), intravascular macrophages, and dendritic cells (present in the bronchial epithelium and seen in small numbers in the interstitium). With the exception of the dendritic cells, these anatomical distinctions may be more perceived than real. Although subtle differences in cell physiology, membrane antigen expression, and function have been observed between, for example, interstitial and alveolar macrophages[3], these differences are likely to be a result of the cells responding to their location, rather than fundamental differences in ontogeny. There is little doubt that interstitial macrophages migrate to the air spaces, thus by location becoming alveolar macrophages. In turn, alveolar or airway macrophages have been shown to travel back into the lung parenchyma and migrate through the tissues or through the lymphatic vessels to the bronchial lymph nodes. There is, therefore, not only a constant recruitment of monocytes into this organ, but also a traffic of macrophages throughout the various compartments of the lung. It is thus clear that the macrophage populations are not sessile, but exhibit a motile capacity that may represent an integral part of their function in this organ.

The dendritic cells form a network of interdigitating cells within the bronchial epithelium — representing, perhaps, the lung equivalent of the Langerhans cells of the skin[4]. There is still debate over the origin of dendritic cells — whether they are also monocyte derived or develop as a separate lineage. Although some studies of fetal material have suggested that they are separate from the "macrophage family", it has been shown *in vitro* that cells with dendritic cell characteristics

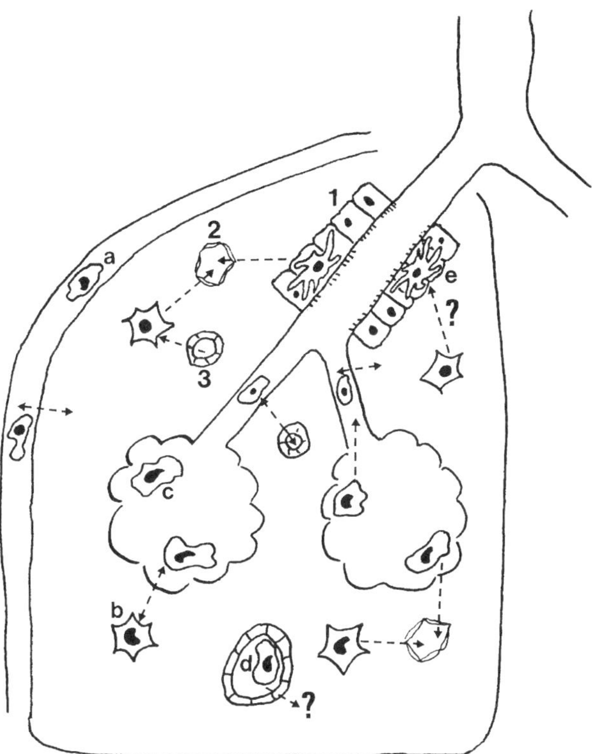

Figure 5.1. Schematic representation of the lung demonstrating the distinct anatomical locations of pulmonary macrophages. a = Pleural macrophages; b = interstitial macrophages; c = alveolar/airway macrophages; d = intravascular macrophages; e = intraepithelial dendritic cells. The likely movement of these cells is indicated by dashed lines and arrowheads. 1 = Epithelium; 2 = lymphatics; 3 = blood vessels. Whether dendritic cells differente from interstitial cells and whether there is traffic of intravascular macrophages out of the vessels is unclear, and thus indicated "?"

can differentiate from monocytes. In the lung, the dendritic cells, in common with the phagocytes, will migrate to lymph nodes, and cells with characteristics of dendritic cells are observed within the alveolar macrophage pool obtained by bronchoalveolar lavage (BAL) and, as stated above, are seen in small numbers distributed throughout the interstitium.

The intravascular macrophages are a population of mature mononuclear phagocytes that are found within the capillaries. These cells are common in the lungs of cattle, sheep, pigs, goats, horses and cats. Under steady state conditions they are absent or only rarely present in man, although there have been suggestions that they might occur in association with some pathological conditions such as biliary cirrhosis or infection. This chapter will not specifically refer to these cells further, as they are well reviewed elsewhere[5], although many of the characteristics described later for interstitial and alveolar macrophages would also apply to these intravascular phagocytes. The focus of this chapter will be on human pulmonary macrophages.

Because pulmonary macrophages represent a "moving target", it is very difficult to determine the lifespan of these cells. It is known that after whole body radiation and bone marrow transplantation the lung macrophage pool is replenished (including dendritic cells) within three months, although under steady state conditions their turnover is probably measured in days or weeks rather than months. There is little doubt, however, that they can exhibit a certain longevity — particularly the macrophages in the airways. These cells, once laden with debris, are expelled by climbing the bronchial tree eventually to be swallowed; this may take weeks.

The overall picture of lung macrophages, therefore, is one of a steady recruitment of monocytes from the circulation maturing into macrophages in the tissue, distributing themselves to particular compartments in the lung, and then taking on appropriate characteristics to function within the respective environment (Fig. 5.1). It is most unlikely that these processes of distribution and differentiation are random, as an appropriate balance of macrophage functional capacity must be sustained at distinct sites. In this regard, there are considerable data indicating that macrophage differentiation and function are regulated by cytokines and growth factors derived from local lymphocytes, epithelial cells and fibroblasts[6].

PHENOTYPIC DISCRIMINATION

The development of monoclonal antibody technology and the use of these reagents in immunohistology and immunocytology have allowed subsets of cells to be discriminated by antigenic phenotype. Many studies have applied such technology to investigations of pulmonary macrophages. There is a great temptation at this point to list the myriad of such monoclonal antibodies, the abbreviated nomenclature, and the relative specificity. This, however, would only tax the memory and add some confusion to a book concentrating on lung defence. To avoid this, comments here are restricted to those reagents that have been found useful in our laboratory. The principle adopted is that phenotype is important when related to maturity or function of cell subsets, as these characteristics are often difficult or impossible to identify by histology alone. A restricted list of monoclonal antibodies we have found of value is presented in Table 5.1. It is important to stress that many other reagents not listed here have been used by other workers studying lung macrophages in man and in rats and mice[7–9].

Several important points emerge from this restricted phenotypic analysis. *First*, CD14 is a cluster of differentiation (CD) marker that can be used to discriminate monocytes from mature macrophages and dendritic cells. The epitope seen by this monoclonal antibody is present on virtually all monocytes, yet is not expressed on mature cells. Interestingly, the number of CD14+ cells in the lung interstitium is relatively low, suggesting that maturation is rapid after these cells emigrate from the capillaries. Furthermore, CD14+ cells are rare in normal BAL samples, although their numbers may increase in some pathological conditions, such as drug induced fibrosis.

Table 5.1. Monoclonal antibody identifying macrophage subsets

Cell type	CD14	CD68	CD35	CD64	αHLA-DR	RFD1	RFD7
Monocytes	+	+	+	+	+/−	−	−
Pleural macrophages	−	+	+	+	+/−	−	+
Intravascular macrophages	Not tested in man						
Interstitial macrophages							
Subset 1	−	+	+	+	+/−	−	+
2	−	+	+	+	+	+	+
3	−	+	+/−	+/−	+	+	−
Alveolar macrophages							
Subset 1	−	+	+	+	+/−	−	+
2	−	+	+	+	+	+	+
3	−	+	+/−	+/−	+	+	−
Dendritic cells	−	+	−	−	+	+	−

− =< 5% of CD68+ cells positive

+ => 90% of CD68+ cells positive

+/− = variable but normally <20% positive.

Second, CD68 appears to be a pan-monocyte/macrophage marker which may also appear on dendritic cells. Detailed descriptions of these intraepithelial dendritic cells, however, have been performed only in rodents, and it is not yet confirmed that the CD68+/RFD1+ cells in human bronchial epithelium are identical to those originally described, although this seems likely. However, virtually all interstitial and alveolar macrophages express CD68.

Third, all dendritic cells and a majority of both interstitial and alveolar macrophages express major histocompatibility complex (MHC) class II HLA-DR. This is true in man, yet in rodents few interstitial macrophages or cells in the airways are the murine equivalent, Ia+, under normal conditions. Such an observation could be taken to imply that a functional capacity to present antigen may exist in a broader population of pulmonary macrophages in man than in rodents. Although most cells are HLA-DR+ in health, lung inflammation is inevitably associated with a quantitative increase in MHC class II expression on these cells. The significance of this is yet to be established, as the functional threshold of HLA-DR expression cannot be determined easily within the tissues.

Fourth, it is clear that, on phenotypic grounds, a heterogeneity exists within both the interstitial and airway macrophage populations. Such an observation is not unique to the use of monoclonal antibodies RFD1 and RFD7 applied here, but has been observed with other reagents[10]. This heterogeneity is of considerable interest, as it appears to reflect functional differences between these subsets of macrophages (Table 5.2). There is evidence that, in addition to "classic" phagocytic effector macrophages, subsets can be identified that stimulate or suppress T cell differentiation[11]. These three subsets are found in variable proportions, one to another, in both the lung interstitium and bronchial lamina propria. All three phenotypically distinct populations are also present in BAL samples.

 L. W. Poulter

Table 5.2. Macrophage subset proportions in the normal lung: percentage of total cells positive for RFD1, RFD7 or both monoclonal antibodies

	RFD1+ Inductive cells	RFD7+ Phagocytes	RFD1/D7+ Suppressive cells
Alveolar/airway macrophages	18* (10–40)	71 (25–85)	11 (5–25)
Interstitial/bronchial wall macrophages	11 (3–19)	44 (17–65)	46 (27–70)

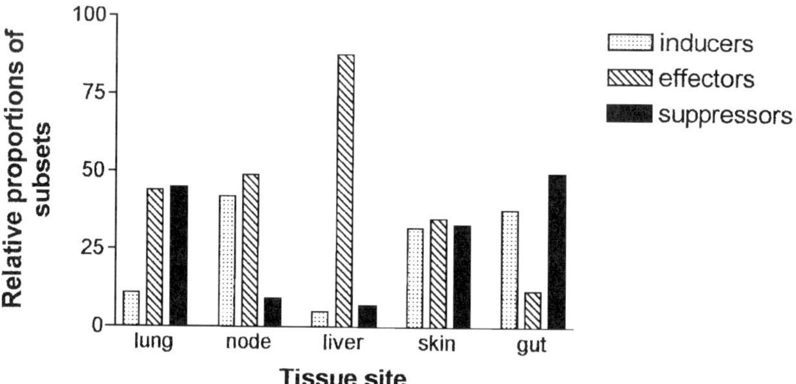

Figure 5.2. The relative proportions of macrophage subsets with inductive, effector or suppressive phenotype in various organs. This summary is based on double immunofluorescence staining with monoclonal antibodies RFD1 and RFD7 in a variety of studies over several years. Mean values are given; there is always a considerable variability (Table 5.2). These data do not reflect total macrophage numbers, which are also variable from one site to another

Comparative studies have shown that the relative balance of these subpopulations in the lung tissue differs from that at other sites in the body, such as the lymph nodes, liver, skin and gut (Fig. 5.2). Interestingly, a relatively high proportion of macrophages with suppressive phenotype occurs only in the lung and gut, possibly implying that this is a mucosa associated phenomenon (see below).

Finally, the distribution of Fc and C3b receptors is seen not surprisingly, to follow, the functional characteristic of phagocytosis. The intraepithelial dendritic cells show either no or very low expression of these receptors and are reported as having very low phagocytic potential. This functional characteristic is also true for the airway macrophages with a T cell stimulatory phenotype (RFD1+) which also appear as poor phagocytes[12]. Levels of expression of receptors FcR and C3bR are, however, variable and thus differences throughout all macrophage subsets may be quantitative rather than qualitative. Further work is clearly required, relating phenotype to function, for it is only with a clear understanding of this relationship that it will be possible to determine the functional capacity of cells identified using immunohistology *in situ*.

MACROPHAGES AND NON-SPECIFIC DEFENCE

It is remarkable that, despite being constantly exposed to the environment, the lung rarely succumbs to infection. The reason for this rests with the efficiency with which the macrophages of the airways can eliminate micro-organisms. Such capacity is part of the non-specific defence mechanisms of the lung, and in this regard the macrophages work in concert with other factors such as surfactant, mucous secretion, and mucociliary clearance to prevent potentially infectious agents invading the tissues of the lung. Any particulate material of a size up to 3 µm can readily reach the alveoli; here, macrophages recognise and phagocytose micro-organisms, particulates, and macromolecular debris. These cells are uniquely designed for this response (Fig. 5.3).

Phagocytosis and digestion occur in stages, beginning with attachment of the microbes to the surface of the macrophages. This process may be mediated by receptors on the macrophage that are selective for terminal mannose sugars, which are commonly found on micro-organisms. Alveolar macrophages also express receptors for C3b and, as the alternate complement pathway is active in the airways, C3b can act as an opsonin, facilitating both attachment and subsequent phagocytosis. Fibronectin receptors are also present on alveolar macrophages. It is believed that these enable the macrophages to "crawl" around the alveoli and bronchial tree, because the epithelial cells of the bronchioli secrete fibronectin. Coating of alveolar macrophages with this substance might thus restrict their movement and enhance the attachment of microbes. Once phagocytosis occurs, the phagosomes fuse with lysosomes in the cytoplasm of the cell: the lysosomes contain large amounts of acid hydrolases that constitute an anaerobic microbicidal pathway. As airway macrophages (unlike monocytes and neutrophils) have very little myeloperoxidase, they do not utilise halide/peroxidase microbicidal mechanisms. They do, however, exhibit a "respiratory burst" producing reactive oxygen intermediates (ROIs) and are thus able to use both aerobic and non-aerobic microbicidal mechanisms. Furthermore, these cells release free oxygen radicals, proteases and acid hydrolases, thus contributing to extracellular killing of micro-organisms. There is good evidence that airway macrophages also produce nitric oxide and release this substance into their immediate environment; however, the studies were performed with rat cells, and although it has been shown that human macrophages can produce nitric oxide, the relevance of this substance to their microbicidal capacity is still debated.

The success of this non-specific phagocytosis and microbicidal capacity is dependent on the dose of infectious agent and on the type of agent involved. In mouse experiments it has been shown that inocula of up to 10^5 organisms can be removed by macrophages alone, whereas greater inocula require recruitment of polymorphonuclear leucocytes or the induction of acquired immunity for their removal[13]. Whereas organisms such as *Staphylococcus aureus* are readily killed by alveolar macrophages, many Gram negative microbes are resistant to macrophage killing. Furthermore, mycobacteria, *Listeria* and *Legionella* are effectively phagocytosed but are resistant to intracellular digestion, and it requires immune activation of the macrophage populations for their removal[14].

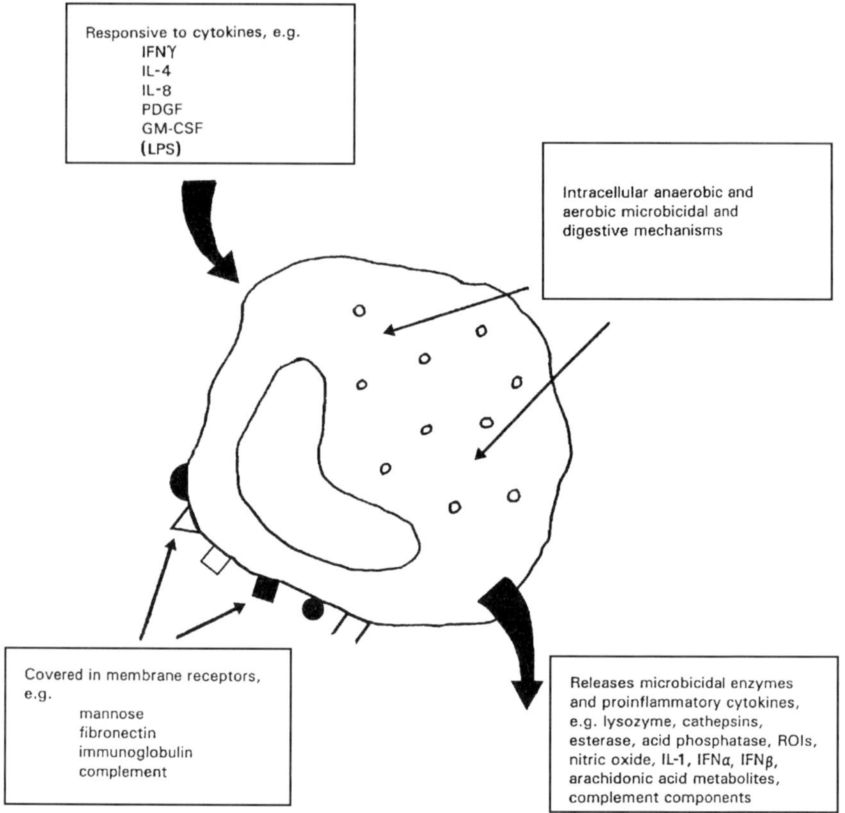

Figure 5.3. The macrophage is ideally designed as an effector cell both in innate and acquired immunological responses. Membrane receptors trap microbes and other foreign materials which are destroyed by powerful intracellular digestive systems. These cells respond to a multitude of signals from their environment and, in turn, can themselves release microbicidal factors and immune regulating mediators. IFN = Interferon; IL = interleukin; PDGF = platelet derived growth factor; GM-CSF = granulocyte macrophage colony stimulating factor; LPS = lipopolysaccharide; ROIs = reactive oxygen intermediates

Alveolar macrophages will also respond to viral infections, although elimination of overt viral infection normally involves an acquired immune response (see below). Virus infected macrophages have been shown to secrete interferons alfa and beta, thus preventing further viral infection of surrounding cells. They are also able to destroy viruses with their complement of hydrolytic enzymes. Virus infection of macrophages, however, does cause a reduced capacity of these cells to produce ROIs. It has been further suggested that airway macrophages may exhibit direct cytotoxic action against virally infected cells. This mechanism may also be enhanced by antibody in antibody dependent cellular cytotoxicity.

Interstitial macrophages appear to be less effective phagocytes and have a lower activity with regards the production of ROIs and nitric oxide. It is important to remember, however, that most data on the functional capacity of these cells have been derived from *in vitro* studies of cell suspensions following tissue disruption and digestion. The impact on cell function of these unavoidable procedures, which are not required for the study of alveolar macrophages, is not known. *In situ*, it would seem likely, however, that the exposure of interstitial macrophages to micro-organisms would occur only when the first line defences of the airway phagocytes, surfactants and epithelium had been breached. Under such circumstances, acquired immunological responses would be initiated and thus the role of these interstitial cells may be expected to be more one of immunocompetent inductive or effector cells rather than non-specific phagocytes[15]. Nevertheless, examination of the lung parenchyma of heavy smokers reveals carbon laden macrophages not only in the airways but also within the interstitium, indicating that these cells can function as non-specific phagocytes. The possibility exists, of course, that these "interstitial" cells have in fact migrated from the airways, although the experimental data indicate that the macrophages of the interstitium function more within the mechanisms of the acquired immune response system[15].

MACROPHAGES IN ACQUIRED IMMUNITY

As elsewhere in the body, the acquired immune response system in the lung involves stages of induction, recall and regulation. There is good evidence to suggest, however, that subtle differences in these mechanisms are unique to mucosal surfaces, including the bronchial mucosa, and these are reflected in part by the role of the macrophage populations of the lung in acquired immunity.

THE INDUCTION OF ACQUIRED IMMUNITY

Alveolar macrophages have been shown capable of migrating to draining bronchial lymph nodes, where they home to the T cell paracortical areas[16]. This in itself is somewhat surprising, as macrophages entering lymph nodes draining other tissues normally appear within the marginal sinus. It is also believed that the dendritic cells of the bronchial epithelium migrate to this area, where they become antigen presenting interdigitating cells[17]. Antigen carried by these cells is thus available for the primary stimulation of appropriate T cell clones within the lymphoid tissue draining the lung.

As the dendritic cells from the lung epithelium may be seen as the constitutive antigen presenting cells, the fact that alveolar macrophages also drain to this site, rather than the marginal sinus, seems unexplained. One possibility is that the alveolar macrophages serve to digest large molecules to the deca- or octapeptides required by the dendritic cells for presentation. It has also been suggested, however, that these airway derived cells act to inhibit or at least regulate T cell stimulation by the dendritic cells[18]. This phenomenon is clearly seen *in vitro*, where alveolar macrophages have been shown to suppress the induction of T cell responses. This mechanism is perhaps more relevant to secondary immune responses in which memory T cells primed to a particular antigen are already a reality. It has been known for some time that alveolar macrophages are very poor stimulators of T cells compared, for example, with peritoneal macrophages or monocyte derived macrophages. Elegant experiments have shown that use of dichloromethylene diphosphonate (a cytotoxic drug) encapsulated in liposomes to destroy phagocytic macrophages of the airways significantly increased the T cell stimulatory capacity of lung macrophages in culture[19].

Thus the normal pool of airway macrophages contains a population of phagocytic suppressive cells that, under normal circumstances, can downregulate T cell reactivity but are destroyed using a selective phagocyte toxin[19]. The interstitial macrophages, however, appear more capable of inducing T cell responses. These cells express larger amounts of MHC class II antigens and secrete greater amounts of interleukin-1 (IL-1). Such characteristics are consistent with T cell stimulation and may be relevant to secondary responses promoted locally in the lung once T cell priming has occurred.

EFFECTOR FUNCTION IN ACQUIRED IMMUNITY

The effector function of the lung macrophage pool rests with the interstitial and alveolar or airway macrophages rather than dendritic cells, which appear to function solely as inducers of T cell responses. This effector function can be seen as an amplification, by local T cell derived cytokines[20], of those inherent mechanisms described above and in Fig. 5.3 as part of the non-specific defensive role of these cells. Interferon gamma (IFNγ), IL-3, IL-4 and granulocyte macrophage colony stimulating factor (GM-CSF) all have been shown to increase the microbicidal capacity of pulmonary macrophages. The release of ROIs by these cells is also enhanced by IFNγ and GM-CSF derived from activated T cells, in addition to platelet derived growth factor, tumour necrosis factor α (TNFα), the leukotriene LTB$_4$, and IgG immune complexes[15]. In addition to exerting direct microbicidal activity, ROIs may also be effective against virus infected cells, and can cause local tissue damage in that they are cytotoxic to fibroblasts. These mediators may thus also play a part in the promotion of inflammation. More detailed reviews of cytokines activating macrophages are available elsewhere[21].

The lung interstitial and airway macrophages may contribute to inflammatory processes by releasing arachidonic acid metabolites. Prostaglandins, thromboxanes and leukotrienes are produced by macrophages on activation, inducing acute inflammatory responses including the recruitment of polymorphonuclear cells. In this regard, it should be noted that complement proteins are also produced by these cells, stimulated either through the alternate pathway as part of the non-specific defence system (see above) or through the classic pathway involving specific immune complexes; complement activation may thus contribute directly to local inflammatory processes.

On activation, alveolar macrophages also secrete IL-8 and macrophage inflammatory proteins (MIP) 1 and 2, all of which exhibit chemotactic activity for polymorphonuclear leucocytes. Other cytokines secreted by these cells have fibrogenic activity. For example, transforming growth factor β (TGFβ), TNFα and fibronectin have all been shown to stimulate fibroblast proliferation. It is not possible here to document fully the entire range of cytokines released by these cells, nor their multiplicity of actions; these details are available in a more directed review[22].

It is important to realise that the stimulation of macrophages as an effector population within an acquired immune response represents a quantitative rather than a qualitative change from the function they exert as part of the non-specific defence system. Indeed, contact with bacterial lipopolysaccaride, which commonly stimulates non-specific defence mechanisms, can amplify much of the essential microbicidal capacity and mediator release in the absence of specific T cell stimulation. Furthermore, the effector function of these cells in both the lung interstitium and the airways is expressed in an antigen independent manner — that is, it is non-specific. One effector mechanism that is more "directed" is the formation of granulomata, a mechanism normally associated with a presence of antigenic material resistant to rapid digestion and elimination by macrophages even when activated after a T cell mediated acquired response. The role of the macrophage is central to the formation of granulomata.

Granuloma formation occurs when tissue macrophages accumulate and further differentiate into secretory epithelioid cells and giant cells. The details of this mechanism are still ill defined, but appear to be associated with the expression of adhesion molecules such as CD11b, CD54 and fibroblast growth factor on the macrophages, and an increased local production of vitronectin[23]. These adhesion molecules may halt the migration of macrophages through the tissues and contribute to development of a sedentary situation which may trigger the further differentiation of these cells to epithelioid cells and lead to fusion, forming giant cells. There is some evidence that this differentiation is orchestrated by CD4+ derived cytokines, as it is common to find this subset of T cells distributed amongst the epithelioid cells of granulomas, whereas CD8+ T cells are noticeably absent from the centre of granulomas (Fig. 5.4)[24]. The terminally differentiated macrophages are poor phagocytes but productive secretory cells, capable of releasing a large repertoire of microbicidal enzymes, inflammatory mediators and growth factors. Giant cells, on the other hand, are avid phagocytes and exhibit powerful digestive capacity, as they contain large numbers of lysosomes and high levels of activity of acid hydrolases. It is, however, the factors secreted by the epithelioid cells that may eventually promote fibrosis and collagen deposition,

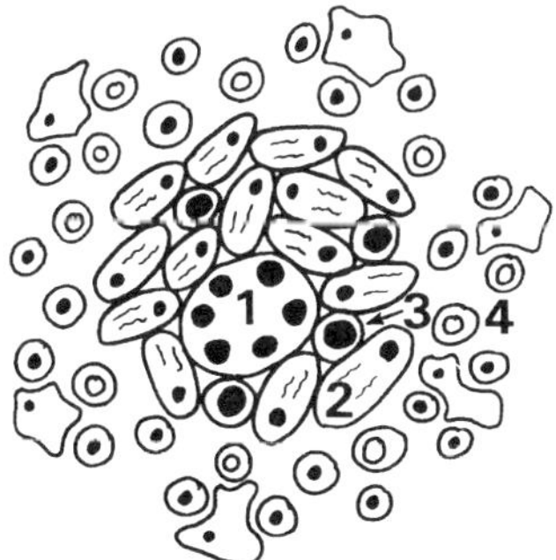

Figure 5.4. Granulomas are characterised by the presence of giant cells (1), epithelioid cells (2), CD4 (3) and CD8 (4) subsets. Often only CD4+ cells appear in the centre. "Non-immune" granulomas do not exhibit any significant mantle of T cells

causing the permanent scarring of lung tissue that is often a consequence of these reactions[23].

There is a continuing debate regarding the pathogenic nature of granulomata. The question of whether their formation is a normal mechanism within the immune defence network or a consequence of dysfunction has yet to be satisfactorily answered. There are clear advantages in evolving a mechanism that can contain and isolate indigestible material until such time that it can be removed. In contrast, the histopathology of granulomatous disease reveals the pathological consequences of granuloma formation, with severe tissue disruption and often fibrosis and the laying down of collagen. A dispassionate view of this apparent paradox, however, leads to the conclusion that granuloma formation is a mechanism evolved within the immune defence network as a protective device in situations in which T cell stimulated macrophages are unable rapidly to remove microbes or other particulate antigens. Because of the potential damaging effects of such tissue reactions, mechanisms have also evolved to dissolve these granulomata once their role has been accomplished (it is recognised that granulomata are often seen as ephemeral). This being the case, the pathology evident in the lung in mycobacterial infection or sarcoidosis, for example, could be viewed as a failure of the *resolving mechanisms* rather than the initial reaction. Under such circumstances of granuloma persistence, the body's defence systems are left with only one course of action — to try and "heal" these disrupted tissues via fibrosis and collagen disposition. It should be emphasised that no hard data exist in support of this conjecture, but it would seem to comply with the current evidence available, and fits with personal observations of both mycobacterial and other granulomatous diseases[25].

LUNG MACROPHAGES AS REGULATORS OF ACQUIRED RESPONSES

The need for protection against a multitude of potential pathogens demands that the effector mechanisms promoted by the acquired immune system are powerful. Such mechanisms could thus be (and sometimes are), damaging to normal tissues and function. Thus strict regulation of these mechanisms is required. This need is arguably greatest at those sites most commonly exposed to foreign material. Unregulated promotion of acquired immune responses in the airways and lung interstitium would inevitably result in a constant state of inflammation. This situation is avoided by an interacting network of regulating mechanisms in which pulmonary macrophages have a significant role.

It has already been mentioned above that both airway and interstitial macrophages are heterogenous populations. Some 15–30% of macrophages obtained from the normal airway by BAL exhibit both phenotypic and functional characteristics of suppressive cells[10]. Partially purified populations of these cells have been shown to be capable of suppressing both autologous and allogeneic T cell stimulation[26]. It seems likely that the presence of these cells may explain why the BAL derived macrophage pool appears to be such a poor stimulator of T cells *in vitro* (an observation reported by several workers). The role of these cells in the lung would thus be to regulate T cell reactions preventing heightened immunological stimulation despite constant exposure to antigen (Fig. 5.5). It is

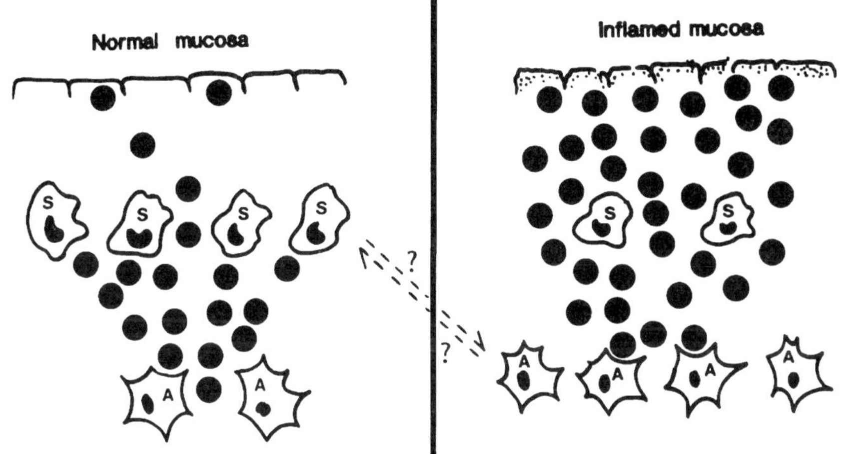

Figure 5.5. In the normal bronchial wall (left), suppressive macrophages (S) downregulate T cell activation promoted by inductive antigen presenting cells (A). Reduced proportions of suppressive macrophages (right), are associated with loss of regulation, possibly resulting in inflammation. Whether inductive and suppressive cells can switch roles is unknown

also likely that these cells are within the population observed draining to lymph nodes and potentially interacting with dendritic cells in the paracortical areas where they may regulate dendritic cell–T cell interaction[17].

In man, the mechanism underlying this suppressive activity is unknown. However, studies in the rat have revealed that culture with a nitric oxide synthetase inhibitor blocks the suppressive effect of lung macrophages, thus strongly implicating nitric oxide as an important mediator of this reaction[18]. BAL derived macrophages also release TGFβ and IL-10. Both these cytokines are known to exhibit suppressive effects on T cells. Of the two, TGFβ is of particular interest as it can preferentially inhibit the expansion of Th2-like T cell clones. This T cell population is responsible, amongst other things, for producing IL-4, the cytokine that promotes IgE class switching in B cells. As allergic responses involving IgE are particularly susceptible to suppression by macrophages in the lung[27], it is tempting to speculate that TGFβ production is associated with the suppressive capacity of alveolar macrophages. Preliminary evidence in our laboratory indicates that, although TGFβ production is not limited to those macrophage populations with suppressive phenotype, these particular cells appear to be the greater producers of this cytokine compared with other phenotypically distinct macrophage subsets.

There is less information regarding interstitial macrophages. In a normal subject, however, subsets of macrophages have been distinguished in the interstitium and the bronchial wall lamina propria that exhibit the phenotype "inductive" (antigen presenting cells), "effector" (phagocytes) or "suppressive" (T cell regulating cells)[26,28]. Indeed, the proportions of macrophages with suppressive phenotype are greater in the tissues and bronchial wall (up to 50%

of the total macrophage pool) than in the airways. Most interestingly, in patients with bronchial asthma, in whom chronic T cell mediated inflammation occurs, a significant reduction in the relative proportions of these suppressive cells is seen[26]. This phenomenon is also observed in the mucosa of the gut, where in normal tissues high proportions of macrophages exhibit a suppressive phenotype, whereas in samples from patients with colitis these populations are significantly reduced[29].

Studies completed in 1996 (VJ Tormey *et al.*, submitted for publication) revealed that the relative proportions of inductive or suppressive macrophages developing from monocytes can be regulated by T cell cytokines. IFNγ and IL-4 promote the differentiation of inductive macrophages, whereas IL-10 promotes development of suppressive cells. There is some evidence that, even when mature, pulmonary macrophages can switch phenotype and function in response to cytokine signals. One might thus consider the intriguing possibility that macrophages exhibit a "plasticity" of phenotype and function. This would be an ideal characteristic for cell populations migrating through quite different environments within the lung: the pleural space, interstitium, bronchial wall, alveoli and airways. Studies to confirm (or deny) this conjecture are eagerly awaited. In the meantime, a better understanding of the complex role of lung macrophages in all aspects of defence of the lung not only will further our knowledge of the diversity of the defence network, but may also offer up the potential of new targets for treatment in many lung diseases associated with immunological dysfunction.

SUMMARY

Pulmonary macrophages are a population of monocyte derived cells that exhibit a ubiquitous distribution, occurring in all compartments of the lung. They have been classified by location into pleural, intravascular, interstitial, alveolar and airway macrophages. All of these cells have similar phenotypic and functional characteristics, although subtle differences can be observed that are unique to certain locations. These differences are likely to reflect signals received from the local environment. Dendritic cells are a unique population in the bronchial epithelium that appear specifically designed for antigen capture and presentation. The airway interstitial and dendritic cells have all been shown capable of migration and drainage to local lymph node, where they characteristicaly home into the paracortical T cell areas.

The major function of the alveolar and airway cells is to act as phagocytes constituting a part of lung innate defences. They also act as phagocytic effector cells in acquired immunity when activated by cytokines produced as a result of T cell stimulation. These specific acquired immune responses significantly enhance both the phagocytic and microbicidal capacity of the macrophages. In this regard, these macrophages can utilise both aerobic and non-aerobic microbicidal mechanisms, using lysosomal acid hydrolases, reactive oxygen intermediates, or both, in addition to nitric oxide to kill infective organisms, both intracellularly and extracellularly. Dendritic cells, by contrast, have little or no phagocytic/microbicidal capacity but are equipped with high expression of class II MHC antigens and interdigitating processes to capture and present antigens to T cells inducing acquired immune responses.

The interstitial cells also appear to exhibit some antigen presenting capacity and are further involved in granuloma formation when stimulated to differentiate into epithelioid cells and giant cells. In these circumstances, cytokines released particularly by the epithelioid cells are also involved in fibrinogenesis and collagen deposition. This process, it is believed, may represent an attempt at local "healing", yet can develop into a devastating tissue process leading to severe loss of function.

Under steady state conditions, all of these defence mechanisms may be dependent on a delicate balance between subsets of pulmonary macrophages identified both in the lung tissues and in the airways. These cells, discriminated by their antigenic phenotype, also exhibit different functional capacity, being able to act as inductive cells, effector cells or suppressive cells within the T cell mediated acquired immune defence system. It appears that to sustain "health", a relatively high proportion of suppressive cells is required in the lung which reduces T cell reactivity to the multitude of antigens likely to enter this particular organ. Pathological conditions are associated with a relative reduction in this population. It is tempting to speculate that regulation of the balance between these subsets, which may be controlled by T cell derived cytokines, is the key to sustaining good defence of the lung without promoting inflammatory hypersensitivity.

ACKNOWLEDGEMENTS

L. W. Poulter's research on lung macrophages is supported by Glaxo Wellcome Research & Development U.K. Ltd.

REFERENCES

1. Van Furth R. 1980. Cells of the mononuclear phagocyte system. Nomenclature in terms of sites and conditions. In: Van Furth R, ed. *Mononuclear Phagocytes. Functional Aspects.* The Hague, Boston, London: Mortinus Nijhoff, 1980; 1–30.
2. Van Furth R. 1988. Development and distribution of mononuclear phagocytes in the normal steady state and inflammation. In: Gallins J I, Goldstein J M, Synderman R, eds. *Inflammation: Basic Principals and Clinical Correlates.* New York: Raven Press, 1988; 281–295.
3. Prokhorova S, Lavnikova N, Laskin D L. Functional characterisation of interstitial macrophages and sub-populations of alveolar macrophages from rat lung. *J Leucoc Biol* 1994; **66:** 141–146.
4. Schon-Hegard M A, Oliver J, McMenamin P G, *et al.* Studies on the density, distribution and surface phenotype of intra epithelial class II major histocompatibility complex [1a] antigen leaving dendritic cells in the conducting airways. *J Exp Med* 1991; **173:** 1345.
5. Staub N C. Pulmonary intravascular macrophages. *Ann Rev Physiol* 1994; **56:** 47–67.
6. Toews G B. Pulmonary defence mechanisms. *Semin Respir Infect* 1993; **8:** 160–167.
7. Kobzik L, Godleski J J, Biondi A, *et al.* Immunohistologic analysis of a human pulmonary alveolar macrophage antigen. *Clin Immunol Immunopathol* 1985; **37:** 213–219.
8. Akiyama J, Chida K, Sato A, *et al.* Four monoclonal antibodies AMH- 1-2-3- and 4 give varied reactivities with monocytes, alveolar macrophages and epithelioid-cell granulomas. *J Clin Immunol* 1988; **8:** 372–380.

9. Nibbering P H, Leigh P C, Van Furth R. Quantitative immunocytochemical characterisation of mononuclear phagocytes I. Monoblasts, promonocytes, monocytes and peritoneal and alveolar macrophages. *Cell Immunol* 1987; **103:** 374–385.

10. Mearlen J, nan Hoorst W, deWit H J, *et al.* Distribution and immunophenotype of mononuclear phagocytes and dendritic cells in the human lung. *Am J Respir Cell Mol Biol* 1994; **10:** 487–492.

11. Spiteri M A, Poulter L W. Characterisation of immune inducer and suppressor macrophages from the normal human lung. *Clin Exp Immunol* 1991; **83:** 157.

12. Spiteri M A, Clarke S W, Poulter L W. The isolation of phenotypically and functionally distinct alveolar macrophages from human broncho-alveolar lavage. *Eur Respir J* 1992; **5:** 717–726.

13. Onofriu H N M, Toews G B, Lipscomb M F, *et al.* Granulocyte/alveolar macrophage interaction in pulmonary clearance of *Staphylococcus aureus. Am Rev Respir Dis* 1983; **127:** 335–342.

14. Horwitz M A, Silverstein S C. Activated human monocytes inhibit the intracellular multiplication of Legionnaires' disease bacteria. *J Exp Med* 1981; **154:** 1618–1627.

15. Lohmann-Matthes M -L, Steinmuller C, Franke-Ullman G. Pulmonary macrophages. *Eur Respir J* 1994; **7:** 1678–1689.

16. Thepen T, Claassen E, Hoeben K, *et al.* Migration of alveolar macrophages from alveolar space to paracortical T cell area of the draining lymph node. *Adv Exp Med Biol* 1993; **329:** 305–310.

17. Thepen T, Kraal G, Holt P G. The role of alveolar macrophages in regulation of lung inflammation. *Ann NY Acad Sci* 1994; **725:** 200–206.

18. Holt P G, Oliver J, Bilyk N, *et al.* Down regulation of the antigen presenting cell function(s) of pulmonary dendritic cells *in vivo* by resident alveolar macrophages. *J Exp Med* 1993; **177:** 397–407.

19. Begg J T, Lee S T, Thepen T, *et al.* Depletion of alveolar macrophages by liposome-encapsulated dichloromethylene diphosphonate. *J Appl Physiol* 1993; **74:** 2812–2819.

20. Skerrett S J, Martin T R. Intratracheal IFN_γ augments pulmonary defences against experimental legionellosis. *Am Rev Respir Dis* 1994; **149:** 50–58.

21. Kelley J. Cytokines of the lung (state of the art). *Am Rev Respir Dis* 1990; **141:** 765–788.

22. Gordon S, Frazer I, Nash D, *et al.* Macrophages in tissues and *in vitro. Curr Opin Immunol* 1992; **4:** 25–32.

23. Marnex J F, Leroux C, Greenland T, *et al.* From granuloma to fibrosis in interstitial lung diseases: molecular and cellular interactions. *Eur Respir J* 1994; **7:** 779–785.

24. Mishra B, Poulter L W, Janossy G, *et al.* The distribution of lymphoid and macrophage-like cell subsets of sarcoid and Kveim granulomata. Possible mechanism of negative PPD reaction in sarcoidosis. *Clin Exp Immunol* 1983; **54:** 705–711.

25. Poulter L W. Immune aspects of sacroidosis. A review. *Postgrad Med J* 1988; **64:** 536–541.

26. Poulter L W, Burke C M. Macrophages and allergic lung disease. *Immunobiology* 1996; **195:** 574–587.

27. Thepen T, Mcmenamin C, Girn B, *et al.* Regulation of IgE production in presensitized arrivals; *in vivo* elimination of alveolar macrophages preferentially increases IgE responses to inhaled allergen. *Clin Exp Allergy* 1992; **22:** 1107–1114.

28. Hutter C, Poulter L W. The balance of macrophage subsets may be customised at mucosal surfaces. *FEMS Microbiol Immunol* 1992; **105:** 309–316.

29. Allison M C, Poulter L W. Changes in phenotypically distinct mucosa macrophage populations may be a prerequisite for the development of inflammatory bowel disease. *Clin Exp Immunol* 1991; **85:** 504–509.

6

The Role of Adhesion Molecules in T Cell Activation and Migration

DAVID H. ADAMS

Queen Elizabeth Hospital, Birmingham, UK

INTRODUCTION

In the past few years there has been an enormous expansion in our understanding of the cell surface receptors that mediate cell–cell and cell–extracellular matrix interactions. Adhesion molecules have been shown to have crucial roles throughout biology, from embryology and reproduction to host defences against invading pathogens. The recognition that adhesion molecules are more than cellular glue, and are capable of signalling and relaying crucial information both from and to the cell, has reinforced the importance of the roles they have in biology.

Leucocytes possess an array of cell surface molecules, many of which are capable of mediating adhesion, and these adhesion molecules play a crucial part in most aspects of immune function. The current chapter will concentrate on the role of adhesion molecules in the regulation of T lymphocyte function, although many of the principles will apply to other cell types.

The efficient working of the immune system depends on its ability to recognise and respond to an almost infinite number of foreign antigens. In order for this to occur lymphocytes must:

(i)   be able to recognise foreign antigen and respond to it appropriately
(ii) have access to tissues to allow continuous surveillance and recruitment to sites of invasion.

Both these aspects of lymphocyte function are crucially dependent upon regulated adhesion, and this chapter will review the role of adhesion molecules in both antigen-dependent and antigen-independent T cell functions.

Pulmonary Defences. Edited by Robert A. Stockley.
© 1997 John Wiley & Sons Ltd.

T CELL ADHESION MOLECULES AND THEIR LIGANDS

T lymphocytes express a large number of cell surface molecules that are capable of mediating adhesion to other cell types and to extracellular matrix. These interactions allow the T cell to be aware of and to respond to its environment, and have a crucial role in cell to cell communication and the activation and regulated function of the immune system[1]. The main T lymphocyte adhesion molecules will be briefly outlined.

INTEGRINS

Integrins are a family of cell surface glycoprotein adhesion molecules that traverse the cell membrane and provide a link between the extracellular environment and the inside of the cell. They are the major receptors for extracellular matrix and are also involved in cell–cell interactions. Each integrin is a heterodimer that consists of a non-covalently linked α and β chain (Fig. 6.1). In man there are at least 15 α chains and eight β chains. The associations between the chains are limited: some α chains will only associate with a single β chain, whereas others will associate with several distinct β chains.

The ability of integrins to interact with their ligands is modulated by conformational changes induced by activation[2]. Thus the functional activity of a given integrin is determined by its state of activation and by its level of cellular expression. This requirement for activation provides a mechanism for rapidly regulating integrin function[3].

Integrins can be divided into broad subfamilies based on their β chains; three of these subfamilies are expressed by leucocytes (Table 6.1).

β_1 Integrins

There are six members of this family that are expressed on T cells. They consist of a common β chain (cluster of differentiation (CD) 29) non-covalently associated with distinct α chains (CD49a–f). They are also termed VLA molecules, as they

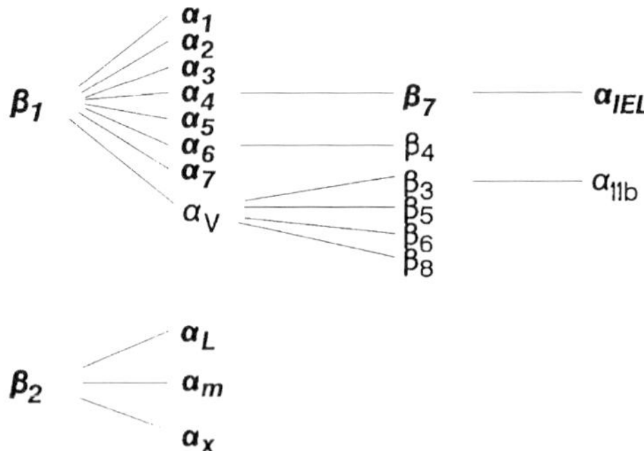

Figure 6.1. The integrin family of adhesion receptors, classified according to their β chains. The molecules in bold italics are those expressed on leucocytes. IEL = Intraepithelial lymphocyte

Table 6.1. Integrins expressed on leucocytes

Receptor	Other names	CD designation	Ligands	Expression
β_1 integrins				
$\alpha_1\beta_1$	VLA-1	CD49a/CD29	Coll, LN	T and B cells
$\alpha_2\beta_1$	VLA-2	CD49b/CD29	Coll, LN, FN	T cells
$\alpha_3\beta_1$	VLA-3	CD49c/CD29	Coll, FN, LN, En, Ep	Leucocytes
$\alpha_4\beta_1$	VLA-4	CD49d/CD29	FN, VCAM-1	T cells, monocytes
$\alpha_5\beta_1$	VLA-5	CD49e/CD29	FN	Leucocytes
$\alpha_6\beta_1$	VLA-6	CD49f/CD29	LN	T cells
β_2 integrins				
$\alpha_1\beta_2$	LFA-1	CD11a/CD18	ICAM-1, -2, -3	Leucocytes
$\alpha_m\beta_2$	Mac-1	CD11b/CD18	C3bi, Fac X, ICAM-1	Leucocytes
$\alpha_x\beta_2$	p150,95	CD11c/CD18	Fb, C3bi	Leucocytes
β_7 integrins				
$\alpha_4\beta_7$			FN, VCAM-1, MAdCAM	Activated T cells
$\alpha_{IEL}\beta_7$		CD103αE	E-cadherin	Epithelial T cells

VLA 1–6 = Very late activation antigens 1–6; Coll = collagen; LN = laminin; FN = fibronectin; En = entactin; Fb = fibrinogen; Ep = epiligrin; VCAM-1 = vascular cell adhesion molecule-1; LFA-1 = lymphocyte function associated antigen-1; ICAM-1 = intercellular adhesion molecule-1; Mac-1 = macrophage-1; MAdCAM = mucosal addressin cell adhesion molecule.

were originally discovered as markers of very late activation on stimulated T cells. VLA-1, -3, -5 and -6 bind to extracellular matrix proteins and are involved in T cell interactions with tissue components. VLA-4 ($\alpha_4\beta_1$) binds both to fibronectin and to a member of the immunoglobulin superfamily, vascular cell adhesion molecule-1 (VCAM-1). VLA-4–VCAM-1 interactions are involved in adhesion to endothelium and in interactions with antigen presenting cells[4].

β_2 Integrins

The expression of β_2 integrins is restricted to leucocytes. They consist of three molecules with a common β chain (CD18) and distinct α chains. T cells express lymphocyte function associated antigen-1 (LFA-1) (CD11a/CD18) and, to a lesser extent, macrophage-1 (Mac-1; CD11b/CD18). Both these integrins bind to intercellular adhesion molecule-1 (ICAM-1) and ICAM-3, and LFA-1 also binds to ICAM-2[1]. Mac-1 is unusual amongst integrins in that cell surface expression can be rapidly increased by translocation from cytoplasmic stores without the need for *de novo* synthesis.

β_7 Integrins

Two β_7 integrins have been described, $\alpha_{IEL}\beta_7$ which is expressed by intraepithelial lymphocytes in the gut and mediates adhesion of T cells to epithelium[5,6], and $\alpha_4\beta_7$ which binds to VCAM-1, the CS-1 fragment of fibronectin or mucosal addressin cell adhesion molecule-1 (MAdCAM-1) (see below) and is associated with gut homing of T cells[7,8].

CELL ADHESION RECEPTORS OF THE IMMUNOGLOBULIN SUPERFAMILY

CD4 and CD8

The T cell receptors CD4 and CD8 mediate antigen specific recognition. CD8+ T cells recognise foreign antigen in the context of self major histocompatibility complex (MHC) class I molecules. CD8+ T cells are usually cytolytic, and are capable of directly killing antigen bearing cells (e.g. virus infected macrophages). CD4+ T cells recognise endogenously processed peptides bound in the groove of MHC class II molecules. CD4+ T cells usually display "helper" functions, being able to secrete cytokines that modulate the recruitment and activity of other T cells, B cells and other effector cells. Both molecules mediate weak but crucial adhesive interactions between T cells and antigen presenting cells (APCs) (CD4) and cytotoxic T cells and target cells (CD8). There is now evidence that CD8 participates in a cascade of adhesive interactions in which inside out signalling influences the strength of binding between cytolytic T lymphocytes (CTLs) and target cells[9] (see below).

CD2/LFA-3 (CD58)

CD2 is one of the first specific T cell markers to appear during development of human T cells in the thymus. Its natural ligand is another immunoglobulin superfamily member, LFA-3. The interaction of CD2 with LFA-3 enhances the adhesion of T cells to other cells, including antigen presenting cells and target cells in cytotoxicity[10].

CD28/CTLA-4

CD28 and its activation dependent homologue, CTLA-4, are expressed on T cells and bind to a family of inducible B cell ligands, B7-1, B7-2 and B7-3. This interaction appears to be particularly important in costimulation of T cell activation, as blockade of the pathway can lead to the induction of anergy[11].

ICAM-1, ICAM-2, ICAM-3

The ICAMs are ligands for the β_2 integrins[1]. ICAM-1 is expressed at low levels on many cells, including leucocytes, endothelium and epithelium, and is upregulated with inflammation. ICAM-2 is largely confined to endothelium, where it is constitutively expressed. ICAM-3 is expressed at high levels on leucocytes and exists in different forms resulting from differential glycosylation[12].

VCAM-1

VCAM-1 is expressed on endothelium and some APCs. Expression on endothelium is increased with cytokine activation. The T cell ligand for VCAM-1 is the β_1 integrin, VLA-4[13].

MAdCAM-1

MAdCAM-1 is a heavily glycosylated member of the immunoglobulin super-family that is expressed on endothelium in the gut. It can mediate both primary and secondary adhesion of T cells to endothelium when it engages the T cell integrin, $\alpha_4\beta_7$. This pathway is involved in homing of T cells to the gut and possibly also to inflamed synovium[8].

CD31

CD31 is expressed on endothelium and by a subset of mainly CD8+ T cells. It mediates homotypic adhesion between endothelial cells and has been proposed as an adhesion trigger for CD31+ T cells, as engagement of CD31 by antibody or homotypic binding can activate T cell integrins[13,14].

SELECTINS

The selectins are a family of three lectin-like adhesion molecules that bind to distinct carbohydrate receptors[15].

E-Selectin

The expression of E-selectin (so-called because it was discovered on endothelium) is confined to endothelial cells. It is upregulated within 1–2 h by proinflammatory cytokines such as tumour necrosis factor α (TNFα) and interleukin-1 (IL-1). It mediates binding to several poorly defined oligosaccharide receptors on leuco-cytes, including a receptor expressed on a subset of CD4 T cells called cutaneous lymphocyte antigen (CLA)[16].

P-Selectin

P-selectin was originally described on platelets, but is also expressed on endothe-lium. It is found in Weibel-Palade bodies in the cytoplasm, from where it can be rapidly mobilised to the cell membrane in response to cytokine activation. A subset of activated T cells bind to P-selectin *in vitro*, although the biological significance of this is as yet unclear[17].

L-Selectin

This is expressed on leucocytes, including lymphocytes. It binds to an endothelial oligosaccharide to support lymphocyte binding to lymph node high endothelial venules. It may also have a role in the binding of T cells to endothelium at other sites, although this remains contentious[18].

OTHER ADHESION MOLECULES

CD43 is widely expressed at high levels on all leucocytes including T cells. It is absent in the Wiskott-Aldrich syndrome of immunodeficiency[19]. CD43 is a sialo-glycoprotein with a strong net negative charge, properties that suggest it might be involved in decreasing adhesion, although several monoclonal antibodies to

CD43 can costimulate T cells and increase homotypic adhesion. Its role in the regulation of adhesion remains unclear[20,21].

CD44 is expressed on T and B cells, monocytes and granulocytes. It is one of several cell surface molecules that are increased on memory T cells compared with naive cells. There are several variants of CD44, produced by variable splicing of at least five different exons; in addition to being expressed on leucocytes, some of these variants are also expressed by epithelium and endothelium. CD44 can carry glycosaminoglycan side chains, allowing it to act as a proteoglycan. It has been proposed that, in this form, endothelial CD44 can present gycosaminoglycan-binding cytokines at the endothelial surface. CD44 has structural homology with the cartilage link protein and can act as a receptor for hyaluronate. It has been shown to mediate binding of T cells to high endothelial venules and to synovial endothelium. Cross linking CD44 on the cell surface of T cells enhances their activation[22].

T CELL DIFFERENTIATION

DEVELOPMENT IN THE THYMUS

T cells develop from bone marrow stem cells that migrate to the thymus where they mature into thymus dependent (T) lymphocytes. In the specialised microenvironment of the thymus, the immature T cells, or thymocytes, undergo a period of intense proliferation and differentiation, passing through a series of discrete phenotypic stages, that can be identified by distinctive patterns of expression of various cell surface proteins. These include the adhesion molecules CD2, LFA-1, VLA-4, VLA-5 and L-selectin. Changes in the functional activation of thymocyte integrins define different stages of thymocyte differentiation and have a vital role in the maturation process[23]. The thymocyte passes through several maturation steps, during which it acquires the specific T cell receptor (TCR) complex associated with CD3 and either CD4 or CD8 cell surface receptors[24–27]. The single positive T cell then exits the thymus as a naive CD4+ or CD8+ T cell.

PERIPHERAL DIFFERENTIATION OF T CELLS DETERMINES THEIR SUBSEQUENT PATTERNS OF RECIRCULATION

Figure 6.2 summarises this stage of T cell differentiation. After completing their development and maturation in the thymus, T cells enter the circulation and recirculate as naive T cells until they encounter their specific antigen. On encountering antigen, the naive T cell is activated and undergoes complex changes before returning to the resting state as a memory T cell that has the ability to respond promptly to subsequent encounters with antigen. Naive T cells circulate continuously between the bloodstream and the secondary lymphoid tissues (lymph nodes, tonsils, Peyer's patches, spleen, gut associated lymphoid tissues and mucosa associated lymphoid tissue)[28]. The traffic of T cells from the circulation into secondary lymphoid tissues is an antigen independent process that is regulated by adhesive interactions with specialised endothelial cells, called high endothelial venules (HEV), within lymphoid tissue[29–31]. This selective recirculation of naive T cells through secondary lymphoid tissue ensures that their initial

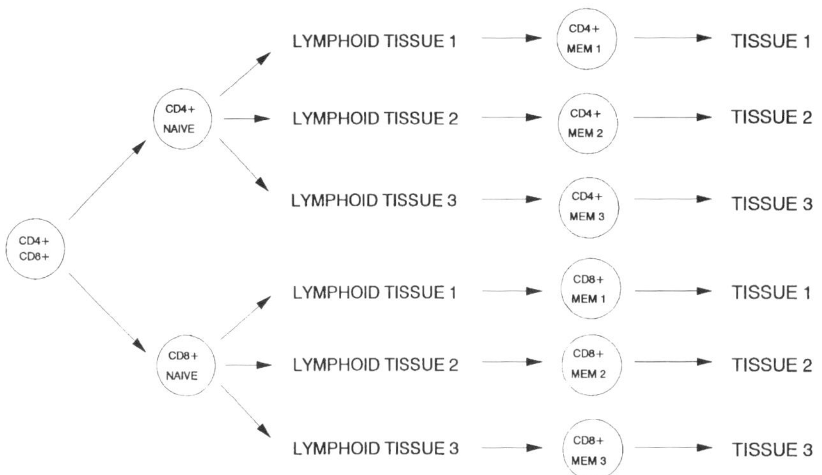

Figure 6.2. Simplified view of the peripheral differentiation of T cells and their patterns of recirculation. T cells exit the thymus as either CD4+ or CD8+ naive cells. They recirculate between the blood and lymphoid tissue until they are activated in the lymph node by antigen. After activation, the T cell returns to the circulation as a memory cell (MEM). The memory T cell shows different patterns of migration depending on where it was activated. Thus a memory cell that was activated in lymphoid tissue draining tissue 1 will subsequently recirculate almost exclusively through tissue 1. This increases the chances of the T cell coming into contact with its specific antigen again

contact with antigen will take place in the specialised environment of the lymph node where they can be optimally activated by APCs[28].

T cells are activated when the TCR–CD4 complex is engaged by antigenic peptides in association with MHC molecules and appropriate costimulatory signals. After such an encounter, the naive T cell undergoes a number of phenotypic and functional changes and differentiates into a memory T cell or an effector cell[32,33]. After activation, memory T cells return to a resting state, but are primed to respond rapidly to a further encounter with antigen. Compared with naive T cells, memory cells show different patterns of recirculation: they do not enter secondary lymph nodes but tend to migrate through tissue and, furthermore, memory T cells have restricted patterns of recirculation that are determined by the tissue in which they were activated. Thus memory T cells activated in lymph nodes draining the skin subsequently migrate almost exclusively through dermal tissues, whereas memory T cells that were exposed to antigen in the gut migrate through intestinal tissues. These restricted patterns of recirculation help to increase the chance of a particular T cell re-encountering antigen and thus improve the efficiency of immune surveillance[34,35].

The transition from naive to memory cell is characterised by distinct phenotypic changes that include alterations in the expression of CD45 isoforms and also altered expression of a number of adhesion molecules. For instance, expression of L-selectin is reduced[29], whereas expression of LFA-1, LFA-3, VLA-4 and CD44 is increased. L-selectin has a particular role in mediating the binding of naive T cells to HEV in lymph nodes, and the lower levels of L-selectin expressed on memory cells compared with naive T cells bias recruitment of memory cells away from lymphoid tissue[29]. The site at which memory T cells are activated determines their expression of other adhesion molecules that confer the ability to migrate to a particular site on the memory T cell. For instance, memory T cells activated in peripheral lymph nodes draining the skin express high levels of the molecule CLA, that allows them subsequently to bind preferentially to E-selectin expressed on dermal endothelium[16,29,30,36], whereas memory T cells that are exposed to antigen in gut associated lymphoid tissue express high levels of the $\alpha_4\beta_7$ integrin that binds to MAdCAM-1 (an endothelial adhesion molecule that is preferentially expressed on gut endothelium) and promotes migration into gut tissues[7,8].

The complement of adhesion molecules expressed by a particular T cell will therefore confer on it the ability to migrate to specific tissues. Peripheral memory T cells should thus be considered as consisting of multiple subsets, each with a distinct pattern of recirculation *in vivo*. To date, "homing" molecules, believed to confer tissue tropism to T cells, have been proposed for recruitment to the synovium, lung and liver, in addition to the gut[37–42].

T CELL ACTIVATION

ANTIGEN PRESENTATION AND COSTIMULATION

Several members of the immunoglobulin superfamily have a crucial role in T cell activation. These include the cell surface molecules CD4 and CD8 that act as receptors for MHC restricted responses; CD3, which is a crucial part of the TCR complex; and the adhesion molecules LFA-3 and CD2 that are involved in adhesion strengthening and also provide costimulation and ICAM-1 and ICAM-3, both of which are ligands for the leucocyte integrin, LFA-1[43].

The initial interaction of an APC with a T cell is mediated by ICAM-1, and possibly ICAM-3 on the APC binding to T cell LFA-1. This is initially a low affinity interaction, but provides sufficient adhesion to facilitate the binding of CD2 on T cells to LFA-3 on the APC. This interaction triggers a conformational change in LFA-1 that results in functional activation of the integrin and adhesion strengthening, allowing the TCR to engage antigen. Occupancy of the TCR leads to further activation of LFA-1 and the generation of a stable conjugate between the APC and T cell[1,43].

In addition to their role in bringing antigen presenting cells and responding T cells into close contact, adhesion molecules also provide costimulatory signals that are required for optimum T cell activation. If the T cell receptor is engaged by antigen in the absence of such costimulatory signals, it will fail to respond to the antigen and may be anergised[43–45]. The enhanced, LFA-1 mediated adhesion that is a consequence of TCR engagement provides costimulation for T cell activation[1,43], as does the binding of CD2 to its counter receptor, LFA-3 (CD58).

Several other intercellular adhesion pathways have been shown to provide co-stimulation, including VLA-4/VCAM-1, CD44[22,43,46,47], and interactions with extracellular matrix components via the $\beta1$ integrins VLA-4, VLA-5 and VLA-6 and the vitronectin receptor, $\alpha_v\beta_3$[48−51].

Attention has focused recently on the role of another adhesion pathway in costimulation: the binding of CD28 and its activation dependent homologue CTLA-4 on T cells to B7 on APCs. This pathway is of particular interest because it can prevent the induction of tolerance[45,52]. CD28 and CTLA-4 belong to the immunoglobulin superfamily and are expressed on T cells. They bind to two inducible ligands on APCs, B7-1 (CD80) and B7-2 (CD86). *In vitro* costimulation via B7 prevents the induction of alloantigen specific tolerance in human T cells, whereas costimulation via ICAM-1 does not. Blockade of B7 in animals using an immunoglobulin–CTLA-4 fusion protein can result in long lasting tolerance to xenografts[52] and profound immunosuppression in cardiac allografts[53,54].

Whereas engagement of CD28 promotes T-cell proliferation, CTLA-4 appears to induce apoptosis and may provide a regulatory mechanism for switching off antigen dependent reactions.

T CELL CYTOTOXICITY

The majority of CTLs are CD8+ T cells that recognise foreign antigen in association with MHC class I molecules. In order to destroy their target structures, CTLs must first adhere to them. This adhesion allows the CTL to make a "lethal hit" by disrupting the cell membrane and injecting proteolytic enzymes such as granzymes that induce internal disintegration and apoptosis in the target cell[55].

CTL adhesion to its target is regulated by sequential adhesive interactions that provide a mechanism for rapid strengthening of adhesion between the two cells[56,57]. Occupation of the TCR and CD8 by antigen in association with MHC class I triggers functional activation of LFA-1 which binds ICAM-1 on the target, resulting in marked adhesion strengthening between the CTL and its target. LFA-1/ICAM-1 mediated adhesion activates other pathways, including CD2/LFA-3, and further enhances engagement of CD8 and the TCR[56]. Thus the antigen dependent interactions act synergistically with LFA-1 mediated adhesion to provide maximal adhesion between the cells. *In vitro* antibodies to both LFA-1 and ICAM-1 can effectively block CTL lysis of target cells[58−60], as can blockade of the interaction between CD2 on CTLs and LFA-3 (CD58) on target cells, although blockade of the latter pathway inhibits killing to a lesser degree[60,61].

There is now evidence that integrin mediated adhesion provides costimulatory signals for cytotoxic T cell activation in addition to promoting cell–cell contact[9,56]. Initial studies suggest that this costimulation is provided by the β_1 integrins VLA-4 and VLA-5, rather than by LFA-1[56].

T CELL ENDOTHELIAL INTERACTIONS AND RECRUITMENT TO TISSUE

The emigration of T cells into lymphoid tissue takes place at the specialised HEVs[62], and entry into non-lymphoid tissue occurs preferentially at the level of

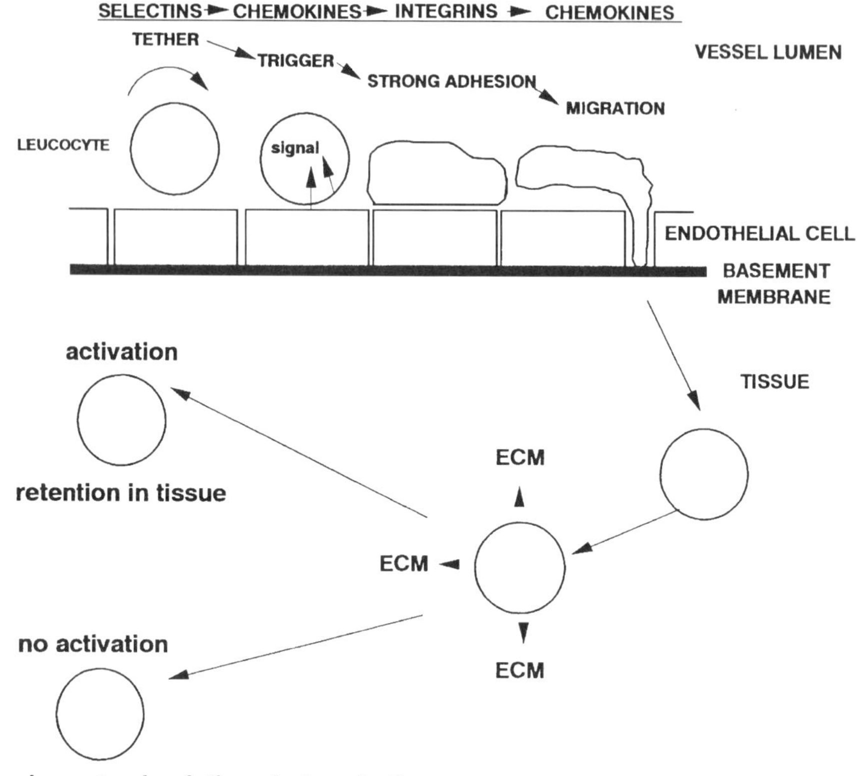

Figure 6.3. T cell interactions with endothelium and emigration into tissue. The flowing T cell is initially tethered to the vessel wall by primary adhesion involving selectins. This causes the cell to roll or bump on the endothelium, where it comes into contact with trigger factors that can activate T cell integrins, thus promoting strong adhesion to endothelial adhesion molecules such as intercellular adhesion molecule-1 and vascular cell adhesion molecule-1. In the presence of a correct chemotactic factor, the T cell will migrate into and through tissue. It interacts with tissue via β_1 integrin binding to extracellular matrix (ECM) and, if it comes into contact with antigen in the context of appropriate costimulatory signals, it is activated, causing a further increase in integrin function and retention in tissue. If it is not activated, it returns to the circulation via the draining lymphatics

the postcapillary venule. In order to extravasate, T cells must first recognise and bind to endothelial adhesion molecules. This process is regulated by sequential adhesive interactions between the T cell and the endothelium in which both cell types have an active role[63-65]. The process can be divided into four steps (Fig. 6.3).

PRIMARY ADHESION OR TETHERING

The initial step, or primary adhesion, is transient binding that causes the flowing T cell to roll or bump along the endothelium. This primary adhesion can be mediated by selectins[15]. L-selectin, which is expressed on all circulating T cells but particularly naive T cells, binds to several poorly defined carbohydrate receptors, including peripheral addressin and glycosylated cell adhesion molecule-1 (GlyCAM-1) on HEVs in lymph nodes[15,66–68]. L-selectin has been proposed as a lymph node homing receptor, although whether it also has a role in mediating primary adhesion to other tissues is not clear[29]. E-selectin is expressed on cytokine activated endothelium and can support adhesion of a subset of CD4+ memory T cells[16,30]. As mentioned above, the binding of CLA on skin homing T cells to E-selectin is believed to have an important role in directing T cell migration to the skin[69]. P-selectin, which is rapidly mobilised from cytoplasmic granules to the surface of activated endothelium and platelets, can mediate binding of a subset of activated T cells *in vitro*, suggesting a possible role for this molecule in T cell endothelial interactions *in vivo*[17].

Each selectin recognises specific carbohydrate sequences and mediates adhesion of particular leucocyte subsets. Selectins are long molecules that extend out of the surrounding glycocalyx, allowing them to capture passing lymphocytes. Furthermore, they mediate transient, activation independent binding, which is ideal for primary adhesion/tethering because it allows the lymphocyte to come into contact with the endothelium but subsequently to disengage if further strong adhesion is not triggered[15].

It was formerly believed that selectins were required for primary adhesion. This hypothesis has now been challenged with the discovery that at least two other non-selectin ligands can mediate primary adhesion of T cells. These are VCAM-1, which can mediate lymphocyte rolling under low flow conditions, and MAdCAM-1[30,70].

ACTIVATION OF T CELL INTEGRINS

Primary adhesion causes the lymphocyte to roll or bump on the vessel wall. This brings it into contact with proadhesive factors that activate secondary adhesion by triggering T cell integrins. The integrins can then bind to counter receptors on activated endothelium, thereby bringing the cell to a complete halt[63–65,71].

The proadhesive factors are crucial to the cascade, as T cell integrins do not bind well to their ligands in the absence of activation[2,3]. Two different categories of adhesion triggers have been described for T cells: cell surface molecules and soluble factors/cytokines. Engagement of the T cell surface molecule CD31 can activate LFA-1 and VLA-4 by inducing a conformational change in the T cell integrins, resulting in increased avidity for their endothelial ligands, ICAM-1 and VCAM-1[14]. CD31 is widely expressed on endothelium and on a restricted subset of T cells. As homotypic adhesion of CD31 can trigger integrins, it is possible that CD31 on the T cell engages CD31 expressed on endothelium. Alternatively, there may be another CD31 ligand on endothelium[14,72–74].

CD31 might be involved in the recruitment of the distinct subset of T cells that expresses CD31, but clearly cannot be the trigger factor for the majority of circulating T cells that are CD31 negative[72]. Other triggers must therefore exist. It has been proposed that engagement of selectins can, under certain circumstances, lead to integrin activation, thereby providing both primary adhesion and the trigger step[75], but most of the interest in adhesion triggering factors in recent years has focused on a family of structurally distinct cytokines, called chemokines[64,65,76,77].

Chemokines are a family of structurally related chemotactic cytokines that are secreted by inflammatory cells including platelets, lymphocytes, monocytes and, under certain circumstances, activated endothelium[78–80]. Approximately 30 human chemokines have been isolated, all of which bind to G protein linked, seven domain transmembrane spanning receptors[81]. Chemokines can be divided into three subfamilies based on their structure: α chemokines include IL-8, *groα* (also known as melanoma stimulating activity) and interferon inducible protein-10 (IP-10); β chemokines include macrophage inflammatory protein-1α (MIP-1α), MIP-1β, RANTES (rapid on activation normal T cell expressed and secreted) and monocyte chemoattractant protein-1 (MCP-1); a novel chemokine, lymphotactin, belongs to a distinct subfamily.

The β chemokine, MIP-1β, was the first cytokine reported to trigger T cell integrins, when it was shown to activate VLA-4 binding to VCAM-1[82]. Since then, several other chemokines have been shown to activate T cell adhesion, including MIP-1α, MCP-1, RANTES, and IP-10[83]. In addition three other, structurally distinct, growth factors have been shown to have proadhesive properties. Two of these, macrophage stimulating protein-1 (MSP-1) and hepatocyte growth factor (HGF) are members of the plasminogen family of growth factors[84,85]. MSP-1 acts on activated macrophages but has no effect on T cells, whereas HGF can trigger integrin mediated adhesion and migration of memory T cells[85]. HGF is better known as an epithelial growth factor, but several properties suggest it might have an important role in the immune system: it can activate immune cells including neutrophils and B lymphocytes[86,87], it is produced by inflammatory cells, and it can be detected on inflamed endothelium[85,88,89]. It has recently been reported that another growth factor, growth hormone, can also trigger T cell adhesion and migration, suggesting that other growth factors/cytokines share these properties[90].

Proadhesive cytokines display preferential activity for particular leucocyte subsets. For instance, the α chemokines IL-8 and *groα* act primarily on neutrophils, whereas the β chemokines tend to act on mononuclear cells, and lymphotactin is specific for lymphocytes[91–93]. Similarly, HGF acts on T cells, whereas MSP-1 only affects macrophages[85]. Furthermore, there is evidence for preferential activity within T cell subsets: for example, MIP-1β acts on naive T cells, whereas RANTES and HGF act only on memory T cells[82,85]. The existence of subset specific adhesion triggers provides another layer of selectivity to endothelial binding and suggests that the recruitment of a particular subset of T cells to a given site will be determined by both local proadhesive cytokines and the expression of the correct leucocyte and endothelial adhesion molecules.

If they are to trigger adhesion effectively, proadhesive factors must be available at the vessel wall to allow interaction with circulating T cells[94]. Recent work suggests that immobilisation on proteoglycans in the endothelial glycocalyx is responsible for the retention of proadhesive cytokines at relevant sites[82,94]. Proadhesive cytokines have glycosaminoglycan binding motifs that would allow them to bind to proteoglycans. In support of this hypothesis, several of the

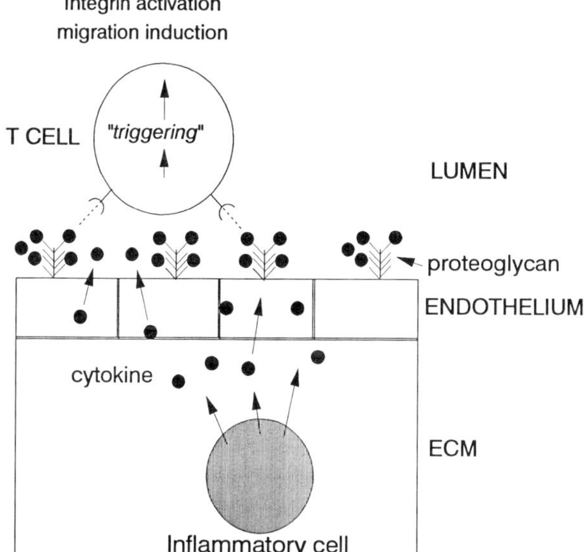

Figure 6.4. Proposed model for the presentation of proadhesive cytokines at the endothelial surface. Proadhesive cytokines, typically chemokines, are secreted by inflammatory cells infiltrating the tissue or by the endothelium itself. They are transported to the luminal surface of the vessel, where they bind to proteoglycans via glycosaminoglycan binding sites, thereby interacting with T cells that have been tethered by primary adhesion. Differential binding of chemokines to proteoglycans, together with site- and activation dependent differences in endothelial proteoglycans, confer potential selectivity to the model. ECM = Extracellular matrix

chemokines, in addition to HGF, have been demonstrated on the luminal surface of endothelium[79,82,85]. There is now evidence that chemokines show differential binding to proteoglycans and, as endothelial proteoglycans vary from site to site and with activation, this could provide a mechanism by which tissues can selectively express a particular proadhesive factor, enabling them to recruit specific leucocyte subsets[95] (Fig. 6.4).

Proadhesive cytokines are transcribed by both inflammatory cells at sites of inflammation and the endothelium itself[78]. Endothelia from different tissues show particular patterns of chemokine secretion and differential responses to proinflammatory cytokines[78]. For instance, lung microvascular endothelial cells secrete both MCP-1 and IL-8 *in vitro*, but their response to proinflammatory cytokines differs, suggesting that the nature of the activating cytokine *in vitro* will determine which proadhesive cytokine is secreted.

STRONG ADHESION

Strong adhesion is mediated by T cell integrins. LFA-1 binds to ICAM-2 on resting endothelium and ICAM-1, which is upregulated on endothelium within a few hours by proinflammatory cytokines such as TNFα and IL-1[96]. VLA-4 binds to VCAM-1, which is also induced on cytokine activated endothelium.

                                    David H. Adams

However, some cytokines, notably IL-4, can upregulate VCAM-1 but not ICAM-1, suggesting that the inflammatory stimulus will determine which endothelial ligands are expressed[97,98]. The exact contribution of LFA-1/ICAM-1 and VLA-4/VCAM-1 to T cell endothelial binding *in vivo* is unclear. VLA-4 seems to be particularly important in the recruitment of T cells to some sites, such as the brain[99,100]. The fact that lymphocytic infiltration of tissues occurs in patients with leucocyte adhesion deficiency type I, in whom LFA-1 is absent, suggests that VLA-4 might have the dominant role in T cell recruitment *in vivo*[101].

MIGRATION

After strong adhesion, the T cell migrates into tissue under the influence of local promigratory factors. Many different cytokines can induce T cell migration *in vitro* and some of these factors display subset specificity[102,103]. All of the proadhesive cytokines described above also induce migration responses, suggesting that the same cytokines might be acting to trigger T cell adhesion and then to promote transendothelial migration into tissue. However, it is also possible that several cytokines participate at different stages of the adhesion cascade during the recruitment of a particular leucocyte subset.

Thus whether a particular T cell is recruited into a specific tissue will depend on:

(i) the adhesion molecules that are expressed on the endothelium (selectins or selectin ligand, ICAM-1, VCAM-1)

(ii) the adhesion molecules expressed on the T cell (selectin or selectin ligand, integrins LFA-1, VLA-4 or $\alpha_4\beta_7$)

(iii) the presence of a relevant proadhesive cytokine and chemotactic factor.

It is likely that these factors act together to determine which leucocyte subsets are recruited[64,65].

CONCLUSIONS

Adhesion molecules are crucial to the efficient functioning of the immune system, where they regulate T cell activation, cytotoxicity and recruitment into tissues. The greater understanding of the molecular mechanisms involved in the regulation and function of adhesion molecules is shedding important light on how the immune system works and suggests the possibility of directing new treatments toward the selective antagonism of particular adhesion pathways involved in lymphocyte mediated tissue damage[104,105]. It remains to be seen, however, whether the important scientific advances outlined above can be converted into clinical treatments.

REFERENCES

1. Springer T A. Adhesion receptors of the immune system. *Nature* 1990; **346:** 425–434.
2. Hynes R O. Integrins: versatility, modulation, and signaling in cell adhesion. *Cell* 1992; **69:** 11–25.

3. Schweighoffer T, Shaw S. Adhesion cascades: diversity through combinatorial strategies. *Curr Opin Cell Biol* 1994; **4**: 824–829.

4. Hemler M E. VLA proteins in the integrin family: structures, functions, and their role on leukocytes. *Annu Rev Immunol* 1990; **8**: 365–400.

5. Parker C M, Cepek K L, Russel G J, *et al*. A family of $\beta 7$ integrins on human mucosal lymphocytes. *Proc Natl Acad Sci USA* 1992; **89**: 1924–1928.

6. Cepek K L, Parker C M, Madara J L, *et al*. Integrin $\alpha E\beta 7$ mediates adhesion of T lymphocytes to epithelial cells. *J Immunol* 1993; **150**: 3459–3470.

7. Schweighoffer T, Tanaka Y, Tidswell M, *et al*. Selective expression of integrin $\alpha 4\beta 7$ on a subset of human CD4+ memory T cells with hallmarks of gut-trophism. *J Immunol* 1993; **151**: 717–729.

8. Berlin C, Berg E L, Briskin M J, *et al*. Alpha 4 beta 7 integrin mediates binding to the mucosal vascular addressin MAdCAM-1. *Cell* 1993; **74**: 185–195.

9. O'Rourke A M, Mescher M F. Cytotoxic T lymphocyte activation involves a cascade of signalling and adhesion events. *Nature* 1992; **358**: 253–255.

10. Makgoba M W, Sanders M E, Shaw S. The CD2-LFA-3 and LFA-1-ICAM-1 pathways: relevance to T-cell recognition. *Immunol Today* 1989; **10**: 417–422.

11. Boussiotis V A, Freeman G J, Gray G, *et al*. B7 but not intercellular adhesion molecule-1 costimulation prevents the induction of human alloantigen-specific tolerance. *J Exp Med* 1993; **178**: 1753–1763.

12. Vazeux R, Hoffman P A, Tomita J K, *et al*. Cloning and characterisation of a new intercellular adhesion molecule ICAM-R. *Nature* 1992; **360**: 485–488.

13. Shimizu Y, Newman W, Tanaka Y, *et al*. Lymphocyte interactions with endothelial cells. *Immunol Today* 1992; **13**: 106–112.

14. Tanaka Y, Albelda S M, Horgan K J, *et al*. CD31 expressed on distinctive T cell subsets is a preferential amplifier of $\beta 1$ integrin-mediated adhesion. *J Exp Med* 1992; **176**: 245–253.

15. Lasky L A. Selectins: interpreters of cell-specific carbohydrate information during inflammation. *Science* 1992; **258**: 964–969.

16. Picker L J, Kishimoto T K, Smith C W, *et al*. ELAM-1 is an adhesion molecule for skin-homing T cells. *Nature* 1991; **349**: 796–799.

17. Damle N K, Klussman K, Dietsch M T, *et al*. GMP-140 (P-selectin/CD62) binds to chronically stimulated but not resting CD4+ T lymphocytes and regulates their production of proinflammatory cytokines. *Eur J Immunol* 1992; **22**: 1789–1793.

18. Camerini D, James S P, Stamenkovic I, *et al*. Leu-8/TQ1 is the human equivalent of the Mel-14 lymph node homing receptor. *Nature* 1989; **342**: 78–82.

19. Mentzer S, Remold-O'Donnell E, Crimmins M, *et al*. Sialophorin, a surface sialoglycoprotein defective in the Wiskott-Aldrich syndrome is involved in human T-lymphocyte proliferation. *J Exp Med* 1987; **165**: 1383–1389.

20. Axelsson B, Youseffi-Etemad R, Hammarstrom S, *et al*. Induction of aggregation and enhancement of proliferation and IL-2 secretion in human T cells by antibodies to CD43. *J Immunol* 1988; **141**: 2912–2917.

21. Ardman B, Sikorski M A, Staunton D E. CD43 interferes with T-lymphocyte adhesion. *Proc Natl Acad Sci USA* 1992; **89**: 5001–5005.

22. Shimizu Y, van Seventer G A, Siraganian R, *et al*. Dual role of the CD44 molecule in T cell adhesion and activation. *J Immunol* 1989; **143**: 2457–2463.

23. Salomon D R, Mojcik C F, Chang A C, *et al*. Constitutive activation of integrin alpha 4-beta-1 defines a unique stage of human thymocyte development. *J Exp Med* 1994; **179**: 1573–1584.

24. Ramarli D, Fox D A, Reinherz E L. Selective inhibition of interleukin 2 gene function following thymocyte antigen/major histocompatibility complex receptor crosslinking: possible thymic selection mechanism. *Proc Natl Acad Sci USA* 1987; **84**: 8598–8602.

25. Singer K H, Haynes B F. Epithelial-thymocyte interactions in human thymus. *Hum Immunol* 1987; **20**: 127–144.

26. Yang S Y, Denning S M, Mizuno S, *et al*. A novel activation pathway for mature thymocytes: costimulation of CD2 (T, p50) and CD28 (T, p44) induces autocrine interleukin 2/interleukin 2 receptor-mediated cell proliferation. *J Exp Med* 1988; **168**: 1457–1468.

27. Haynes B F, Denning S M, Singer K H, *et al*. Ontogeny of T-cell precursors: a model for the initial stages of human T-cell development. *Immunol Today* 1989; **10**: 87–91.

28. Picker L J, Butcher E C. Physiologic and molecular mechanisms of lymphocyte homing. *Annu Rev Immunol* 1992; **10:** 561.

29. Picker L J, Treer J R, Ferguson-Darnell B, *et al*. Control of lymphocyte recirculation in man: I. Differential regulation of the peripheral lymph node homing receptor L-selectin on T cells during the virgin to memory cell transition. *J Immunol* 1993; **150:** 1105–1121.

30. Picker L J. Control of lymphocyte homing. *Curr Opin Immunol* 1994; **6:** 394–406.

31. Mackay C R. Homing of naive, memory and effector lymphocytes. *Curr Opin Immunol* 1993; **5:** 423–427.

32. Sanders M E, Makgoba M W, Sharrow S O, *et al*. Human memory T lymphocytes express increased levels of three cell adhesion molecules (LFA-3, CD2, and LFA-1) and three other molecules (UCHL1, CDw29, and Pgp-1) and have enhanced IFN-gamma production. *J Immunol* 1988; **140:** 1401–1407.

33. Sanders M E, Makgoba M W, Shaw S. Human naive and memory T cells: reinterpretation of helper-inducer and suppressor-inducer subsets. *Immunol Today* 1988; **9:** 195–199.

34. Mackay C R, Marston W L, Dudler L, *et al*. Tissue-specific migration pathways by phenotypically distinct subpopulations of memory T cells. *Eur J Immunol* 1992; **22:** 887–895.

35. Mackay C R. Migration pathways and immunologic memory among T lymphocytes. *Semin Immunol* 1992; **4:** 51.

36. Picker L J, Treer J R, Ferguson-Darnell B, *et al*. Control of lymphocyte recirculation in man. II. Differential regulation of the cutaneous lymphocyte-associated antigen, a tissue-selective homing receptor for skin-homing T cells. *J Immunol* 1993; **1500:** 1122–1136.

37. McNab G, Reeves J L, Salmi M, *et al*. Vascular adhesion protein-1 (VAP-1) mediates binding of human T cells to human hepatic endothelium. *Gastroenterology* 1996; **110:** 522–528.

38. Salmi M, Jalkanen S. A 90-kilodalton endothelial cell molecule mediating lymphocyte binding in humans. *Science* 1992; **257:** 1407–1409.

39. Salmi M, Kalimo K, Jalkanen S. Induction and function of vascular adhesion protein-1 at sites of inflammation. *J Exp Med* 1993; **178:** 2255–2260.

40. Saltini C, Hemler M E, Crystal R G. T lymphocytes compartmentalized on the epithelial surface of the lower respiratory tract express the very late activation antigen complex VLA-1. *Clin Immunol Immunopathol* 1988; **46:** 221–233.

41. Zhu D Z, Cheng C F, Pauli B U. Mediation of lung metastasis of murine melanomas by a lung-specific endothelial cell adhesion molecule. *Proc Natl Acad Sci USA* 1991; **88:** 9568–9572.

42. Furfaro S, Berman J S. The relation between cell migration and activation in inflammation: beyond adherence. *Am J Respir Cell Mol Biol* 1992; **7:** 248–250.

43. van Seventer G A, Shimizu Y, Shaw S. Roles of multiple accessory molecules in T-cell activation. *Curr Opin Immunol* 1991; **3:** 294–303.

44. Schwartz R H. Acquisition of immunologic self-tolerance. *Cell* 1989; **57:** 1073–1081.

45. Schwartz R H. Costimulation of T lymphocytes: the role of CD28, CTLA-4, and B7/BB1 in interleukin-2 production and immunotherapy. *Cell* 1992; **71:** 1065–1068.

46. van Seventer G A, Shimizu Y, Horgan K J, *et al*. The LFA-1 ligand ICAM-1 provides an important costimulatory signal for T cell receptor-mediated activation of resting T cells. *J Immunol* 1990; **144:** 4579–4586.

47. Webb D S, Shimizu Y, van Seventer G A, *et al*. LFA-3, CD44, and CD45: physiologic triggers of human monocyte TNF and IL-1 release. *Science* 1990; **249:** 1295–1297.

48. Juliano R L, Haskill S. Signal transduction from the extracellular matrix. *J Cell Biol* 1993; **120:** 577–585.

49. Shimizu Y, Mobley J L. Distinct divalent-cation requirements for integrin-mediated CD4+ T-lymphocyte adhesion to ICAM-1, fibronectin, VCAM-1, and invasin. *J Immunol* 1993; **151:** 4106–4115.

50. Shimizu Y, van Seventer G A, Horgan K J, *et al*. Roles of adhesion molecules in T cell recognition: fundamental similarities between four integrins on resting human T cells (LFA-1, VLA-4, VLA-5, VLA-6) in expression, binding, and costimulation. *Immunol Rev* 1990; **114:** 109–143.

51. Shimizu Y, Shaw S. Lymphocyte interactions with extracellular matrix. *FASEB J* 1991; **5:** 2292–2299.

52. Boussiotis V A, Gribben J G, Freeman G J, *et al.* Blockade of the CD28 co-stimulatory pathway: a means to induce tolerance. *Curr Opin Immunol* 1994; **6:** 797–807.

53. Lenschow D J, Bluestone J A. T cell co-stimulation and *in vivo* tolerance. *Curr Opin Immunol* 1993; **5:** 747–752.

54. Turka L A, Linsley P S, Lin H, *et al.* T-cell activation by the CD28 ligand B7 is required for cardiac allograft rejection *in vivo. Proc Natl Acad Sci USA* 1992; **89:** 11102–11105.

55. Sarin A, Adams D H, Henkart P A. Protease inhibitors selectively block T-cell receptor-triggered programmed cell-death in a murine T-cell hybridoma and activated peripheral T-cells. *J Exp Med* 1993; **178:** 1693–1700.

56. Argov S, Poros A, Klein E. Cation requirement in natural, *in vitro* generated, and antibody dependent killing exerted by human lymphocytes. *Immunobiology* 1979; **156:** 25–34.

57. Schweighoffer T, Shaw S. Adhesion cascades: diversity through combinatorial strategies. *Curr Opin Cell Biol* 1992; **4:** 824–829.

58. Blanchard D, Van Els C, Borst J, *et al.* The role of the T cell receptor, CD8 and LFA-1 in different stages of the cytolytic reaction mediated by alloreactive T lymphocyte clones. *J Immunol* 1987; **138:** 2417–2421.

59. Makgoba M W, Sanders M E, Luce G E, *et al.* Functional evidence that intercellular adhesion molecule-1 (ICAM-1) is a ligand for LFA-1 in cytotoxic T cell recognition. *Eur J Immunol* 1988; **18:** 637–640.

60. Makgoba M W, Sanders M E, Luce G E, *et al.* Intercellular adhesion molecule-1 (ICAM-1) monoclonal antibody inhibits cytotoxic T lymphocyte recognition. *Ann NY Acad Sci* 1988; **532:** 427–428.

61. Shaw S, Luce G E G, Quinones R, *et al.* Two antigen-independent adhesion pathways used by human cytotoxic T cell clones. *Nature* 1986; **323:** 262–264.

62. Anderson A O, Shaw S. T cell adhesion to endothelium: the FRC conduit system and other anatomic and molecular features which facilitate the adhesion cascade in lymph node. *Semin Immunol* 1993; **5:** 271–282.

63. Adams D H, Shaw S. Leucocyte endothelial interactions and regulation of leucocyte migration. *Lancet* 1994; **343:** 831–836.

64. Springer T A. Traffic signals for lymphocyte recirculation and leukocyte emigration: the multi-step paradigm. *Cell* 1994; **76:** 301–314.

65. Butcher E C. Leukocyte-endothelial cell recognition: three (or more) steps to specificity and diversity. *Cell* 1991; **67:** 1033–1036.

66. Mebius R E, Breve J, Kraal G, *et al.* Developmental regulation of vascular addressin expression: a possible role for site-associated environments. *Int Immunol* 1993; **5:** 443–449.

67. Lasky L A, Singer M S, Dowbenko D, *et al.* An endothelial ligand for L-selectin is a novel mucin-like molecule. *Cell* 1992; **69:** 927–938.

68. Imai Y, Lasky L A, Rosen S D. Sulphation requirement for GlyCAM-1, an endothelial ligand for L-selectin. *Nature* 1993; **361:** 555–557.

69. Berg E L, Yoshino T, Rott L S, *et al.* The cutaneous lymphocyte antigen is a skin lymphocyte homing receptor for the vascular lectin endothelial cell-leukocyte adhesion molecule 1. *J Exp Med* 1991; **174:** 1461–1466.

70. Jones D A, McIntire L V, Smith C W, *et al.* A 2-step adhesion cascade for T-cell endothelial-cell interactions under flow conditions. *J Clin Invest* 1994; **94:** 2443–2450.

71. Hathaway M, Burnett D, Elias E, *et al.* Secretion of soluble chemotactic factors including interleukin-6. a mechanism for the recruitment of CD8+ T lymphocytes to human liver allografts during rejection. *Hepatology* 1993; **18:** 511–519.

72. Albelda S M, Muller W A, Buck C A, *et al.* Molecular and cellular properties of PECAM-1 (endoCAM/CD31): a novel vascular cell-cell adhesion molecule. *J Cell Biol* 1991; **114:** 1059–1068.

73 Delisser H M, Muller W A, Newman P J, *et al.* PECAM-1 (CD31) mediates heterophilic cell-cell adhesion. *J Cell Biol* 1991; **115:** 70A.

74. Tanaka Y, Shaw S. T cell adhesion cascades: general considerations and illustration with CD31. *Adv Exp Med Biol* 1992; **323:** 157–162.

75. Lo S K, Lee S, Ramos R A, *et al.* Endothelial-leukocyte adhesion molecule 1 stimulates the adhesive activity of leukocyte integrin CR3 (CD11b/CD18, Mac-1, $\alpha\beta$) on human neutrophils. *J Exp Med* 1991; **173:** 1493–1500.

76. Oppenheim J J, Zachariae C O C, Mukaida N, *et al*. Properties of the novel proinflammatory supergene "intercrine" cytokine family. *Annu Rev Immunol* 1991; **9:** 617–648.

77. Schall T J. Biology of the RANTES/SIS cytokine family. *Cytokine* 1991; **3:** 165–183.

78. Brown Z, Gerritsen M E, Carley W W, *et al*. Chemokine gene expression and secretion by cytokine-activated human microvascular endothelial cells. Differential regulation of MCP-1 and IL-8 in response to gamma interferon. *Am J Pathol* 1994; **145:** 913–921.

79. Adams D H, Hubscher S, Fear J, *et al*. Hepatic expression of MIP-1α and MIP-1β after liver transplantation. *Transplantation* 1996; **61:** 817–825.

80. Miller M D, Krangel M S. Biology and biochemistry of the chemokines: a family of chemotactic and inflammatory cytokines. *CRC Crit Rev Immunol* 1992; **12:** 17–46.

81. Murphy P M. The molecular-biology of leukocyte chemoattractant receptors. *Annu Rev Immunol* 1994; **12:** 593–633.

82. Tanaka Y, Adams D H, Hubscher S, *et al*. T-cell adhesion induced by proteoglycan-immobilized cytokine MIP-1β. *Nature* 1993; **361:** 79–82.

83. Taub D D, Conlon K, Lloyd A R, *et al*. Preferential migration of activated human CD4+ and CD8+ T cells in response to MIP-1α and MIP-1β. *Science* 1993; **260:** 355–358.

84. Skeel A, Yoshimura T, Showalter S D, *et al*. Macrophage stimulating protein: purification, partial amino acid sequence and cellular activity. *J Exp Med* 1991; **173:** 1227–1234.

85. Adams D H, Harvath L, Bottaro D P, *et al*. Hepatocyte growth factor and macrophage inflammatory protein-1β: structurally distinct cytokines that induce rapid cytoskeletal changes and subset-preferential migration in T cell. *Proc Natl Acad Sci USA* 1994; **91:** 7144–7148.

86. Jiang W, Puntis M C A, Nakamura T, *et al*. Neutrophil priming by hepatocyte growth factor, a novel cytokine. *Immunology* 1992; **77:** 147–149.

87. Kmiecik T E, Keller J R, Rosen E, *et al*. Hepatocyte growth factor is a synergistic factor for the growth of hematopoietic progenitor cells. *Blood* 1992; **80:** 2454–2457.

88. Rubin J S, Chan A M-L, Bottaro D P, *et al*. A broad spectrum human lung fibroblast-derived mitogen is a variant of hepatocyte growth factor. *Proc Natl Acad Sci USA* 1991; **88:** 415–419.

89. Michalopoulos G, Zarnegar R. Hepatocyte growth factor. *Hepatology* 1992; **15:** 149–156.

90. Taub D D, Tsarfaty G, Lloyd A R, *et al*. Growth hormone promotes human T cell adhesion and migration to both human and murine matrix proteins *in vitro* and directly promotes xenogenic engraftment. *J Clin Invest* 1994; **94:** 293–300.

91. Kelner G S, Kennedy J, Bacon K B, *et al*. Lymphotactin—a cytokine that represents a new class of chemokine. *Science* 1994; **266:** 1395–1399.

92. Schall T J, Bacon K, Toy K J, *et al*. Selective attraction of monocytes and T lymphocytes of the memory phenotype by cytokine RANTES. *Nature* 1990; **347:** 669–671.

93. Schall T J, Bacon K, Camp R D, *et al*. Human macrophage inflammatory protein alpha (MIP-1alpha) and MIP-1beta chemokines attract distinct populations of lymphocytes. *J Exp Med* 1993; **177:** 1821–1826.

94. Tanaka Y, Adams D H, Shaw S. Proteoglycans on endothelial cells present adhesion-inducing cytokines to leukocytes. *Immunol Today* 1993; **14:** 111–114.

95. Witt D P, Lander A D. Differential binding of chemokines to glycosaminoglycan subpopulations. *Curr Biol* 1994; **4:** 394–400.

96. Pober J S, Gimbrone M A Jr, Lapierre L A, *et al*. Overlapping patterns of activation of human endothelial cells by interleukin 1, tumor necrosis factor, and immune interferon. *J Immunol* 1986; **137:** 1893–1896.

97. Chin Y H, Cai J P, Xu XM. Transforming growth factor-β1 and IL-4 regulate the adhesiveness of Peyer's patch high endothelial venule cells for lymphocytes. *J Immunol* 1992; **148:** 1106–1112.

98. Briscoe D M, Cotran R S, Pober J S. Effects of tumor necrosis factor, lipopolysaccharide, and IL-4 on the expression of vascular cell adhesion molecule-1 in vivo. Correlation with CD3+ T cell infiltration. *J Immunol* 1992; **149:** 2954–2960.

99. Baron J L, Madri J A, Ruddle N H, *et al*. Surface expression of alpha4 integrin by CD4 T cells is required for their entry into brain parenchyma. *J Exp Med* 1993; **177:** 57–68.

100. Yednock T A, Cannon C, Fritz L C, *et al*. Prevention of experimental autoimmune encephalomyelitis by antibodies against alpha4beta1 integrin. *Nature* 1992; **356:** 63–66.

101. Anderson D C, Springer T A. Leukocyte adhesion deficiency: an inherited defect in the Mac-1, LFA-1, and p150,95 glycoproteins. *Annu Rev Med* 1987; **38:** 175–194.

102. Adams D H, Hathaway M, Shaw J, *et al.* Transforming growth factor-β induces human T lymphocyte migration *in vitro. J Immunol* 1991; **147:** 609–612.
103. Bacon K B, Gearing A, Camp R. Induction of *in vitro* human lymphocyte migration by IL-3, IL-4 and IL-6. *Cytokine* 1990; **2:** 100–105.
104. Adams D H. Therapeutic potential of inhibiting the ICAM-1/LFA-1 pathway of leukocyte adhesion in transplantation. In: Salomon DR, ed. *Recent Developments in Transplantation Medicine. New Immunosuppressive Agents II—Adhesion Molecules and Monoclonal Antibodies.* University of Wisconsin: Bioliterature Inc., 1995.
105. Adams D H. Adhesion molecules and liver transplantation: new strategies for therapeutic intervention. *J Hepatol* 1995; **23:** 225–231.

7

Neutrophils

DAVID BURNETT

Institute of Research and Development, Birmingham, UK

INTRODUCTION

Neutrophils have a key role in the secondary defence of the lung. Small numbers can be found within the airways in health but, once local defences have been overwhelmed, large numbers of neutrophils are recruited from the circulation to protect the lung from invasive organisms (Fig. 7.1). In order to achieve this primary function of killing micro-organisms, neutrophils have a sophisticated system of cellular proteins and enzymes enabling them to detect and move to areas of infection, where they ingest and destroy the micro-organisms.

The importance of this cell type in the defence of the lung is highlighted by the recurrence and severity of infections when neutrophil numbers are suppressed or genetic defects impair their functions. This chapter describes the origins, recruitment and functions of neutrophils, outlining the importance of these cells in host defence.

NEUTROPHIL ORIGINS

Neutrophils are myelopoietic cells of the granulocyte lineage, which also includes eosinophils, basophils and mast cells. Neutrophils are also often called polymorphonuclear leucocytes because of their characteristic multi-lobed nuclei. This feature makes them probably the most readily identified cells in the blood under the microscope. They are the most abundant type of leucocyte in the body; the numbers normally found in the circulation exceed 5×10^{11}.

In common with other haemopoietic cells, neutrophils are produced in the bone marrow. The differentiation of neutrophils takes place entirely in the marrow and characteristic stages in this process, from stem cell to the mature neutrophil, have been recognised[1] (Fig. 7.2). The first of these is the myeloblast, which has an oval, unlobed nucleus and no cytoplasmic granules. The second characterised stage is the promyelocyte. The primary or azurophil granules are produced at

Pulmonary Defences. Edited by Robert A. Stockley.
© 1997 John Wiley & Sons Ltd.

                                 D. Burnett

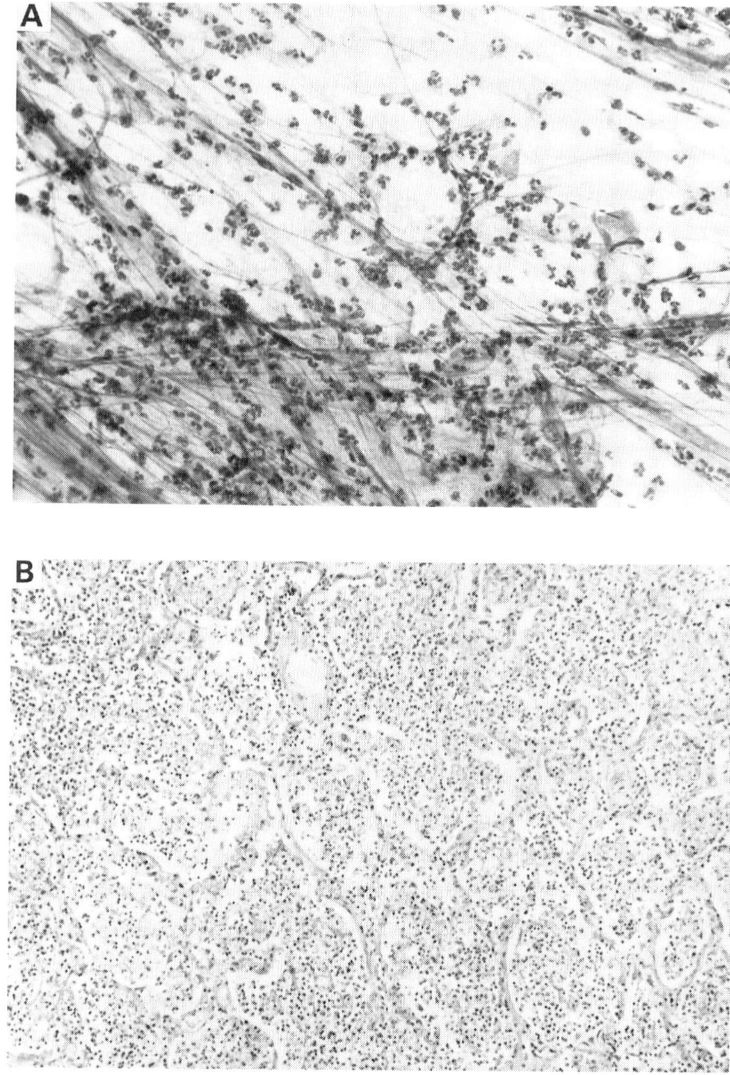

Figure 7.1. A: Neutrophils in sputum from a patient with bronchiectasis (courtesy of Dr Anita Pye, University of Birmingham).   **B:** Neutrophil infiltrate in a patient with lobar pneumonia (courtesy of Dr C. Newman, Department of Pathology, Birmingham Heartlands Hospital)

this stage and the ultimate contents of these granules synthesised and packaged also[1]. The cell proceeds to the third stage, the myelocyte, which also contains the newly formed secondary or specific granules and their contents. Cell divisions have ensured that all cells contain a full complement of granules. By the fourth recognised stage of differentiation, the metamyelocyte, granule production and synthesis of their components has ceased and there is no longer cell division.

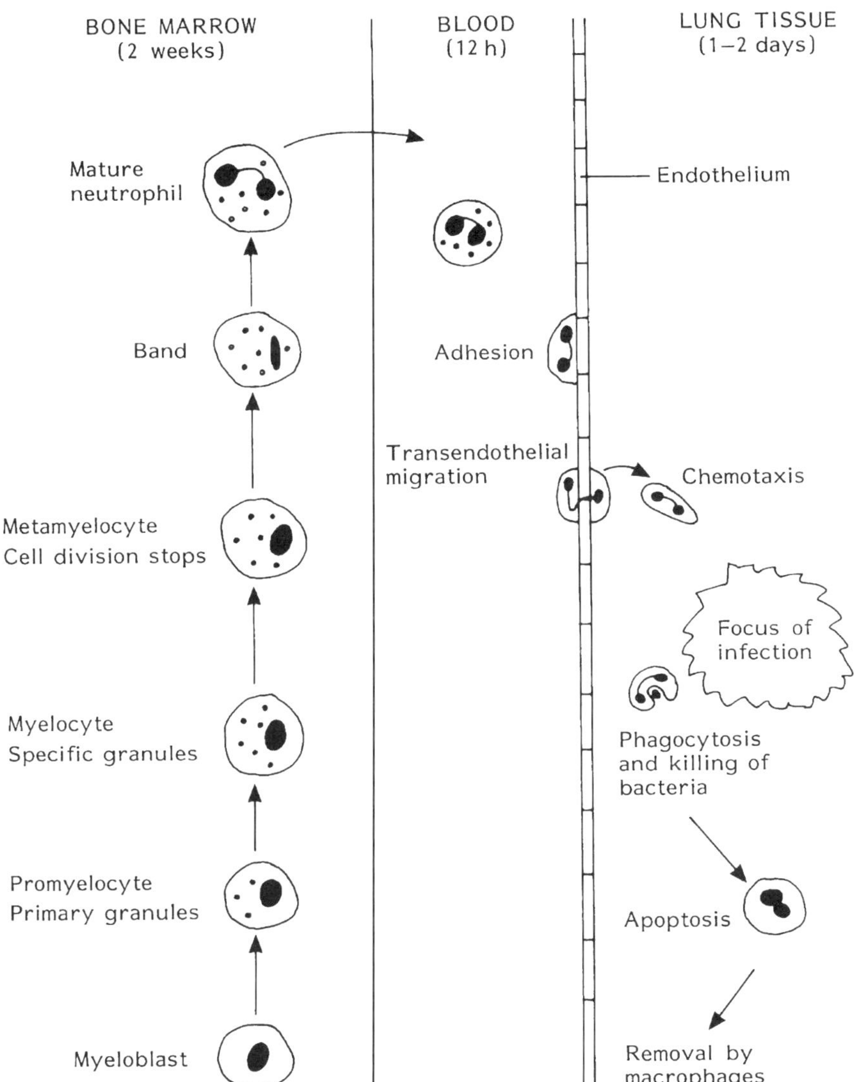

Figure 7.2. Schematic demonstration of the possible stages in the existence of neutrophils. Maturation occurs over about 2 weeks in the bone marrow. After terminal differentiation into a mature neutrophil, the cell migrates to the blood, where it remains for a short time only before removal and destruction. If, during this period, the cell encounters signals resulting from inflamed tissue, it may adhere to activated endothelium and migrate to the inflammatory focus. Here, neutrophils engulf bacteria and kill them by a variety of methods. Neutrophils in the tissues may become apoptotic and are then recognised and engulfed by macrophages. Sometimes, however, huge numbers of neutrophils may accumulate at infected sites and many will die by necrosis, releasing harmful granule contents

                          D. Burnett

The cells differentiate further via the "band" nucleus stage to mature neutrophils, which have the characteristic multi-lobed nuclei. The process of differentiation takes about 2 weeks and these mature cells remain in the marrow for approximately 2 days before being released into the blood, where they do not survive long (their half life being approximately 8 h).

About half the neutrophils in the circulation are believed to be "marginated", that is "parked" on endothelium. These cells can be mobilised rapidly. This mobilisation, coupled with increased granulopoiesis during episodes of infection[2], results in the neutrophilia which makes large numbers of these cells available to combat infectious agents.

NEUTROPHIL RECRUITMENT TO THE LUNGS

Because mature neutrophils are not capable of division, all of these cells found within lung tissues will be derived directly from the blood. Once in the tissues, neutrophils do not recirculate, but are believed to undergo programmed cell death, or apoptosis, after which they are destroyed by macrophages. The process of neutrophil recruitment to infected and damaged lung tissue comprises a complex series of events involving specific signals from the tissues, to which the blood neutrophils respond by

(i)   adhesion to endothelial cells
(ii) migration through endothelium into lung tissues.

NEUTROPHIL ADHESION TO ENDOTHELIUM

Adhesion of circulating neutrophils to the endothelial cells of postcapillary venules is a prerequisite for subsequent transendothelial migration. The process of adhesion has been defined, as for other leucocytes, in terms of a model system which can be identified conveniently as constituting three steps: *tethering, triggering* and *strong adhesion*[3,4]. These steps are sequential, but overlapping.

Tethering

Tethering is the first crucial step in halting the progress of neutrophils as they flow along the venule. Under normal shear stresses associated with blood flow, the cells tend to move at the edges of the vessel lumen, making contact with the endothelial cells. Tethering of the cells is brought about by at least three cell surface receptors, called *selectins*. The selectin family of adhesion molecules bind to sialylated carbohydrate groups on their *counter receptors* and are therefore lectin-like receptors. Neutrophils express L-selectin constitutively and the counter receptor is expressed on endothelial cells. Endothelial cells themselves express two selectins, E-selectin and P-selectin. The molecules of P-selectin are stored within the Weibel-Palade bodies in endothelial cells and translocate rapidly to the plasma membrane under the influence of inflammatory mediators, including histamine. In contrast, E-selectin is not prestored, but is synthesised rapidly by endothelial cells and transported to the plasma membrane in response to inflammatory cytokines including interleukin-1 (IL-1), interleukin-8 (IL-8) and tumour necrosis factor α (TNFα).

The importance of the selectin mediated tethering step in neutrophil adherence is demonstrated by leucocyte adhesion deficiency-II (LAD-II), which is characterised by a failure to express sialyl Lewis X, the counter receptor for E-selectin and P-selectin. The consequence of LAD-II is a failure of neutrophil migration to inflammatory foci[5,6], resulting in recurrent bacterial infections.

Thus weak selectin mediated attachment of neutrophils to endothelium will occur selectively at sites where inflammatory mediators are being expressed. The interactions of the selectins with their counter receptors are not strong, and the bonds are broken easily under the influence of shear stress forces. The result is that these initial adhesion events are transitory, causing rolling of the cells along the endothelial surface. Permanent, strong, adhesion requires the second step, *triggering*.

Triggering and Strong Adhesion

Tethering of neutrophils will have the effect of bringing the cells into close, relatively prolonged, contact with endothelial cells at regions of inflammation, and consequently into contact also with factors that trigger or activate the neutrophil receptors — *integrins*, responsible for strong adhesion. The integrins are a family of transmembrane glycoproteins. They are heterodimeric proteins, each consisting of one α subunit and one β subunit, which are bound non-covalently. Subfamilies of integrins share common β subunits and different subfamily members have distinct α subunits. Thus the most important neutrophil integrin, macrophage-1 (Mac-1), is a member of the leucocyte cellular adhesion molecule (LeuCAM) subfamily, or β_2 integrins, which have β_2 subunits (CD18). The α subunit of Mac-1 is $\alpha 1$ (CD11b). Thus Mac-1 is designated under the "cluster of differentiation" (CD) nomenclature as CD18/CD11b (it is also known as CR3 or Mo1). Another β_2 integrin, lymphocyte function associated antigen-1 (LFA-1) (CD18/CD11a), is expressed by neutrophils, but is probably less important than Mac-1 for strong binding.

The importance of the β_2 integrins in the process of neutrophil recruitment is illustrated by the inherited condition, LAD-I. Patients with LAD-I suffer from recurrent infections; although the neutrophils demonstrate normal effector functions, they are unable to migrate to infected tissues. This condition has been shown to be due to reduced or absent expression of the β_2 integrins[7]. The counter receptors on endothelial cells for the β_2 integrins are the intercellular adhesion molecules, or ICAMs. Mac-1 binds to ICAM-1 (CD54) and LFA-1 binds to ICAM-1, ICAM-2 and ICAM-3[4]; the domains on ICAM-1 bound by LFA-1 and Mac-1 are different. One amino acid sequence known to be recognised by Mac-1 and LFA-1 is Arg-Gly-Asp, the RGD ligand, which is found on several proteins including C3bi. Mac-1 also has a (different) binding site for bacterial lipopolysaccharide[8].

Another family of integrins, the β_1 integrins, or VLA (very late activating antigens), is also represented on neutrophils, which express VLA-5 ($\beta_1\alpha_5$) and VLA-6 ($\beta_1\alpha_6$). VLA-5 binds to fibronectin and VLA-6 to laminin. Neutrophils have other receptors for connective tissue proteins; for instance they can bind to vitronectin by a mechanism referred to as the urokinase dependent system.

The expression of integrins and ICAMs is modulated by a variety of proinflammatory factors; it is this feature which underlies the "triggering" phase necessary for strong adhesion.

Integrin adhesiveness is increased on neutrophils by many factors, including host cell derived cytokines such as IL-8 and also by compounds derived from micro-organisms, such as *N*-formyl-methionyl-leucyl-phenylalanine (fMLP) and other formylated peptides. The increased adhesive properties of integrins on triggered neutrophils are not the result of the presence of a larger number of integrin molecules on the cell surface. Triggering results in conformational changes in a proportion of the integrin molecules, which induces a greater affinity for the counter receptors. Similarly, endothelial cells are subject to activation by proinflammatory agents. Whereas ICAM-2 appears to be expressed constitutively by endothelial cells and synthesis is believed not to be regulated, ICAM-1 expression can be increased. This induction of ICAM-1 expression appears to be influenced differently in various tissues. Endothelial expression of ICAM-1 is increased by cytokines such as IL-1 and TNFα and by bacterial lipopolysaccharide. Thus strong adhesion of neutrophils to endothelial cells, through integrin–ICAM interactions and associated changes in neutrophil shape (flattening and spreading), is regulated by proinflammatory factors, presumably ensuring that this process is confined to areas of tissue where the cells are required. This regulation clearly must be reversible if the cells are to be able to enter the next stage, *transendothelial migration*.

NEUTROPHIL MIGRATION

Neutrophils have been shown to migrate in response to a large number of chemotactic factors. Chemotaxis is defined as directional movement along a concentration gradient of a chemotactic factor. Typically, *in vitro* systems demonstrate neutrophil migration in response to concentrations of a soluble chemotactic factor, such as fMLP, over several orders of magnitude (Fig. 7.3), with a maximum motility at the optimum concentration but decreased movement at lower or higher concentrations. It should be noted that blood neutrophils are not homogeneous with respect to their chemotactic responses. There appear to be two subpopulations, one responsive, the other not[10]. Chemotaxis in responsive cells is extremely sensitive: neutrophils can "detect" a concentration gradient of fMLP that changes only by 1–2% of the cell's length[11]. The nature of the neutrophil response to a chemotactic gradient may be important *in vivo*. The chemotactic signal will be greatest at the source of the factor's release and decrease with distance. The exquisite sensitivity of the cell to a changing concentration gradient will ensure movement in the direction of the signal, but the rate of movement will decrease after the optimum concentration is encountered. Thus neutrophils will accumulate at or near the appropriate site. Also, neutrophils adapt to uniform concentrations of a chemotactic factor, such that movement eventually diminishes. The cell will then continue moving only if the concentration changes, or in response to a different chemotactic signal. Interestingly, adhesion molecule expression has

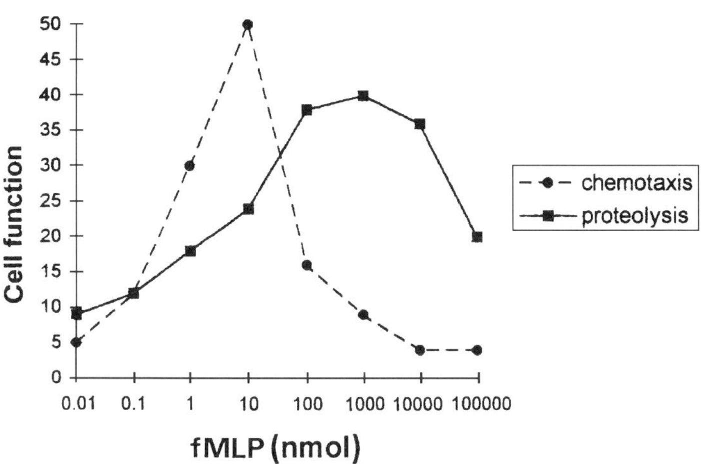

Figure 7.3. Neutrophils can be activated with formylated peptides, such as *N*-formyl-methionyl-leucyl-phenylalanine (fMLP) (see text). The response is proportional to increasing concentrations of fMLP until an optimal concentration is reached, when the response declines. The optimal concentration may be different for various functions. This graph shows that, in an assay for neutrophil chemotaxis in response to fMLP, a maximum effect is seen at a concentration of about 10 nmol. The ability to hydrolyse a protein substrate (extracellular proteolysis of fibronectin[9]) reaches a maximum response at a greater concentration of fMLP

been shown to be downregulated on neutrophils that have migrated in response to a chemotactic signal *in vitro*[12]. This altered expression might represent the breaking of cell adhesion in order for migration to occur.

The response of neutrophils to chemotactic factors is effected through specific receptors on the plasma membrane, typically pertussis toxin-sensitive G protein coupled receptors with seven transmembrane domains. When the cell adheres, it also polarises and the surface receptors, such as LFA-1 and those for immunoglobulin Fc, fMLP and cytokines are expressed on the adherent surface and tend to predominate on the "front" edge of the moving cells[13]. This redistribution of receptors is often associated with changes in receptor affinity for ligand, as demonstrated by LFA-1 during cell triggering.

The processes involved in neutrophil recruitment to infected tissues are complex. They involve a sequence of events that must take place in the correct order and will result from a multitude of signals. The paradigm for neutrophil recruitment is relevant to other cells, such as lymphocytes (see Chapter 6). Although some of the elements responsible for leucocyte recruitment are recognised by a variety of cells, many are selective for a particular set or subset of leucocyte. Thus the adhesion molecules involved in neutrophil attachment to endothelium are different from those responsible for lymphocyte adhesion. Similarly, the factors responsible for triggering and migration of various cells differ. For instance, fMLP and leukotriene B_4 (LTB_4) affect a variety of cell types including neutrophils and lymphocytes. Neutrophils, however, respond particularly to some factors, such as IL-8, which have little effect on lymphocytes. IL-8 is one of a number of related cytokines designated *chemokines*, which are relatively small polypeptides and divided into three subfamilies; IL-8 and *groα*, which are both chemotactic for neutrophils, belong to the α subfamily. A multitude of compounds have now been shown to be chemotactic/activating factors for neutrophils. Some agonists may prime the neutrophil — that is, render the cell susceptible to activation by another factor. Characteristically, activating factors are produced at sites of infection and inflammatory damage. Several of the neutrophil chemotactic factors, notably LTB_4 and the cytokines including TNFα and IL-8, are produced by inflammatory cells and activated endothelium. Others are protein and peptide components of damaged extracellular matrix, such as collagen[14] and laminin[15]. The activation of complement results in the release of chemotactic peptides such as $C5a$[16], and antigen–antibody complexes are also chemotactic for neutrophils[17]. Infecting micro-organisms themselves produce factors including the formyl peptides such as fMLP. Another component of Gram negative bacteria, lipopolysaccharide (LPS) or endotoxin, can prime neutrophil functions, including the respiratory burst, adhesion, phagocytosis and chemotactic responses. Neutrophils express the LPS binding receptor, CD14, but the cells respond to lower concentrations of LPS bound to a serum LPS binding protein.

NEUTROPHIL EFFECTOR FUNCTIONS

Many chemotactic factors have wider effects on neutrophils. Not only do they induce and direct cell movement, but often they also activate cell effector functions responsible for killing and elimination of micro-organisms. Frequently, however, a concentration inducing maximum chemotaxis may be different from that resulting in maximum activation of other functions; for fMLP this difference is two orders of magnitude. This suggests a mechanism allowing the attraction of neutrophils without the activation of potentially tissue damaging functions until the cells are at the infected site.

Activated neutrophils eliminate micro-organisms by means of a range of mechanisms, which generally fall into three categories: phagocytosis, the respiratory burst, and cytotoxic peptides and proteins.

PHAGOCYTOSIS

The recognition and phagocytosis of bacteria by neutrophils is a necessary prelude to intracellular killing, which is undoubtedly the primary defensive expression of these cells. Bacteria which are opsonised by immunoglobulin, complement, or both are particularly "attractive" to neutrophils. The recognition of opsonised bacteria is mediated through immunoglobulin receptors and binding of C3 by Mac-1. The role of immunoglobulin A (IgA) in opsonisation has been the subject of controversy but IgA, for which neutrophils possess Fc receptors, can opsonise bacteria for neutrophil phagocytosis[18]. This property may be particularly important at mucosal sites such as the major bronchi in the lungs, where IgA represents the major class of immunoglobulin. Neutrophils, however, can also recognise unopsonised bacteria and other particles, and have been shown to phagocytose bacteria in response to "recognition" of protein and carbohydrate components of bacteria, although little is known about this mechanism. Many intracellular pathogens, such as *Echovirus*, adenoviruses, *Yersinia* and *Leishmania*, express surface receptors for integrins and these are important for intracellular invasion[19]. It is likely that the recognition of many micro-organisms by neutrophils is also mediated by adhesion molecules, including integrins[20]. The process of phagocytosis traps the bacteria within the phagocyte, but micro-organisms which have been phagocytosed and encapsulated within phagolysosomes must be killed and degraded. Killing is achieved by a combination of the respiratory burst and the action of cytotoxic proteins which are stored in the cytoplasm and granules.

THE RESPIRATORY BURST

The products of the respiratory burst (see below) are oxidative products, originating from the membrane bound NADPH oxidase system. The importance of this process which, as the name suggests, requires oxygen and glucose, is illustrated by chronic granulomatous disease: affected individuals are susceptible to bacterial infections because their phagocytic cells are unable to generate the products of the respiratory burst[21]. Some of the steps in the generation and removal of oxidative molecules resulting from the "respiratory burst" are as follows:

1. Superoxide radical can be produced via the hexose monophosphate shunt or NADPH oxidase shunt:

$$2NADPH + 2O_2 \longrightarrow 2NADP + 2H^+ + 2O_2^-$$

2. Superoxide is converted to hydrogen peroxide by spontaneous dismutation or with catalysis by superoxide dismutase:

$$O_2^- + O_2^- + 2H^+ \longrightarrow O_2 + H_2O_2$$

3. Hydrogen peroxide is
   a) catalytically broken down by catalase:

$$H_2O_2 \longrightarrow H_2O + O_2$$

   b) catalytically broken down by glutathione peroxidase in the presence of reduced glutathione (Gl–SH) to produce oxidised glutathione (Gl) and water:

$$H_2O_2 + 2Gl\text{-}SH \longrightarrow 2Gl + 2H_2O$$

   c) converted, in the presence of superoxide radical and free iron or copper ions, to hydroxyl radical by the Haber–Weiss reaction:

$$H_2O_2 + O_2^- \longrightarrow OH + OH^- + O_2$$

   d) converted, in the presence of Fe^{++} or Cu^{++}, to hydroxyl radical by the Fenton reaction:

$$H_2O_2 + Fe^{2+} \longrightarrow Fe^{3+} + OH + OH^-$$

The production of superoxides begins with the reduction of oxygen by NADPH oxidase to form superoxide radical ($O_2{}^-$). Superoxide radicals can react spontaneously (dismute) to produce molecular oxygen and hydrogen peroxide, but this reaction is catalysed by superoxide dismutase. The reduction of hydrogen peroxide to water or to hypochlorous acid in the presence of chloride, is catalysed by the enzyme myeloperoxidase, a constituent of azurophil granules.

Another potential toxic byproduct of the respiratory burst is hydroxyl radical, produced by the Haber-Weiss and Fenton reactions, from superoxide radical or hydrogen peroxide in the presence of free iron. As these reactive species are extremely toxic to host cells and to micro-organisms, it is significant that they are short lived or catabolised rapidly. Thus superoxide anion dismutes spontaneously or under the influence of superoxide dismutase. Peroxides are removed by myeloperoxidase or catalase. Furthermore, such highly oxidative species will be effectively chelated by "bystander" molecules such as free amino acids. Clearly, however, the components of healthy tissues would also be susceptible to damage if these oxidants were available. Indeed, tissue damage caused by oxidants derived from inflammatory cells such as neutrophils has been proposed as an important factor in the pathogenesis of several pulmonary diseases.

NEUTROPHIL GRANULES

Neutrophils contain at least two, and possibly four, distinct granule populations. The primary granules (also known as azurophil or peroxidase positive granules) are non-secretory — that is, their contents are not released in appreciable amounts from living neutrophils, even when the cells are "activated". The primary granules are those which fuse with phagocytosed bacteria (in phagosomes) to form the phagolysosome. They contain the major proportion of bactericidal proteins and enzymes, including myeloperoxidase (hence the name peroxidase positive granule). A second major type of granule is the secondary (specific or peroxidase negative) granule, the contents of which are released from the cell upon activation.

Two other granule populations have now been identified: gelatinase granules and secretory vesicles. It has been proposed that, not only are the matrix components of these granules released from activated neutrophils, but in addition the membranes of these granules contain components, including receptors, which are rapidly incorporated into the plasma membrane of the cell as required[22]. Although most of the bactericidal components of the neutrophil are found in the granules, especially the primary granules, the cell cytoplasm does also contain calprotectin, originally known as L1 protein. Calprotectin is a calcium binding protein with an M_r of 36 kDa and comprises two polypeptide chains: the heavy chain, $L1_H$ and the light chain, $L1_L$, the latter being identical in sequence to a protein termed the cystic fibrosis antigen[23]. Calprotectin is present in the neutrophil cytosol and has been demonstrated to have antibacterial and antinematodal properties[23].

In addition to the cytotoxic effects of the respiratory burst, there is an array of molecular components in the granules that have the ability to kill and degrade micro-organisms. Carbohydrate components of bacteria are attacked by enzymes such as sialidase, α-mannosidase, β-glucuronidase, N-acetyl-β-glucosaminidase and lysozyme, which hydrolyse carbohydrate bonds in bacterial walls. Other peptides and proteins, which may conveniently be called "cytotoxic proteins", have the ability to damage the integrity of bacterial membranes by mechanisms which are poorly understood at the molecular level, but are believed to result in the production of lytic pores.

CYTOTOXIC PROTEINS

Defensins

The defensins, located in azurophil granules, are a family of four cyclic, single chain peptides with molecular weights of about 4000. All are similar in amino acid sequence and structure, each having three intrachain disulphide bonds. Three of them, human neutrophil peptides (HNP) 1–3, differ only in their final N-terminal amino acids[24]; HNP-4 has less homology. Defensins are toxic to fungi and enveloped viruses in addition to bacteria.

Azurocidin and CAP 57

Two other cytotoxic azurophil proteins are CAP 57[25] and azurocidin, also known as CAP 37. Although having no proteolytic activity, azurocidin shares considerable structural homology with the proteinases elastase, cathepsin G, proteinase 3 and granzymes (see below).

PROTEINASES

Proteinases are found within the primary (azurophil) and specific granules, but with the interesting distinction that, whereas the specific granules contain two metalloproteinases, the primary granules contain serine proteinases.

Serine proteinases

There are at least three identified serine proteinases in neutrophil primary granules: elastase, cathepsin G and proteinase 3 (also known as Wegeners autoantigen, P29 or APG7). They, together with azurocidin (not a proteinase), the lymphocyte granzymes and mast cell chymase, comprise a superfamily of proteins that share considerable amino acid homology, especially in their N-terminal regions (Table 7.1).

The neutrophil serine proteinases are all synthesised at the promyelocytic stage of cell development, in the bone marrow. They are translated as pre-pro-proteins.

Table 7.1. The pro-protein N-terminal sequences of proteins of the neutrophil azurophil granules. Removal of the pro-dipeptide results in the mature proteins which, in the case of elastase, proteinase 3 and cathepsin G, are active proteinases. Note the homology in sequences of all four proteins

Protein	Propeptide		N-terminus of mature protein																
Elastase	S	E	I	V	G	G	R	R	A	R	P	H	A	W	P	F	M	V	S	L
Proteinase 3	A	E	I	V	G	G	H	E	A	Q	P	H	S	R	P	Y	M	A	S	L
Azurocidin	?	?	I	V	G	G	R	K	A	R	P	H	Q	F	P	F	L	A	S	I
Cathepsin G	G	E	I	I	G	G	R	E	S	R	P	H	S	R	P	Y	M	A	Y	L

The removal of a signal peptide at the N-terminus results in a pro-protein, which is converted to the active enzyme by cleavage of a terminal dipeptide (Table 7.1). The homology of the superfamily members in this region suggests that a single dipeptidylpeptidase is responsible for this process; this is believed to be dipeptidylpeptidase II (cathepsin C). The enzymes are transported to and stored in the primary granules in this potentially active form and, as a result of their highly basic charge, are bound to the sulphated glycosaminoglycans of the granule matrix, but they have proteolytic activity at neutral pH, while that in the primary granule is acidic. The appropriate conditions for proteolytic activity occur after fusion of the granules with phagolysosomes, when the pH increases for a short time[26]. The importance of these proteinases in the bactericidal activity of neutrophils is demonstrated by the Chediak-Higashi syndrome. This autosomal recessive condition is associated with abnormal granules in a number of cell types and affected individuals suffer from recurrent infections. The neutrophil phagocytic activity and respiratory burst are normal, but bacterial killing is not. The blood neutrophils contain no elastase, cathepsin G or proteinase 3, although other primary granule proteins are present. Evidence to date suggests that, although the proteins of the elastase/cathepsin G superfamily are synthesised in the marrow promyelocytes of patients with Chediak-Higashi disease, the granules cannot package the proteins; they are therefore absent from mature neutrophils[27].

Elastase is so called because of its ability to hydrolyse elastin, a component of connective tissue that is resistant to hydrolysis by many other proteinases. Nevertheless, elastin can also hydrolyse a wide range of other proteins and peptides, and probably has a major role in degrading the protein components of microorganisms. Neutrophils contain about 1 pg of elastase per cell and the molar concentration in each granule is extremely high.

Cathepsin G has a "chymotrypsin-like" proteolytic activity and will contribute to the hydrolysis of the proteins of micro-organisms. In addition, however, cathepsin G contains two peptide domains, IIGGR and HPQYNQR, which are antimicrobial. This activity is not related to the proteolytic activity of the enzyme. Elastase contains no such identified sequence, but appears to be able to co-operate with cathepsin G in this non-proteolytic killing in a way which is not understood.

Proteinase 3 has a "preference" for target peptides and proteins (including elastin) similar to that of elastase, but a pH optimum of about 6.5, in contrast to that of elastase, which is between 8 and 9.

Metalloproteinases

Neutrophils contain two identified metalloproteinases: a "collagenase" and gelatinase. Both enzymes are stored as zymogens or pro-enzymes, and enzyme activity is expressed after activation; this might be mediated by other proteases, but they have been shown also to be activated *in vitro* by oxidants including hypochlorous acid[28]; these proteinases would therefore be rendered proteolytic during neutrophil activation. Both pro-collagenase and pro-gelatinase are stored in the matrix of specific granules, and pro-gelatinase is also located in the matrix of gelatinase granules. It is likely, therefore, that these enzymes are released from neutrophils during cell activation.

DO NEUTROPHIL PRODUCTS KILL EXTRACELLULAR MICRO-ORGANISMS?

Neutrophils are not strictly secretory cells, as are mast cells, for example. The latter degranulate readily upon activation, releasing proteinases and other cytotoxic products believed to be important in the killing of parasites. The neutrophil appears to be a cell designed primarily for the phagocytosis and intracellular disposal of bacteria. Nevertheless, the release of the contents of secondary and gelatinase granules and secretory vesicles would result in some cytotoxic elements and metalloproteinases being present outside the cell, where they could contribute to microbial killing. In contrast, even potent neutrophil activating agents such as phorbol esters, bacterial components (LPS and formyl peptides) and cytokines do not result in the release of significant amounts of azurophil contents from the cell *in vitro*, although there is some release at the site of contact between cell and substrate[9] and perhaps, therefore, also where the neutrophil is in contact with a micro-organism during phagocytosis. Azurophil granule contents including elastase are, nevertheless, present in lung secretions during episodes of acute and chronic infection associated with the presence of large numbers of neutrophils. Indeed, the green colour of purulent sputum is attributable to the large amounts of neutrophil myeloperoxidase, which is a green protein. Much of this material is present inside the neutrophils, but a considerable amount can be detected in solution after removal of cells by centrifugation[29]. These products are probably released from cells which have died; the contribution they make to microbial killing at infected sites is not known, although this may be potentially important.

Neutrophils are undoubtedly efficient antimicrobial cells. They possess many mechanisms and molecules which, together, can remove and destroy pathogens. The wide range of mechanisms suggests considerable redundancy in the system. Nevertheless, the results of deficiencies of individual components, such as those seen in chronic granulomatous disease, Chediak-Higashi syndrome and the adhesion molecule deficiencies, demonstrate how important each of these must be in the efficient functioning of these inflammatory cells.

REFERENCES

1. Bainton D F, Ullyot J L, Farquhar M G. The development of neutrophilic polymorphonuclear leucocytes in human bone marrow: origin and content of azurophil and specific granules. *J Exp Med* 1971; **134:** 907–934.

2. Athens J W, Haab O P, Raab S O, *et al.* Leukokinetic studies.XI. Blood granulocyte kinetics in polycythemia vera, infection and myelofibrosis. *J Clin Invest* 1965; **44:** 778–788.

3. Adams D H, Shaw S. Leucocyte–endothelial interactions and regulation of leucocyte migration. *Lancet* 1994; **343:** 831–836.

4. Springer T A. Traffic signals for lymphocyte recirculation and leukocyte emigration: the multistep paradigm. *Cell* 1994; **76:** 301–314.

5. Etzioni A, Frydman M, Pollack S, *et al.* Brief report: recurrent severe infections caused by a novel leukocyte adhesion deficiency. *N Engl J Med* 1992; **327:** 1789–1792.

6. von Andrian U H, Berger E M, Ramezani L, *et al. In vivo* behaviour of neutrophils from two patients with distinct inherited leukocyte adhesion deficiency syndromes. *J Clin Invest* 1993; **91:** 2893–2897.

7. Anderson D C, Springer T A. Leukocyte adhesion deficiency: an inherited defect in the Mac-1, LFA-1, and p150,95 glycoproteins. *Annu Rev Med* 1987; **38:** 175–194.

8. Wright S D, Levin S M, Jong M T C, *et al.* CR3 (CD11b/CD18) expresses one binding site for Arg-Gly-Asp-containing peptides and a second site for bacterial lipopolysaccharide. *J Exp Med* 1989; **169**: 175–183.

9. Chamba A, Afford S C, Stockley R A, *et al.* Extracellular proteolysis of fibronectin by neutrophils: characterization and the effects of recombinant cytokines. *Am J Respir Cell Mol Biol* 1991; **4**: 330–337.

10. Harvath L, Leonard E J. Two neutrophil populations in human blood with different chemotactic activities: separation and chemoattractant binding. *Infect Immun* 1982; **36**: 443–449.

11. Zigmond S H. Chemotactic response of neutrophils. *Am J Respir Cell Mol Biol* 1989; **1**: 451–453.

12. Harvath L, Brownson N E, Terle D A. Downregulation of human neutrophil adhesion molecule surface expression after chemotaxis. In: Schlossman S F, Boumsell L, Gilks W, *et al.*, eds. *Leukocyte Typing V: White Cell Differentiation Antigens*. Proceedings of the fifth International Workshop and Conference, 1993, Boston. Oxford: Oxford University Press, 1995; 1602–1604.

13. Shield J M, Haston W S. Behaviour of neutrophil leucocytes in uniform concentrations of chemotactic factors: contraction waves, cell polarity and persistence. *J Cell Sci* 1985; **74**: 75–93.

14. Senior R M, Hinek A, Griffin G L, *et al.* Neutrophils show chemotaxis to type IV collagen and its 7S domain and contain a 67kD type IV collagen-binding protein with pectin properties. *Am J Respir Cell Mol Biol* 1989; **1**: 479–487.

15. Bryant G, Rao C N, Brentani M, *et al.* A role for the laminin receptor in leukocyte chemotaxis. *J Leucoc Biol* 1987; **41**: 220–227.

16. Toews G B, Vial W C. The role of C5 in polymorphonuclear leukocyte recruitment in response to *Streptococcus pneumoniae*. *Am Rev Respir Dis* 1984; **129**: 82–86.

17. Boyden S. The chemotactic effect of antibody and antigen on polymorphonuclear leukocytes. *J Exp Med* 1962; **115**: 453–466.

18. Burnett D, Chamba A, Stockley R A, *et al.* The effects of recombinant GMCSF and IgA opsonization on neutrophil phagocytosis of latex beads coated with P6 outer membrane protein from *Haemophilus influenzae*. *Thorax* 1993; **48**: 638–642.

19. Isberg R R, Van Nhieu G T. Binding and internalization of microorganisms by integrin receptors. *Trends Microbiol* 1994; **2**: 10–14.

20. Hogg N. The leukocyte integrins. *Immunol Today* 1989; **10**: 111–114.

21. Curnette J T, Whitten D M, Babior B M. Defective superoxide production by granulocytes from patients with chronic granulomatous disease. *N Engl J Med* 1974; **290**: 593–597.

22. Borregaard N, Kjeldsen L, Lollike K, *et al.* Granules and vesicles of human neutrophils. The role of endomembranes as source of plasma membrane proteins. *Eur J Haematol* 1993; **51**: 318–322.

23. Fagerhol M K. Nomenclature for proteins: is calprotectin a proper name for the elusive myelomonocytic protein?. *J Clin Pathol Clin Mol Pathol* 1996; **49**: M74–M79.

24. Selsted M E, Harwig S S L, Granz T, *et al.* Primary structure of three human neutrophil defensins. *J Clin Invest* 1985; **76**: 1436–1439.

25. Pereira H A, Spitznaegel J K, Winton E F, *et al.* The ontogeny of a 57-kD cationic antimicrobial protein of human polymorphonuclear leukocytes: localization to a novel granule population. *Blood* 1990; **76**: 825–834.

26. Segal A W, Geisow M, Garcia R, *et al.* The respiratory burst of phagocytic cells is associated with a rise in vacuolar pH. *Nature* 1981; **290**: 406–409.

27. Burnett D, Ward C J, Stockley R A, *et al.* Neutrophil elastase and cathepsin G protein and messenger RNA expression in bone marrow from a patient with Chediak-Higashi syndrome. *J Clin Pathol Mol Pathol* 1995; **48**: M28–M34.

28. Peppin G J, Weiss S J. Activation of the endogenous metalloproteinase, gelatinase, by triggered human neutrophils. *Proc Natl Acad Sci USA* 1986; **83**: 4322–4326.

29. Buttle D J, Burnett D, Abrahamson M. Levels of neutrophil elastase and cathepsin B activities, and cystatins in human sputum: relationship to inflammation. *Scand J Clin Lab Invest* 1990; **50**: 509–516.

8

Eosinophils

G. M. WALSH AND A. J. WARDLAW

Leicester University Medical School, Leicester, UK

INTRODUCTION

The eosinophil is one of the most striking of cells, readily identified in haematoxylin and eosin stained sections by the bilobed nuclei and bright red granules, and it is closely associated with two of the most common and universal of diseases, namely asthma and parasitic infection. The characteristic appearance of the eosinophil resulted in its early identification by Ehrlich in 1879, and its association with asthma and allergic disease was soon recognised[1]. Curiosity about the role of the eosinophil in asthma and other diseases has persisted ever since. In recent years, there has been an explosion of interest in these cells, reflected in an exponential increase in the number of published papers and books devoted to the subject[2-5]. This interest has been mainly the result of increasing evidence that the eosinophil may be responsible for much of the tissue damage seen in asthma, and the hope that modulation of eosinophil function may be an effective therapy for the disease.

MORPHOLOGY AND ULTRASTRUCTURE

Eosinophils are non-dividing granulated cells with a diameter of approximately 8 μm (Fig. 8.1). The membrane bound specific granules, of which there are about 20 per human eosinophil, are one of their most characteristic features. They are spherical or ovoid and contain a crystalline core surrounded by a less electron dense matrix. The core is comprised of major basic protein (MBP) and the matrix contains the other three basic granule proteins: eosinophil cationic protein (ECP), eosinophil peroxidase (EPO) and eosinophil derived neurotoxin (EDN or EPX). These basic proteins stain avidly with analine dyes such as the eosin from which the cell gained its name. Eosinophils also contain lipid bodies, which are non-membrane-bound organelles and the principal store of arachidonic acid esterified

Pulmonary Defences. Edited by Robert A. Stockley.
© 1997 John Wiley & Sons Ltd.

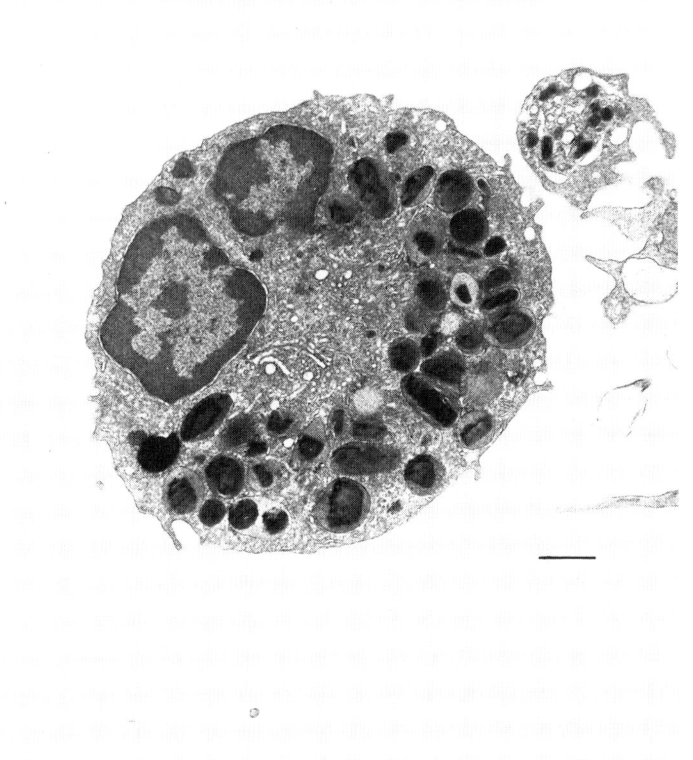

Figure 8.1. Transmission electron micrograph of an eosinophil showing the characteristic specific granules with their electron dense core. Horizontal bar represents 1 µm. (Courtesy of Dr A Dewar, National Heart and Lung Institute)

into glycerophospholipids. Eosinophil primary granules are a third type of intracellular organelle and contain Charcot-Leyden crystal protein (CLC protein). CLC protein is also found diffusely in the nucleus and cytoplasm in activated eosinophils. Primary granules make up approximately 5% of eosinophil granules, are recognised by the absence of a core and are of variable size, being often larger than the specific granules. Basic proteins derived from the specific granules are believed to be important in immunity to parasites and also contribute to the tissue damage associated with allergic inflammation[6].

EOSINOPHIL PRODUCTION

In common with all leucocytes, eosinophils differentiate from stem cell precursors in the bone marrow. They then migrate into the peripheral blood where they circulate with a half life of about 18 h before migrating into tissue. Normal human adult bone marrow contains about 3% eosinophils, of which one third are mature and two thirds are myelocytic precursors. Eosinophilic myelocytes are large cells with a single lobed nucleus, expanded Golgi and extensive dilated cisterns of rough endoplasmic reticulum. They become identifiable when they develop the core containing specific granules which, initially, are interspersed with large numbers of homogenous dense granules.

There is now substantial evidence that the eosinophilia associated with helminthic parasitic infection is T cell dependent[7]. Three T cell derived cytokines have been shown to promote eosinophil growth and differentiation: interleukins 3 and 5 (IL-3, IL-5) and granulocyte macrophage colony stimulating factor (GM-CSF). IL-5 is a disulphide-linked homodimeric glycoprotein with a molecular mass of 40–45 kDa. Culture of mouse bone marrow suggested that IL-5 was a late differentiation factor and could not support eosinophil growth from early precursors. These earlier steps appeared to require other cytokines such as IL-3 and GM-CSF. However, IL-5 transgenic mice have a marked peripheral blood and tissue eosinophilia, with increased numbers of eosinophil precursors in their bone marrow. Despite their marked eosinophilia, these mice have no obvious pathological defect and are essentially healthy. The observation that IL-5 alone was sufficient to generate an eosinophilia is consistent with the fact that increases in numbers of eosinophils are often seen without expansion of the other myeloid lineages[8]. Although IL-5 has been detected in mast cells and eosinophils[9], it is likely that T lymphocytes are the principal source of this cytokine.

In addition to division into subsets on the basis of their receptor phenotype, T cells can also be distinguished by their cytokine profile. Thus Th1 cells produce IL-2 and interferon gamma (IFNγ) and Th2 cells produce IL-4 and IL-5, whereas GM-CSF and IL-3 are products of both cell types[10]. T cells with a Th2 profile of cytokine production are found in allergic and eosinophilic parasitic disease[11]. Eosinophilia in many diseases, therefore, appears to be caused by a specific type of T cell response to certain types of antigen — for example, allergens in allergic disease and parasitic antigens in helminthic infections — whereas drug induced eosinophilia may be due to the drug acting as a hapten for a Th2 response.

EOSINOPHIL ACCUMULATION

Eosinophils are primarily tissue dwelling cells, with about one blood eosinophil for every 100 tissue eosinophils[12]. A critical aspect of eosinophil function is migration from the vascular space into extracellular tissue. The initial step in this process is adherence to postcapillary venular endothelium, which is mediated by binding of adhesion receptors on the surface of leucocytes to their ligands or counterstructures on endothelium. Adhesion receptors are grouped into several gene superfamilies, and include the integrin superfamily, members of the immunoglobulin superfamily, and the selectins[13,14]. Integrins bind to members of the immunoglobulin receptor family and selectins bind, via their lectin domain, to carbohydrate counterstructures that include the moiety sialyl Lewis X. Transmigration through vascular endothelium is a staged process in which the leucocyte is first tethered to the endothelial cell by binding of a selectin receptor to its carbohydrate ligand. The binding affinity of this interaction is relatively weak and the leucocyte rolls along the surface of the endothelium until it comes into contact with a priming stimulus such as a chemotactic mediator. This allows the leucocyte integrin receptor to bind to its corresponding immunoglobulin-like ligand. The resultant bond is much firmer than the selectin carbohydrate bond, and results in the leucocyte flattening and transmigrating between endothelial cells. Three events are therefore required for migration to occur: engagement of a selectin and its receptor, leucocyte activation, and engagement of the integrin–immunoglobulin receptor bond. Having transmigrated through the endothelium, the leucocyte interacts with the extracellular matrix proteins via integrin and other adhesion receptors. Adhesion receptors and their ligands potentially involved in eosinophil function are summarised in Table 8.1.

One potential mechanism for preferential localisation of eosinophils (as opposed to neutrophils) at inflammatory foci might thus be a selective adhesion pathway. IL-5 and IL-3 increase eosinophil, but not neutrophil, adhesion to cultured unstimulated human umbilical vein endothelial cells (HUVECs)[15]. Eosinophils, but not neutrophils, can utilise the very late activating antigen-4/vascular cell adhesion molecule-1 (VLA-4/VCAM-1) pathway for adhesion to cytokine stimulated HUVECs[16]. VCAM-1 expression is selectively upregulated by IL-4[17] and IL-4 is generated at sites of allergic inflammation[18]. IL-4 transgenic mice have a tissue eosinophilia and manifest an inflammatory condition in the eye similar to allergic conjunctivitis[19]. Monoclonal antibody to VLA-4 inhibited eosinophil migration into tissue in guineapigs[20] and prevented antigen

Table 8.1. Eosinophil adhesion receptors and their counter structures

Eosinophil receptor	Endothelial receptor	Matrix protein
Integrin		
VLA-4 ($\alpha_4\beta_1$)	VCAM-1	Fibronectin
VLA-6 ($\alpha_6\beta_1$)		Laminin
α_4/β_7	MAdCAM-1/VCAM-1	Fibronectin
LFA-1	ICAM-1, ICAM-2	
Mac-1	ICAM-1	Fibrinogen
p150,95	Not known	
Immunoglobulin like		
PECAM	PECAM/$\alpha_v\beta_3$	Glycosaminoglycans
ICAM-3 (binds LFA-1)		
Selectins		
L-selectin	*GlyCAM-1, CD34, MAdCAM-1	
Carbohydrate		
PSGL-1	P-selectin/E-selectin	
ESL-1	E-selectin	
Others		
CD44		Hyaluronate

(1) VLA-4 = very late activating antigen 4; (2) VCAM-1 = vascular cell adhesion molecule 1; (3) MAdCAM-1 = mucosal addressin cell adhesion molecule 1; (4) LFA-1 = lymphocyte function associated receptor; (5) ICAM-1 = Intercellular adhesion molecule 1; (6) Mac-1 = macrophage 1; (7) PECAM = platelet endothelial cell adhesion molecule; (8) GlyCAM-1 = glycosylated cell adhesion molecule 1 (*this receptor is secreted); (9) PSGL-1 = P-selectin glycoprotein ligand 1; (10) ESL-1 = E-selectin ligand 1.

induced bronchial hyperreactivity and cellular infiltration in the airways[21], and blocking of VLA-4 or VCAM-1 inhibited eosinophil infiltration into antigen challenged mouse trachea[22]. In contrast, VCAM-1 expression in eosinophilic tissue such as nasal biopsy specimens, nasal polyps, endobronchial biopsy specimens from asthmatic individuals and in the skin of allergic individuals after allergen challenge is very weak or non-existent, despite strong expression of other endothelial adhesion molecules[23,24]. As with neutrophils, eosinophils express L-selectin, which is shed following stimulation. Bronchoalveolar lavage (BAL) samples of eosinophils that have migrated into the airways express very little L-selectin[25]. Eosinophils and neutrophils both use L-selectin to bind to stimulated endothelial cells *in vitro* under conditions that simulate flow. However, a monoclonal antibody to L-selectin (leucocyte adhesion molecule, LAM1-11) blocked eosinophil, but not neutrophil, adhesion — suggesting differences in the functional epitopes on L-selectin expressed by the two cell types[26]. P-selectin has also been shown to have the dominant role in the binding of eosinophils to human nasal polyp endothelium[27] and may be involved in selective recruitment.

Once eosinophils have adhered to the endothelium, they migrate through the tight junctions between the endothelial cells and into the tissues. Thus selective

Table 8.2. Eosinophil chemoattractants and priming agents

Type	Effectiveness (unprimed)	Comments
Lipids		
PAF	High	Non-selective
LTB$_4$	Low	Non-selective
LTE$_4$	Not known	Activity reported *in vivo* only
18s,15s,diHETE	Moderate	Part of guineapig ECF-A
Small molecular wt peptides		
C5a	High	Non-selective
fMLP	Low	Non-selective
Growth factors		
IL-5	Low	Active only on cells from normal
IL-3	Low	subjects. Effective priming agents
GM-CSF	Low	
IL-2	Low	Probably mainly chemokinetic
LCF		
Chemokines		
C-C family (not active neutrophils)		
RANTES	High	Active *in vivo* and *in vitro*
MIP-1α	Low/moderate	Histamine releasers
MCP-3	Moderate	Histamine releasers
Eotaxin	High	Only characterised in guineapigs at present. Active *in vivo* and *in vitro*
C-X-C family		
IL-8	Low	Only active in primed cells

PAF = Platelet activating factor; LT(B$_4$etc) = leukotriene; HETE = hydroxy—eicosatetraenoic acid; ECF-A = eosinophil chemotactic factor of anaphylaxis; fMLP = *N*-formyl-methionyl-leucyl-phenylalanine; IL = interleukin; GM-CSF = granulocyte macrophage colony stimulating factor; LCF = lymphocyte chemoattractant factor; MIP = macrophage inflammatory protein; MCP = monocyte chemoattractant protein.

transendothelial migration may also provide an additional selective pathway for eosinophil, as opposed to neutrophil, accumulation. This can be measured in the laboratory by growing endothelial cells on cellulose filter supports. Using this approach, IL-4 was shown to enhance eosinophil transmigration through endothelium in a VLA-4/VCAM-1 dependent manner[28] and GM-CSF induced selective eosinophil transendothelial migration across unstimulated HUVECs[29]. The chemokine RANTES (rapid on activation normal T cell expressed and secreted; see below) has recently been shown selectively to induce eosinophil transendothelial migration without increasing the numbers of eosinophils adherent to HUVECs[30].

After eosinophils have left the vascular compartment, the next phase of their migration to sites of inflammation maybe under the control of locally produced chemoattractants. A number of eosinophil chemotaxins have been described (Table 8.2, p. 131), although few are both effective and specific. It has been reported that the C-C chemokine, RANTES, is an effective and selective (in the sense of having no activity for neutrophils) chemoattractant for eosinophils[31]. In a guineapig model of allergic inflammation, bronchial challenge of sensitised animals resulted in the generation of "eotaxin", a potent C-C chemoattractant for both human and guineapig eosinophils[32]. *In vivo*, platelet activating factor (PAF) injected into the skin caused the accumulation of eosinophils in atopic individuals, whereas neutrophils were predominant in non-atopic subjects[33]. Increased numbers of neutrophils, but not eosinophils, appeared in BAL fluid 4–6 h after the inhalation of PAF in a group of eight normal subjects, three of whom were atopic[34]. Finally, inhalation of leukotriene E_4 produced eosinophil migration into the airways[35]. The mechanism of these differential effects is not clear.

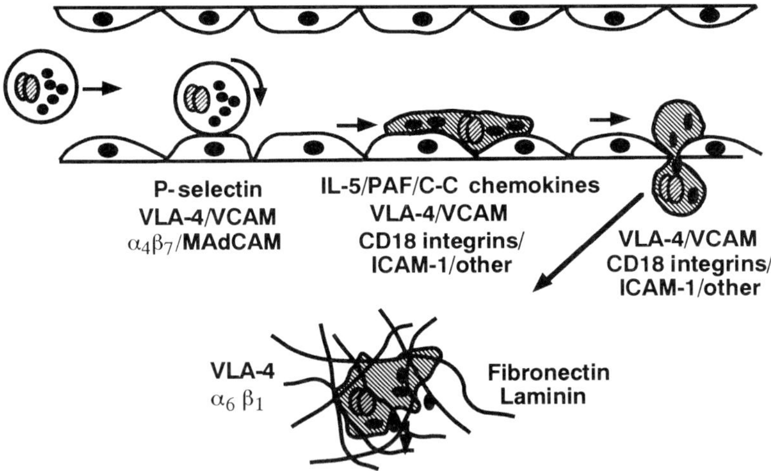

Figure 8.2. Schematic diagram illustrating the possible role of adhesion receptors and chemoattractants in mediating eosinophil migration into tissue and their subsequent interaction with the extracellular matrix. VLA = Very late activating antigen; VCAM = vascular cell adhesion molecule; MAdCAM = mucosal addressin cell adhesion molecule; IL = interleukin; PAF = platelet activating factor; ICAM = intercellular adhesion molecule

Eosinophils can interact with the proteins that make up the extracellular matrix between cells. For example, fibronectin binds to eosinophils through VLA-4, laminin through VLA-6[36] and hyaluronate through CD44. Adhesion to these matrix proteins results in priming for increased release of hydrogen peroxide, leukotriene C_4 (LTC4) and EPO[37-39]. Eosinophils also survive for prolonged periods when cultured on fibronectin, as a result of autocrine stimulation of IL-3 and GM-CSF production[40]. This represents a possible mechanism for prolonged survival of tissue eosinophils in both health and disease; their ultimate removal appears to be largely the result of programmed cell death (apoptosis) and subsequent phagocytosis of the senescent cell by macrophages[41]. Interestingly, transforming growth factor β (TGF β) abrogates the ability of IL-3 and GM-CSF to promote eosinophil viability in culture and induces apoptosis in these cells[42]. The adhesion receptors and chemoattractants potentially involved in eosinophil migration are summarised in Fig. 8.2.

OTHER EOSINOPHIL RECEPTORS

In addition to expressing receptors crucial for their accumulation in allergic inflammation, eosinophils also express receptors important for other functions, including mediator release (Table 8.3). There are three receptors for IgG: the high affinity receptor, $Fc_\gamma R1$ (cluster of differentiation (CD) 64), and two low affinity receptors, $Fc_\gamma RII$ (CD32) and $Fc_\gamma RIII$ (CD16). Only CD32 is constitutively expressed by eosinophils to any significant degree[43]. A number of eosinophil functions are mediated via this receptor, including schistosomula killing, phagocytosis, the secretion of granule proteins, and the generation of newly formed, membrane derived lipid mediators such as PAF and LTC_4. After stimulation for 2 days *in vitro* with IFNγ, eosinophils express CD16 and CD64, in addition to CD32[44]. The eosinophil also binds IgE and eosinophils can undertake a number of IgE dependent functions, including killing of schistosomes opsonised with specific IgE[45]. It was believed that the eosinophil IgE receptor was related to the low affinity IgE receptor found on B lymphocytes, platelets and macrophages $Fc_\varepsilon RII$ (CD23)[46]. However, peripheral blood eosinophils inconsistently express

Table 8.3. Functionally relevant eosinophil receptors other than adhesion molecules

---

Immunoglobulin receptors:
    $Fc_\alpha R$, $Fc_\varepsilon R^*$, $Fc_\gamma RII$ (CD32)

Mediator receptors:
    IL-5*, IL-3*, GM-CSF, RANTES*, Eotaxin*, C5a, PAF, fMLP, LTB_4

Cytokine induced receptors:
    IL-2 (CD25), $Fc_\gamma RIII$(CD16), CD4*, ICAM-1, HLA-DR, CD69

Other receptors
    CR1, CR3 (Mac-1), Mac-2, CD9*, CD45

---

*Not expressed on neutrophils.
RANTES = Rapid on activation normal T cell expressed and secreted chemokine.
Other abbreviations as in Tables 8.1 and 8.2.

messenger RNA (mRNA) for CD23 and do not stain with a panel of monoclonal antibodies directed against this receptor. Eosinophils express the IgE binding protein macrophage-2 (Mac-2), but so do neutrophils which lack IgE dependent functions[47]. More recently, eosinophils have been shown to express the high affinity IgE receptor, which is believed to be involved in host defence against parasites[48]. IgA receptors are also present on eosinophils and these have enhanced expression in allergic individuals. Moreover, eosinophil IgA receptors have a glycosylation pattern that differs from that seen for neutrophil IgA receptors[49]. Incubation of eosinophils with IgA-coated Sepharose beads will trigger substantial release of eosinophil granule proteins[50].

An interesting feature of the eosinophil is its ability to express receptors *de novo* after prolonged (>48 h) culture in a number of cytokines. For example, after culture in GM-CSF, eosinophils express HLA-DR antigens and increased amounts of intercellular adhesion molecule-1 (ICAM-1) which are associated with an *in vitro* capacity to present antigen to T cells[51]. Peripheral blood eosinophils express the early activation antigen CD69 after cytokine stimulation *in vitro*, as do BAL eosinophils from patients with asthma and pulmonary eosinophilia[52,53].

EOSINOPHIL SECRETION AND ACTIVATION

Eosinophils have the capacity to secrete a number of potent mediators (Fig. 8.3). These include basic proteins stored in eosinophil granules, lipid mediators newly formed after eosinophil activation, cytokines, various eosinophil proteases, and components of the oxygen burst, including superoxide and hydrogen peroxide (Fig. 8.3).

MBP has a molecular mass of 13.8 kDa with a pI of 10.9, and contains 17 arginine residues, accounting for its basic charge. It is initially synthesised as an acidic proprotein which may neutralise the toxicity of MBP as it is processed in the Golgi. The pro-portion is shed before MBP becomes stored in the granule[54]. Purified MBP was shown to be cytotoxic for the schistosomula of *Schistosoma mansoni*, and adherence of eosinophils to IgG-coated schistosomula resulted in the secretion of MBP onto the integument of the larvae[55]. MBP at concentrations as low as $10 \mu g \cdot ml^{-1}$ has also been shown to be toxic for both guineapig and human respiratory epithelial cells[56]. The inhalation of MBP, albeit at high concentrations ($1 mg \cdot ml^{-1}$), produced increased bronchial hyperresponsiveness in monkeys[57]. MBP and EPO were shown to be strong agonists for platelet activation, in addition to inducing the non-cytolytic activation of mast cells, basophils and neutrophils[58]. The mechanism of action of MBP is likely to be related to its hydrophobicity and strong negative charge.

EPO is a haem-containing protein composed of a 14 kDa (light) and a 58 kDa (heavy) subunit derived from the same strand of mRNA and subsequently cleaved. The cDNA also demonstrates the presence of a pro-sequence[59]. EPO shares a 68% amino acid identity with human neutrophil myeloperoxidase, in addition to other peroxidase enzymes. EPO is toxic for parasites, respiratory epithelium, and pneumocytes, either alone or (more potently) when combined with hydrogen peroxide (H_2O_2) and halide, especially bromide. However, it appears that thiocyanate, a

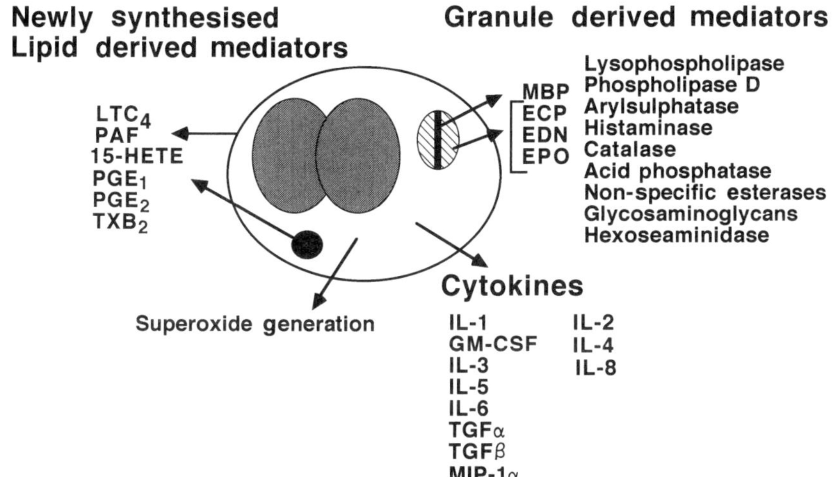

Figure 8.3. Schematic diagram illustrating the source of principal eosinophil derived mediators. LTC4 = Leukotriene C_4; PAF = platelet activating factor; HETE = hydroxy eicosatetraenoic acid; PGE_1, PGE_2 = prostaglandins E_1, E_2; TxB_2 = thromboxane B_2; MBP = major basic protein; ECP = eosinophil cationic protein; EDN = eosinophil derived neurotoxin; EPO = eosinophil peroxidase; IL = interleukin; GM-CSF = granulocyte macrophage colony stimulating factor; TGF = transforming growth factor; MIP = macrophage inflammatory protein

pseudohalide, at physiological concentrations is able to compete for EPO and inhibit the effects of bromide and iodide, even when the halide is present in marked excess[60]. The weak oxidant hypothiocyanous acid may therefore be the major product of EPO reactions *in vivo*. Thus the studies demonstrating the cytotoxic effects of EPO through the H_2O_2–halide system may need revision.

ECP is an arginine rich protein with a pI of 10.8, having 133 amino acids with a molecular mass of 15.6 kDa. ECP shows 66% amino acid homology with EDN and 31% homology with human pancreatic ribonuclease[61]. It has low ribonuclease activity compared with EDN. It appears to be expressed only in eosinophils or eosinophilic cell lines. ECP is toxic for helminthic parasites, isolated myocardial cells, and guineapig tracheal epithelium. ECP also inhibits lymphocyte proliferation *in vitro*. Both ECP and EDN produce neurotoxicity (the Gordon phenomenon) when injected into the cerebrospinal fluid of experimental animals. The secreted form of ECP differs structurally and antigenically from the stored form. This difference has been used to differentiate between resting eosinophils and activated eosinophils in which active secretion is occurring: the monoclonal antibody EG1 recognises the stored form and EG2 recognises the activated state[62].

EDN (also called EPX) is a 16 kDa, glycosylated protein possessing marked ribonuclease activity. In common with ECP, it is a member of a ribonuclease multigene family[63] and is probably secreted by the liver. EDN expression is not restricted to eosinophils, as it is found in mononuclear cells and, possibly, neutrophils. It does not appear to be toxic to parasites or mammalian cells, and its only known function, other than its ribonuclease activity, is the neurotoxicity exhibited in the Gordon phenomenon.

Eosinophils generate an array of lipid mediators—principally eicosanoids, PAF and mediators of the cyclo-oxygenase pathway, including prostaglandins (PG) E_1 and E_2 and thromboxane B_2 (TxB_2). Eosinophils can generate relatively large amounts (up to 70 ng per 10^6 cells) of the sulphidopeptide, LTC_4, after stimulation with the calcium ionophore, but only negligible amounts of LTB_4[64]. This is in contrast to neutrophils, which can produce large amounts of LTB_4, but little LTC_4. LTC_4 generation by human eosinophils is also observed both after stimulation with opsonised zymosan and via an $Fc_\gamma II$ dependent mechanism using Sepharose beads coated with IgG[65]. Eosinophils also generate PAF after stimulation with calcium ionophore or IgG-coated Sepharose beads[66].

Eosinophils can synthesise an array of cytokines. Activated eosinophils have been shown to secrete significant amounts of $TGF\alpha$[67]. After stimulation with calcium ionophore, eosinophils can also generate GM-CSF and IL-3, which prolong eosinophil survival[68,69]. Eosinophils in allergic tissue express mRNA for IL-5[70,71] and tumour necrosis factor α ($TNF\alpha$)[72], and eosinophils have been shown to generate significant quantities of $TGF\beta$, IL-6 and IL-8[73-75]. IL-1 has also been detected in human eosinophils.

The eosinophil contains a number of granule stored enzymes, for which the role in eosinophil function is not clear[2]. They include acid phosphatase (large amounts of which have been isolated from eosinophils), collagenase, arylsulphatase B, histaminase, phospholipase D, catalase, non-specific esterases, vitamin B12 binding proteins, and glycosaminoglycans.

Eosinophils can undergo a respiratory burst with release of superoxide ion and H_2O_2 in response to stimulation. Pretreatment of eosinophils with GM-CSF, IL-3 and IL-5 enhanced the respiratory burst induced by opsonised particles which was accompanied by induction of tyrosine kinase activity[76]. In addition, RANTES appears to be a specific activator of eosinophil oxidative metabolism[77].

A striking feature of eosinophil-rich inflammatory reactions is the marked deposition of granule proteins, often in the presence of relatively small numbers of intact eosinophils. The mechanism of eosinophil secretion *in vivo* is still poorly understood. Eosinophils are cytotoxic for the larvae of helminthic parasites such as schistosomula of *S. mansoni*, but only when the larvae have been opsonised with either complement or IgG. Thus triggering of eosinophil secretion might be dependent on perturbation of Fc_γ or complement receptors, particularly Mac-1. Eosinophils preferentially secrete their mediators onto a large surface—a process described as frustrated phagocytosis. Opsonised zymosan interacts with eosinophils, triggering generation of H_2O_2 and PAF through Mac-1[78]. The ability of eosinophils to secrete their mediators is markedly enhanced by priming with soluble mediators such as chemotactic factors and cytokines. Chemotactic agents can also elicit the direct secretion of both granule proteins and lipid mediators, although soluble mediators are generally ineffective secretogogues, except with highly activated eosinophils or when used in conjunction with cytochalasin B, which inhibits cytoskeletal assembly[79]. Differential secretion of granule proteins, depending on the stimulus, has been reported. IgG complexes induced the secretion of ECP but not EPO, whereas IgE complexes induced secretion of EPO but not ECP[80]; however, secretion was low in both instances. Eosinophils release their granule components by exocytosis, individual granules fusing with the plasma membrane. This process involves a GTP binding protein and is modulated by the intracellular calcium concentration[81]. Priming of eosinophils involves an increase in intracellular calcium and triggering of phosphatidylinositol turnover. As is the case with degranulation, the signal transduction pathways involved in priming appear broadly similar to those described for mast cells and neutrophils[82].

EOSINOPHIL HETEROGENEITY

A proportion of eosinophils from individuals with an increased eosinophil count are less dense than eosinophils from normal subjects[83]. The mechanism for this heterogeneity is unclear. Hypodense eosinophils appear to be vacuolated and contain smaller sized granules, although equal in number to those in normal density eosinophils[84]. It is generally considered that hypodense eosinophils represent an activated phenotype, with demonstration of increased oxygen consumption, cytotoxicity towards helminths and LTC_4 production[85]. They release less PAF after stimulation with IgG Sepharose beads, but this appears to be the result of increased acetyl hydrolase activity. Stimulation of eosinophils either in the short term with PAF or in long term culture with cytokines results in a hypodense phenotype and enhanced effector function[86]. In contrast, hypodense eosinophils have a profile of leucocyte integrin and Fc_γ receptor expression similar to those of normal density cells[43] and normal density cells from individuals with an eosinophilia are also primed. Nonetheless, the weight of evidence suggests that hypodensity represents a primed or partially activated phenotype.

EOSINOPHILS AND DISEASE

THE ROLE OF EOSINOPHILS

Views on the role of eosinophils in health and disease have changed with time. For many years they were believed to ameliorate inflammatory responses; now they are believed to have a tissue damaging role[52,87]. Even more recently, it has become apparent that eosinophils are the source of a range of cytokines, several of which are believed to have a homeostatic, rather than proinflammatory, function. For example, the observation that eosinophils secrete TGFα, together with studies showing increased numbers of eosinophils at the edges of healing wounds, suggests that they may be important in wound healing[88]. Cytokine stimulated eosinophils secrete IL-1, express HLA class II receptors and can present antigen to T cells *in vitro*, suggesting they may be important as accessory cells in T cell mediated reactions. There is evidence that eosinophils slow the rate of progression of solid tumours, presumably by being cytotoxic against tumour cells[89]. Nonetheless, there is also little doubt that eosinophils can cause severe tissue damage under certain circumstances. Persistently high eosinophil counts from many causes, including drug reactions, parasitic infections, eosinophilic leukaemia and hypereosinophilic syndrome (HES), are associated with endomyocardial fibrosis—a condition that presents with heart failure and signs consistent with a restrictive cardiomyopathy. The ventricle is thickened, and histologically there are areas of fibrosis, thrombus formation and inflammation in the endomyocardium, with large numbers of both intact and degranulating eosinophils. Eosinophil granule products are deposited adjacent to myocytes and, *in vitro* have been shown to be toxic for cardiac myocytes. HES, a condition in which there is a high eosinophil count of unknown aetiology, is associated with several features that could be ascribed to the toxic properties of eosinophils[90].

Much of the work on eosinophils undertaken in recent years has been in association with allergic disease and parasitic infection. The observation, in the mid 1970s, that eosinophils could kill parasite targets led to the hypothesis that the teleological role of eosinophils was to counter certain parasitic infections, in particular those associated with helminthic worms[91]. The realisation that eosinophils could release proinflammatory mediators such as PAF and eicosanoids, and the observation that eosinophil basic proteins were toxic for airway epithelium, have led to a consensus that eosinophils are a major effector cell for tissue damage in asthma and could cause many of the pathological features of the disease. These conditions are the most important eosinophilic diseases in terms of numbers of affected individuals. They provide a useful model with which to study eosinophil involvement in disease processes, and will therefore be discussed in some detail.

EOSINOPHILS AND ASTHMA

It is well established that large numbers of eosinophils, together with mononuclear cells, are frequently found in and around the bronchi of patients who have died of asthma. The immunostaining of bronchial tissue from such patients has revealed the existence of large amounts of MBP deposited in the airways[92]. The presence of increased numbers of peripheral blood eosinophils in both atopic and non-atopic chronic asthma is well known, although this increase is not as great as that seen in other eosinophil associated diseases, and the peripheral blood eosinophil count is often normal. One longitudinal study of 14 oral-corticosteroid-dependent asthmatic patients being treated at a chest clinic found, on 44 separate occasions, that eosinophil counts correlated with several measurements of airflow obstruction[93]. Others have found that the degree of bronchial hyperreactivity correlated inversely with the peripheral blood eosinophil count in patients developing a late phase response after antigen challenge[94], and these observations were supported by findings of a similar correlation from a cross sectional study of asthmatic patients seen at a routine chest clinic[95].

Full appreciation of the extent of eosinophil involvement in asthma has come with the use of fibreoptic bronchoscopy to obtain BAL fluid and endobronchial biopsy specimens from the airways of patients with mild to moderate asthma. Aerosolised challenge of sensitised asthmatic subjects with allergen results in an influx to the airways of inflammatory cells consisting of eosinophils, neutrophils and mononuclear cells, and an increase in the amount of eosinophil granule proteins in lavage fluid[96]. A similar picture has been observed after challenge with agents that cause occupational asthma[97,98]. The eosinophilia associated with segmental challenge via the bronchoscope is even more dramatic, up to 50% of the lavage cells being eosinophils[99] with an activated phenotype after 24 h[100]. Similar findings have been made after allergen challenge to the skin and nose[101,102].

An almost invariable increase in the number of eosinophils, in association with increased numbers of mast cells and epithelial cells, has been observed in BAL fluid and endobronchial biopsy specimens from clinical asthmatic patients compared with normal controls[103–106]. A lesser, but often significant increase in airway eosinophils is seen in atopic non-asthmatic subjects or seasonal asthmatic patients out of season. Airway eosinophils in asthma are activated as determined by staining with the monoclonal antibody, EG2, and expression of the activation receptor, CD69[52,107]. Eosinophil infiltration is accompanied by increased numbers of activated CD25 positive T lymphocytes which have a Th2-like profile of cytokine secretion[108] and evidence of epithelial desquamation, with increased numbers of epithelial cells in BAL fluid and signs of epithelial fragility in bronchial biopsy specimens[109]. The increase in eosinophils has been noted in intrinsic and occupational asthma in addition to atopic asthma[110,111]. A BAL eosinophilia is relatively specific to asthma, although it is also seen in pulmonary eosinophilia and some patients with fibrosing alveolitis[112]. The numbers of eosinophils in BAL fluid in asthma are generally only modestly increased, ranging from 1 to 5% (normal value <1%), although occasionally eosinophil counts can be in the range of 30–50%. However, there is a general correlation between the numbers of airway eosinophils and the severity of asthma[113]. Furthermore, inhibition of an airway eosinophilia by disodium chromoglycate[114] or, more effectively, corticosteroids[115,116] is associated with an improvement in bronchial hyperresponsiveness, symptoms and lung function. In addition, inhibition of migration of eosinophils into the airways of allergen challenged non-human primates, using a monoclonal antibody directed against the adhesion molecule ICAM-1, also inhibits the development of airway hyperresponsiveness[117]. However, none of these treatments is specific to the eosinophil: glucocorticoids, for example, probably act to a large extent through inhibition of the release of eosinophil active cytokines from T cells and monocytes[118]. Airway eosinophilia can also occur without asthma or airways hyperresponsiveness[119]. In order that eosinophils cause tissue damage in the airways, they need to be actively secreting their mediators. Measurements of eosinophilic basic proteins may therefore be better than eosinophil numbers as a guide to the degree of eosinophilic inflammation. For example, Adelroth *et al.* found that inhaled corticosteroids had no effect on the number of eosinophils in BAL fluid from asthmatics, but the drugs markedly reduced the amounts of ECP in lavage fluid[120]. The current hypothesis concerning the role of eosinophils in the pathogenesis of asthma is summarised in Fig. 8.4.

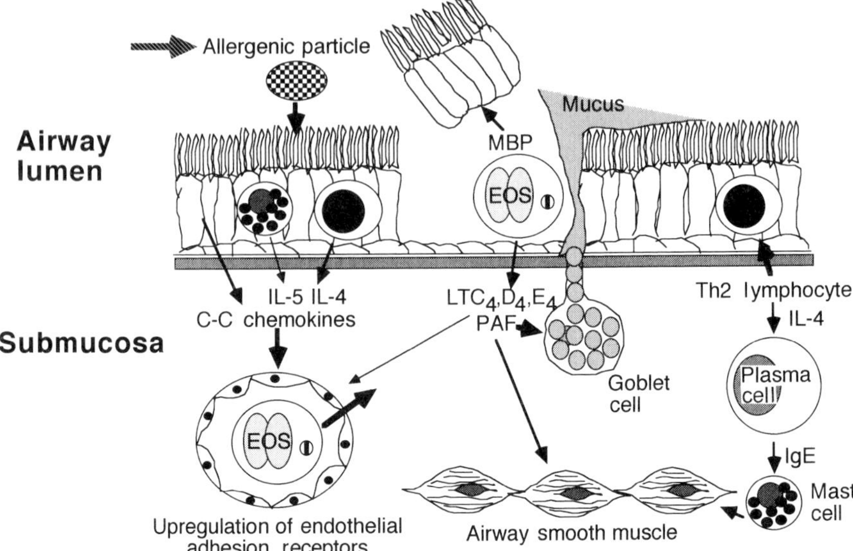

Figure 8.4. Illustration of the current hypothesis concerning the role of eosinophils in asthma. Antigenic particles, in most cases allergens such as house dust mite faecal pellets, are inhaled and interact with Th2 type, antigen specific lymphocytes and intraepithelial mast cells with bound specific IgE. This results in release of chemoattractants such as RANTES, and cytokines such as IL-4 and IL-5, which promote selective eosinophil (EOS) migration from the bronchial circulation. Eosinophils migrate into the submucosa and epithelium, where they release granule proteins which cause epithelial damage and lipid derived mediators which cause mucus hypersecretion and bronchoconstriction in addition to further supporting eosinophil recruitment. Mast cell derived mediators contribute to smooth muscle spasm, and epithelial derived mediators including chemokines and cytokines such as granulocyte macrophage colony stimulating factor serve to amplify the inflammatory response. Abbreviations as in Fig. 8.3

EOSINOPHILS AND PARASITIC DISEASE

Although infection with helminths is by far the commonest cause of a moderate to high eosinophilia in association with parasites, eosinophilia in association with protozoan infections has been described, and ectoparasites such as head lice and scabies can produce a local eosinophilic reaction[121,122]. Eosinophils have been shown to be able to kill a number of opsonised parasites, including new born larvae of *Trichinella spiralis*, larvae of *Nippostrongylus brasiliensis* (a gut parasite in the rat) and *Fasciola hepatica*, in addition to schistosomula of *S. mansoni*[123]. *In vivo*, parasite larvae become coated with specific IgG and IgE antibodies and can activate complement. Dead larvae of *Schistosoma haematobium* and other parasites have been detected surrounded by eosinophils and eosinophil granule products in the skin[124] and antibodies against IL-5 abolish the eosinophilia in parasitised animals[125]. Adult worms both *in vitro* and *in vivo* appear resistant to eosinophil mediated damage. Despite this circumstantial evidence for eosinophils being involved in host defence against parasites, there remains some doubt about their role. Except for one study in the Gambia[126], there is no obvious correlation between the degree of eosinophilia and protection against infection or reinfection. Moreover, treatment of mice infected with *N. brasiliensis* or *S. mansoni* with neutralising monoclonal antibody to IL-5 abolished the eosinophilia without modulating the disease process[127].

OTHER EOSINOPHILIC DISORDERS

More unusual eosinophilic disorders include pulmonary eosinophilia, idiopathic HES, eosinophil leukaemia and Churg Strauss syndrome. The last of these is a life-threatening condition characterised by eosinophilic vasculitis, asthma and a peripheral blood eosinophilia[128]. These conditions are of unknown aetiology. Management generally consists of treatment with high dose oral glucocorticoids, supplemented by chemotherapy if the condition is only partially responsive, as is generally the case in HES and Churg-Strauss syndrome. More recently, treatment with interferons α and γ has been used with anecdotal success in HES. IL-5 antagonists, when they become available, may also be effective.

SUMMARY AND CONCLUSIONS

Eosinophils are characterised by their unique crystalloid granules which contain four basic proteins, MBP, ECP, EDN and EPO. The cell has many features in common with neutrophils but, unlike that cell type, eosinophils utilise VLA-4/VCAM-1 as an adherence pathway and have a number of other receptors not shared by neutrophils. These include recognition units for IgE (distinct from CD23), and receptors for IL-5, IL-3 and RANTES. After stimulation with a variety of agents, eosinophils preferentially elaborate LTC_4 as the major 5-lipoxygenase product of arachidonic acid, produce substantial amounts of PAF and synthesise a number of cytokines. Thus eosinophils have marked proinflammatory potential. There is now convincing evidence that eosinophilia is T cell dependent. The Th2-type cell, which selectively secretes IL-5 and IL-4, seems particularly involved. IL-5, IL-3 and GM-CSF are required for eosinophil maturation, and also activate and prolong the survival of mature cells in culture. IL-5 is unique in that it promotes terminal differentiation of the committed eosinophil precursor and, in mice, appears to be sufficient to promote eosinophil growth from uncommitted stem cells. IL-4 selectively upregulates VCAM-1 expression on endothelial cells *in vitro*, potentially augmenting VLA-4 dependent eosinophil adhesion. The role of eosinophils in disease is complex, but in general their numbers are increased in helminthic parasitic disease, atopic allergy and asthma. Eosinophil products can provoke many of the pathological features of asthma, and helminthic larvae coated with immunoglobulin or complement are particularly susceptible to eosinophil mediated cytotoxicity.

REFERENCES

1. Ehrlich P. Ueber die specifischen granulationen des Blutes. *Arch Anat Physiol Lpz* 1879; **3:** 571–579.
2. Spry C J F. *Eosinophils, a Comprehensive Review and Guide to the Medical Literature.* Oxford: Oxford University Press, 1988.
3. Smith H, Cook R M, eds. *Immunopharmacology of Eosinophils.* London: Academic Press, 1993.
4. Gleich G J, Kay A B, eds *Eosinophils in Allergy and Inflammation.* New York: Marcel Dekker Inc, 1994.
5. Makino S, Fukuda T, eds *Eosinophils. Biological and Clinical Aspects.* Boca Raton: CRC Press, 1993.
6. Dvorak A M, Ishizaka T, Weller P F, *et al.* Ultrastructural contributions to the understanding of the cell biology of human eosinophils. In: Makino S, Fukuda T, eds *Eosinophils. Biological and Clinical Aspects*, chapter 2. Boca Raton: CRC Press, 1993; 13–32.
7. Baston A, Beeson P B. Mechanism of eosinophilia. II Role of the lymphocyte. *J Exp Med* 1970; **131:** 1288.
8. Sanderson C J. Interleukin-5, eosinophils and disease. *Blood* 1992; **79:** 3101.
9. Desreumaux P, Janin A, Colombel J F, *et al.* Interleukin 5 messenger RNA expression by eosinophils in the intestinal mucosa of patients with coeliac disease. *J Exp Med* 1992; **175:** 293.
10. Mossman R, Coffman R L. Th1 and Th2 cells: different patterns of lymphokine secretion lead to different functional properties. *Annu Rev Immunol* 1989; **7:** 145.
11. Corrigan C, Kay A B. T cells and eosinophils in the pathogenesis of asthma. *Immunol Today* 1992; **13:** 501.
12. Spry C J F. The natural history of eosinophils. In: Smith H, Cook R M, eds. *The Immunopharmacology of Eosinophils.* London: Academic Press, 1993; 1–9.
13. Hynes R O. Integrins: versatility, modulation and signaling in cell adhesion. *Cell* 1992; **69:** 11–25.
14. Springer T A. Adhesion receptors of the immune system. *Nature* 1990; **346:** 425–434.
15. Walsh G M, Hartnell A, Wardlaw A J, *et al.* IL-5 enhances the *in vitro* adhesion of human eosinophils, but not neutrophils, in a leukocyte integrin (CD11/18)-dependent manner. *Immunology* 1990; **71:** 258.
16. Walsh G M, Hartnell A, Mermod J-J, *et al.* Human eosinophil but not neutrophil adherence to IL-1 stimulated HUVEC is $\alpha 4/\beta 1$ dependent. *J Immunol* 1991; **146:** 3419–3423.
17. Thornhill M H, Kyan-Aung U, Haskard D O. IL-4 increases human endothelial cell adhesiveness for T cells but not neutrophils. *J Immunol* 1990; **144:** 3060.
18. Kay A B, Sun-Ying, Varney V, *et al.* Messenger RNA expression of the cytokine gene cluster IL-3, IL-4, IL-5 and GM-CSF in allergen-induced late-phase cutaneous reactions in atopic subjects. *J Exp Med* 1991; **173:** 775–778.
19. Tepper R I, Levinson D A, Stanger B Z, *et al.* IL-4 induces allergic-like inflammatory disease and alters T cell development in transgenic mice. *Cell* 1990; **62:** 457.
20. Weg V B, Williams T J, Lobb R R, *et al.* A monoclonal antibody recognizing very late antigen-4 inhibits eosinophil accumulation *in vivo. J Exp Med* 1993; **177:** 561.
21. Pretolani M, Ruffie C, Silva J, *et al.* Antibody to very late activation antigen 4 prevents antigen-induced bronchial hyperreactivity and cellular infiltration in the guinea pig airways. *J Exp Med* 1994; **180:** 795.
22. Nakajima H, Sano H, Nishimura T, *et al.* Role of vascular cell adhesion molecule 1/very late activation antigen 4 and intercellular adhesion molecule 1/lymphocyte function-associated antigen 1 interactions in antigen induced eosinophil and T cell recruitment into the tissue. *J Exp Med* 1994; **179:** 1145.
23. Kyan-Aung U, Haskard D O, Poston R N, *et al.* Endothelial leukocyte adhesion molecule-1 and intercellular adhesion molecule-1 mediate adhesion of eosinophils to endothelial cells *in vitro* and are expressed by endothelium in allergic cutaneous inflammation *in vivo. J Immunol* 1991; **146:** 521.

24. Bentley A M, Robinson D S, Menz G, *et al*. Expression of the endothelial and leukocyte adhesion molecules ICAM-1, E-selectin and VCAM-1 in the bronchial mucosa in steady state and allergen induced asthma. *J Allergy Clin Immunol* 1993; **92:** 857.
25. Georas S N, Liu M C, Newman W, *et al*. Altered adhesion molecule expression and endothelial cell activation accompany the recruitment of human granulocytes to the lung after segmental antigen challenge. *Am J Respir Cell Biol* 1994; **7:** 261.
26. Knol E F, Tackey F, Tedder T F, *et al*. Comparison of human eosinophil and neutrophil adhesion to endothelial cells under nonstatic conditions. Role of L-selectin. *J Immunol* 1994; **153:** 2161.
27. Symon F A, Walsh G M, Watson S R, *et al*. Eosinophil adhesion to nasal polyp endothelium is P-selectin-dependent. *J Exp Med* 1994; **180:** 371.
28. Moser R, Fehr J, Bruijnzeel P B. IL-4 controls the selective endothelium-driven transmigration of eosinophils from allergic individuals. *J Immunol* 1992; **149:** 1432.
29. Ebisawa M, Liu M C, Yamada T, *et al*. Eosinophil transendothelial migration induced by cytokines. II. Potentiation of eosinophil transendothelial migration by eosinophil-active cytokines. *J Immunol* 1993; **152:** 4590.
30. Ebisawa M, Yamada T, Bickel C, *et al*. Eosinophil transendothelial migration by cytokines. III. Effect of the chemokine RANTES. *J Immunol* 1994; **153:** 2153.
31. Kameyoshi Y, Dorschner A, Mallet A I, *et al*. Cytokine RANTES released by thrombin stimulated platelets is a potent attractant for human eosinophils. *J Exp Med* 1992; **176:** 587.
32. Jose P J, Griffiths-Johnson D A, Collins P D, *et al*. Eotaxin: a potent eosinophil chemoattractant cytokine detected in a guinea pig model of allergic airways inflammation. *J Exp Med* 1994; **179:** 881.
33. Henocq E, Vaargaftig B B. Accumulation of eosinophils in response to intracutaneous PAF-acether and allergens in man. *Lancet* 1986; **1:** 1378.
34. Wardlaw A J, Chung K F, Moqbel R, *et al*. Effects of inhaled PAF in human on circulating and bronchoalveolar lavage fluid neutrophils. *Am Rev Respir Dis* 1990; **141:** 386.
35. Laitinen L A, Laitinen A, Haahtela T, *et al*. Leukotriene E4 and granulocytic infiltration into asthmatic airways. *Lancet* 1993; **341:** 989.
36. Georas S N, McIntyre B W, Ebisawa M, *et al*. Expression of a functional laminin receptor ($\alpha6\beta1$, very late activation antigen-6) on human eosinophils. *Blood* 1993; **82:** 2872.
37. Dri P, Cramer R, Spessotto R, *et al*. Eosinophil activation on biological surfaces. Production of O_2 in response to physiologic soluble stimuli is differentially modulated by extracellular matrix components and endothelial cells. *J Immunol* 1991; **147:** 613.
38. Anwar A R E, Walsh G M, Cromwell O, *et al*. Adhesion to fibronectin primes eosinophils via $\alpha4\beta1$ (VLA-4). *Immunol* 1994; **82:** 222.
39. Neeley S P, Hamann K J, Dowling T L, *et al*. Augmentation of stimulated eosinophil degranulation by VLA-4 (CD49d)-mediated adhesion to fibronectin. *Am J Respir Cell Mol Biol* 1994; **11:** 206.
40. Anwar A R E, Moqbel R, Walsh G M, *et al*. Adhesion to fibronectin prolongs eosinophil survival. *J Exp Med* 1993; **177:** 839.
41. Yamaguchi Y, Suda T, Ohta S, *et al*. Analysis of the survival of mature human eosinophils: interleukin-5. *Blood* 1991; **78:** 2542–2547.
42. Alam R, Forsythe P, Stafford S, *et al*. Transforming growth factor-β abrogates the effects of hematopoietins on eosinophils and induces their apoptosis. *J Exp Med* 1994; **179:** 1041.
43. Hartnell A, Moqbel R, Walsh G M, *et al*. Fcγ and CD11/18 receptor expression on normal density and low density human eosinophils. *Immunology* 1990; **69:** 264.
44. Hartnell A, Kay A B, Wardlaw A J. IFN-g induces expression of FcγRIII(CD16) on human eosinophils. *J Immunol* 1992; **148:** 1471.
45. Capron M, Capron A, Dessaint J-P, *et al*. Fc receptors for IgE on human and rat eosinophils. *J Immunol* 1981; **126:** 2087.
46. Capron M, Joualt T, Prin L, *et al*. Functional study of a monoclonal antibody to IgE Fc receptor (FcεR2) of eosinophils, platelets and macrophages. *J Exp Med* 1986; **164:** 72.
47. Capron M, Troung M-J, Desreumaux P, *et al*. Eosinophil membrane receptors: function of IgE and IgA binding molecules. In: Gleich G J, Kay A B, eds. *Eosinophils: Immunological and Clinical Aspects*. New York: Marcel Dekker, in press.

48. Gounni A S, Lamkhioed B, Ochiai K, *et al.* High affinity IgE receptor on eosinophils is involved in defence against parasites. *Nature* 1994; **367:** 183.

49. Monteiro R C, Hostoffer R W, Cooper M D, *et al.* Definition of immunoglobulin A receptors on eosinophils and their enhanced expression in allergic individuals. *J Clin Invest* 1993; **92:** 1681.

50. Abu-Ghazaleh R I, Fujisawa T, Mestecky J, *et al.* IgA-induced eosinophil degranulation. *J Immunol* 1989; **142:** 2393.

51. Weller P F, Rand T H, Barrett T, *et al.* Accessory cell function of human eosinophils. HLA-DR-dependent, MHC-restricted antigen-presentation and IL-1 alpha expression. *J Immunol* 1993; **150:** 2554.

52. Nishikawa K, Morii T, Ako H, *et al. In vivo* expression of CD69 on lung eosinophils in eosinophilic pneumonia: CD69 as a possible activation marker for eosinophils. *J Allergy Clin Immunol* 1992; **90:** 169.

53. Hartnell A, Robinson D S, Kay A B, *et al.* CD69 is expressed by human eosinophils activated *in vivo* in asthma and *in vitro* by cytokines. *Immunology* 1993; **80:** 281.

54. Barker R L, Gleich G J, Pease L R. Acidic precursor revealed in human eosinophil granule major basic protein cDNA. *J Exp Med* 1988; **168:** 1493.

55. Butterworth A E, Wassom D L, Gleich G J, *et al.* Damage to schistosomula of *S. mansoni* induced directly by eosinophil major basic protein. *J Immunol* 1979; **122:** 221.

56. Gleich G J. The eosinophil and bronchial asthma: current understanding. *J Allergy Clin Immunol* 1986; **85:** 422.

57. Gundel R H, Letts L G, Gleich G J. Human eosinophil major basic protein induces airway constriction and airway hyperresponsiveness in primates. *J Clin Invest* 1991; **87:** 1470.

58. Rohrbach M S, Wheatley C L, Slifman N R, *et al.* Activation of platelets by eosinophil granule proteins. *J Exp Med* 1990; **172:** 1271.

59. Ten R M, Pease L R, McKean D J, *et al.* Molecular cloning of the human eosinophil peroxidase. *J Exp Med* 1989; **169:** 1757.

60. Slungaard A, Mahoney J R Jr. Thiocyanate is the major substrate for eosinophil peroxidase in physiological fluids: implications for cytotoxicity. *J Biol Chem* 1991; **266:** 4903.

61. Rosenburg H F, Ackerman S J, Tenen D G. Human eosinophil cationic protein. Molecular cloning of a cytotoxin and helminthotoxin with ribonuclease activity. *J Exp Med* 1989; **170:** 163.

62. Tai P C, Spry C J F, Peterson C, *et al.* Monoclonal antibodies distinguish between storage and secreted forms of eosinophil cationic protein. *Nature* 1984; **309:** 182.

63. Rosenburg H F, Tenen D G, Ackerman S J. Molecular cloning of the human eosinophil-derived neurotoxin: a member of the ribonuclease gene family. *Proc Natl Acad Sci USA* 1989; **86:** 4460.

64. Weller P F. Eicosanoids, cytokines and other mediators elaborated by eosinophils. In: Makino S, Fukuda T, eds. *Eosinophils, Biological and Clinical Aspects.* Boca Raton: CRC Press, 1993; 125–154.

65. Shaw R J, Walsh G M, Cromwell O, *et al.* Activated human eosinophils generate SRS-A leukotrienes following physiological (IgG dependent) stimulation. *Nature* 1985; **316:** 150.

66. Cromwell O, Wardlaw A J, Champion A, *et al.* IgG-dependent generation of platelet activating factor by normal and low density eosinophils. *J Immunol* 1990; **145:** 3862.

67. Wong D T, Weller P F, Galli S J, *et al.* Human eosinophils express transforming growth factor α. *J Exp Med* 1990; **172:** 673.

68. Leary A G, Ogawa M. Identification of pure and mixed basophil colonies in culture of human peripheral blood and marrow cells. *Blood* 1984; **64:** 78.

69. Moqbel R, Hamid Q, Sun-Ying, *et al.* Expression of mRNA and immunoreactivity for the granulocyte/macrophage-colony stimulating factor (GM-CSF) in activated human eosinophils. *J Exp Med* 1991; **174:** 749.

70. Hamid Q, Azzawi M, Sun-Ying, *et al.* Expression of mRNA for interleukin-5 in mucosal bronchial biopsies from asthma. *J Clin Invest* 1991; **87:** 1541.

71. Brodie D H, Paine M M, Firestein G S. Eosinophils express interleukin 5 and granulocyte macrophage-colony-stimulating factor mRNA at sites of allergic inflammation in asthmatics. *J Clin Invest* 1992; **90:** 1414–1424.

72. Finotto S, Ohno I, Marshall J S, *et al.* TNF-α production by eosinophils in upper airways inflammation (nasal polyposis). *J Immunol* 1994; **153:** 2278.

73. Wong D T W, Elovic A, Matossian K. Eosinophils from patients with blood eosinophilia express transforming growth factor β1. *Blood* 1991; **78:** 2702.

74. Hamid Q, Barkans J, Meng Q, *et al.* Human eosinophils synthesize and secrete interleukin-6, *in vitro*. *Blood* 1992; **80:** 1496.

75. Braun R K, Franchini M, Erard F, *et al.* Human peripheral blood eosinophils produce and release interleukin-8 on stimulation with calcium ionophore. *Eur J Immunol* 1993; **23:** 956.

76. Van der Bruggen T, Kok P T M, Raaijmakers J A M, *et al.* Cytokine priming of the respiratory burst in human eosinophils is Ca^{2+} independent and accompanied by induction of tyrosine kinase activity. *J Leucoc Biol* 1993; **53:** 347.

77. Kapp A, Zeck-Kapp G, Czech W, *et al.* The chemokine RANTES is more than a chemoattractant: characterisation of its effect on human eosinophil oxidative metabolism and morphology in comparison with IL-5 and GM-CSF. *J Invest Dermatol* 1994; **102:** 906.

78. Yazdanbakhsh M, Eckmann C M, Roos D. Characterization of the interaction of human eosinophils and neutrophils with opsonized particles. *J Immunol* 1985; **135:** 1378.

79. Kroegel C, Yukawa T, Dent G, *et al.* Stimulation of degranulation from human eosinophils by platelet activating factor. *J Immunol* 1989; **142:** 3518.

80. Khaliffe J, Capron M, Cesbron J Y, *et al.* Role of specific IgE antibodies in peroxidase (EPO) release from human eosinophils. *J Immunol* 1986; **137:** 1659.

81. Nusse O, Lindau M, Cromwell O, *et al.* Intracellular application of guanosine-5'-O-(3-thiotriphosphate) induces exocytic granule fusion in guinea pig eosinophils. *J Exp Med* 1990; **171:** 775.

82. Giembycz M A, Barnes P J. Stimulus–response coupling in eosinophils: receptors, signal transduction and pharmacological modulation. In: Smith H, Cook R M, eds. *Immunopharmacology of Eosinophils*. London: Academic Press, 1993; 91–118.

83. Bass D A, Grover W H, Lewis J C, *et al.* Comparison of human eosinophils from normals and patients with eosinophilia. *J Clin Invest* 1980; **66:** 1265.

84. Caulfield J P, Hein A, Rothenburg M E, *et al.* A morphometric study of normodense and hypodense human eosinophils that are derived *in vivo* and *in vitro*. *Am J Pathol* 1991; **137:** 27.

85. Fukuda T, Makino S. Heterogeneity and activation, In: Makino S, Fukuda T, eds. *Eosinophils, Biological and Clinical Aspects*, chapter 7. Boca Raton: CRC Press, 1993; 156–170.

86. Owen W F, Rothenburg M E, Silberstein D S. Regulation of human eosinophil viability, density and function by granulocyte/macrophage colony stimulating factor in the presence of 3T3 fibroblasts. *J Exp Med* 1987; **166:** 129.

87. Weller P F, Goetzl E J. The regulatory and effector roles of eosinophils. *Adv Immunol* 1979; **27:** 339.

88. Todd R, Donoff B R, Chiang T. The eosinophil as a cellular source of transforming growth factor alpha in healing cutaneous wounds. *Am J Pathol* 1991; **138:** 1307.

89. Lowe D, Jorizzo J, Hutt M S R. Tumour associated eosinophilia, a review. *J Clin Path* 1981; **34:** 1343.

90. Spry C J F. The idiopathic hypereosinophilic syndrome. In: Makino S, Fukuda T, eds. *Eosinophils: Biological and Clinical Aspects*, chapter 22. Boca Raton: CRC Press, 1993; 403–420.

91. Butterworth A E. Cell mediated damage to helminths. *Adv Parasitol* 1984; **23:** 143.

92. Filley W V, Holley K E, Kephart G M, *et al.* Identification by immunofluorescence of eosinophil under granule major basic protein in lung tissue of patients with bronchial asthma. *Lancet* 1982; **2:** 11.

93. Horn B R, Robin E D, Theodore J, *et al.* Total eosinophil counts in the management of bronchial asthma. *N Engl J Med* 1975; **292:** 1152.

94. Durham S R, Kay A B. Eosinophils, bronchial hyperreactivity and late-phase asthmatic reactions. *Clin Allergy* 1985; **15:** 411.

95. Taylor K J, Luksza A R. Peripheral blood eosinophil counts and bronchial hyperresponsiveness. *Thorax* 1987; **42:** 452.

96. De Monchy J G R, Kauffman H F, Venge P, *et al.* Bronchoalveolar eosinophilia during allergen-induced late asthmatic reactions. *Am Rev Respir Dis* 1985; **139:** 1383.

97. Lam S, LeRichie J, Phillips D, *et al*. Cellular and protein changes in bronchial lavage fluid after late asthmatic reaction in patients with red cedar wood asthma. *J Allergy Clin Immunol* 1987; **80:** 44.

98. Fabbri L M, Boschetto P, Zocca E. Bronchoalveolar neutrophilia during late asthmatic reactions induced by toluene diisocyanate. *Am Rev Respir Dis* 1987; **136:** 36.

99. Metzger W J, Zavala D, Richerson H B, *et al*. Local allergen challenge and bronchoalveolar lavage of allergic asthmatic lungs: description of the model and local airway inflammation. *Am Rev Respir Dis* 1987; **135:** 433.

100. Kroegel C, Liu M C, Hubbard W C, *et al*. Blood and bronchoalveolar eosinophils in allergic subjects after segmental antigen challenge: surface phenotype, density heterogeneity and prostanoid production. *J Allergy Clin Immunol* 1994; **93:** 725.

101. Frew A J, Kay A B. The relationship between infiltrating CD4+ lymphocytes, activated eosinophils and the magnitude of the allergen induced late-phase response in man. *J Immunol* 1988; **141:** 4158.

102. Bentley A M, Jacobson M R, Cumberworth V, *et al*. Immunohistology of the nasal mucosa in seasonal allergic rhinitis: increase in activated eosinophils and epithelial mast cells. *J Allergy Clin Immunol* 1992; **89:** 877.

103. Godard P, Chaintreuil J, Damon M, *et al*. Functional assessment of alveolar macrophages comparison of cells from asthmatics and normal subjects. *J Allergy Clin Immunol* 1982; **70:** 88.

104. Flint K C, Leung K B, Hudspith B N, *et al*. Bronchoalveolar mast cells in extrinsic asthma: a mechanism for the initiation of antigen specific bronchoconstriction. *BMJ* 1985; **291:** 923.

105. Tomioka M, Ida S, Shindoh Y, *et al*. Mast cells in bronchoalveolar lumen of patients with bronchial asthma. *Am Rev Respir Dis* 1984; **129:** 1000.

106. Wardlaw A J, Dunnette S, Gleich G J, *et al*. Eosinophils and mast cells in bronchoalveolar lavage fluid and mild asthma: relationship to bronchial hyperreactivity. *Am Rev Respir Dis* 1988; **137:** 62.

107. Azzawi M, Bradley B, Jeffery P K *et al*. Identification of activated T lymphocytes and eosinophils in bronchial biopsies in stable atopic asthma. *Am Rev Respir Dis* 1990; **142:** 1407-1413.

108. Robinson D S, Hamid Q, Sun-Ying. Evidence for a predominant Th2-type bronchoalveolar lavage T lymphocyte population in atopic asthma. *N Engl J Med* 1992; **326:** 298.

109. Jeffery P K, Wardlaw A J, Nelson F C, *et al*. Bronchial biopsies in asthma: an ultrastructural, quantitative study and correlation with hyperreactivity. *Am Rev Respir Dis* 1990; **140:** 1745.

110. Bentley A M, Maestrelli P, Saetta M, *et al*. Activated T lymphocytes and eosinophils in the bronchial mucosa in isocyanate-induced asthma. *J Allergy Clin Immunol* 1992; **89:** 821.

111. Bentley A M, Menz G, Storz C H R, *et al*. Identification of T lymphocytes, macrophages and activated eosinophils in the bronchial mucosa in intrinsic asthma: relationship to symptoms and bronchial responsiveness. *Am Rev Respir Dis* 1992; **146:** 500.

112. Allen J N, Davis W B, Pacht E R. Diagnostic significance of increased bronchoalveolar lavage fluid eosinophils. *Am Rev Respir Dis* 1990; **142:** 642.

113. Bousquet J, Chanez P, Lacoste J Y, *et al*. Eosinophilic inflammation in asthma. *N Engl J Med* 1990; **323:** 1033.

114. Diaz P, Galleguillos F R, Gonzales M C, *et al*. Bronchoalveolar lavage in asthma: the effect of disodium cromoglycate (cromolyn) on leukocyte counts, immunoglobulins and complement. *J Allergy Clin Immunol* 1984; **74:** 41.

115. Schleimer R F. Effects of gluocorticosteroids on inflammatory cells relevant to their therapeutic applications in asthma. *Am Rev Respir Dis* 1990; **141:** S59.

116. Juniper E F, Kline P A, Vanzieleghem A, *et al*. Effect of long term treatment with an inhaled corticosteroid (budesonide) on airway hyperresponsiveness and clinical asthma in non steroid dependent asthmatics. *Am Rev Respir Dis* 1990; **142:** 832.

117. Wegner C D, Gundel R H, Reilly P, *et al*. Intercellular adhesion molecule-1 (ICAM-1) in the pathogenesis of asthma. *Science* 1990; **247:** 456.

118. Taylor I K, Shaw R J. The mechanism of action of corticosteroids in asthma. *Respir Med* 1993; **87:** 261.

119. Gibson P G, Manning P J, O'Byrne P M. Chronic cough; eosinophilic bronchitis without asthma. *Lancet* 1989; **1:** 1346.

120. Adelroth E, Rosenhall L, Johansson S, *et al.* Inflammatory cells and esoinophilic activity in asthma investigated by bronchoalveolar lavage. The effects of anti-asthmatic treatment with budesonide or terbutaline. *Am Rev Respir Dis* 1990; **142:** 91.

121. Kojima S. Eosinophils in parasitic diseases. In: Makino S, Fukuda T, eds. *Eosinophils, Biological and Clinical Aspects*, chapter 21. Boca Raton: CRC Press, 1993; 391–402.

122. Butterworth A E, Thorne K J I. Eosinophils and parasitic diseases. In: Smith H, Cook R, eds. *Immunopharmacology of Eosinophils*. London: Academic Press, 1993; 119.

123. Gleich G J, Adolphson C R. The eosinophil leukocyte: structure and function. *Adv Immunol* 1986; **39:** 177.

124. Kephart G M, Gleich G J, Connor D H, *et al.* Deposition of eosinophil granule major basic protein onto micofilariae of Onchocerca volvulus in the skin of patients treated with diethylcarbamazine. *Lab Invest* 1984; **50:** 51.

125. Coffman R L, Seymour B W, Hudak S, *et al.* Antibody to interleukin-5 inhibits helminth-induced eosinophilia in mice. *Science* 1989; **245:** 308.

126. Hagan P, Wilkins H A, Blumenthal U J, *et al.* Eosinophilia and resistance to *Schistosoma haematobium* in man. *Parasite Immunol* 1985; **7:** 625.

127. Sher A, Coffman R L, Hieny S, *et al.* Ablation of eosinophil and IgE responses with anti-IL-5 and anti-IL-4 antibodies fails to affect immunity against *Schistosoma mansoni* larvae in the mouse. *J Immunol* 1990; **145:** 3911.

128. Guillevin L, Guittard T, Bletry O, *et al.* Systemic necrotizing angiitis with asthma: causes and precipitating factors in 43 cases. *Lung* 1987; **165:** 165.

9

Human Mast Cells

YOSHIMICHI OKAYAMA AND MARTIN K. CHURCH

Southampton General Hospital, Southampton, UK

INTRODUCTION

While, in the western world, the mast cell is considered mainly as a cell responsible for the initiation of the allergic response, its role in individuals in underdeveloped countries appears to be predominantly one of defence against recurrent parasitic infection. The increase in mast cell numbers at the site of parasitic infection and the systemic increase in immunoglobulin E (IgE) levels is well documented. On subsequent infestation, the IgE dependent release of mast cell mediators, including histamine, proteases, prostaglandin $(PG)D_2$ and leukotriene $(LT)C_4$ induces a number of local inflammatory changes which make the environment hostile for the parasite. These responses include smooth muscle contraction, responsible for bronchoconstriction in the airways and increased gastrointestinal motility, and vasodilatation, oedema and mucus secretion, which are prevalent at all mucosal surfaces. Another feature of parasite induced inflammation, and indeed allergic inflammation, is the influx of large numbers of eosinophils. This suggests a special relationship between the mast cell and the eosinophil. Consequently, in addition to considering the mast cell derived mediators of the immediate response, it is also pertinent to discuss the potential of mast cells to initiate and support chronic inflammation, particularly by their generation of cytokines. Thus we will first describe human mast cell development and heterogeneity in order to understand mast cell biology. Second, we will discuss the observations which suggest the involvement of mast cells in disease. Finally, we review mast cell cytokine production which may have a very important role in initiating and maintaining allergic inflammation as part of the role of mast cells in host defence.

Pulmonary Defences. Edited by Robert A. Stockley.
© 1997 John Wiley & Sons Ltd.

DEVELOPMENT AND HETEROGENEITY OF HUMAN MAST CELLS

DEVELOPMENT OF HUMAN MAST CELLS

The study of the development of mast cells from their precursors is notoriously difficult because it is not easy to identify a cell as a mast cell until it matures in the tissues and expresses its characteristic granules and its high affinity $Fc_\varepsilon RI$ receptor for IgE. Mast cell precursors are haemopoietic in origin (Fig. 9.1), being derived from bone marrow stem cells, and enter the circulation as mononuclear cells which may be only tentatively recognised by their expression of the receptor for stem cell factor (SCF) or Steel factor (*c-kit*) and the mRNA for SCF. From the blood, the precursors enter the tissues, where they undergo the final phase of their differentiation in peripheral mucosal or connective tissue microenvironments rich in fibroblasts or stromal cells[1]. Immunocytochemical studies have shown the presence in the tissues of two mast cell (MC) phenotypes distinguishable by their neutral protease content: the MC_T phenotype containing only tryptase and the MC_{TC} phenotype containing both tryptase and chymase[2,3]. Variable amounts of both mast cell types are usually present in a tissue, and their relative abundance probably changes with tissue inflammation or fibrosis, thus making it impossible to base a subtype designation on location alone. However, some rules are evident. MC_T are found predominantly at mucosal surfaces and at areas of T lymphocyte proliferation. Their numbers increase locally during allergic reactions and parasitic infections. Thus they appear to be primarily "immune system related" cells with a role in host defence. Evidence for dependence of MC_T on functional T lymphocytes comes from the analysis of gastrointestinal tissue from subjects with congenital or acquired immunodeficiency disorders, AIDS

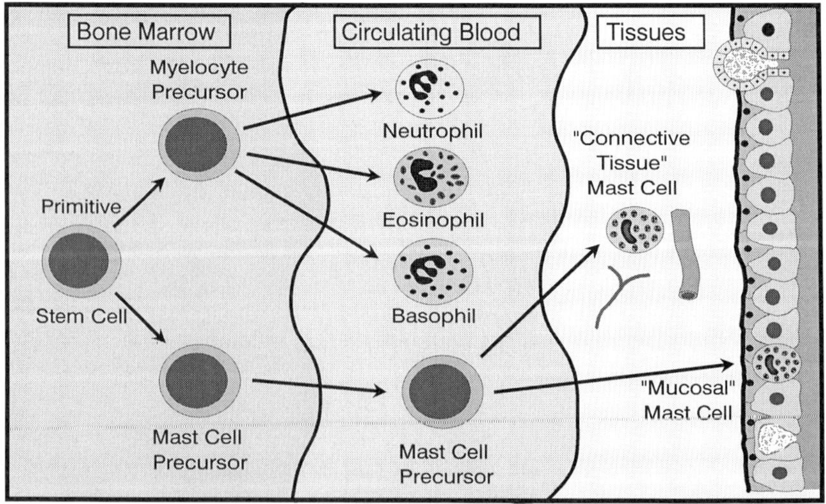

Figure 9.1. The development of human mast cells

or combined immunodeficiency, in whom a marked and selective depletion of MC_T cells is seen[4]. In contrast, MC_{TC} are preferentially sited within connective tissues and do not appear to be dependent on T lymphocyte growth factors for their development, as indicated by the observation of normal or possibly slightly increased numbers in immunodeficiency disorders[4]. The primary role of this cell group is more likely to be one of angiogenesis and tissue reconstruction rather than immunological protection. However, it should be remembered that both phenotypes express $Fc_\varepsilon RI$ and may, therefore, participate fully in IgE dependent allergic or parasitic reactions.

In vitro, cocultures of human cord blood mononuclear cells[1] and fetal liver cells[5] with mouse 3T3 fibroblasts have been found to result predominantly in growth of mast cells, of which 80–90% are MC_{TC}, but with some basophils. Culture of human cluster of differentiation (CD)34+ pluripotent progenitor cells in the presence of both recombinant human interleukin-3 (rhIL-3) and recombinant human stem cell factor (rhSCF) gives rise to cultures containing increased numbers of basophils and mast cells, with the mast cells exhibiting a variety of granular morphologies more reminiscent of mature mast cells[6,7]. Studies of immature mast cells show that both cell types are present at or before the stage at which granule formation begins[8]. Culture of human peripheral mononuclear cells from patients undergoing a severe asthma attack with supernatant from Balb/c 3T3 fibroblasts has been found to produce mast cell-like cells which contain tryptase. However, similar culture of peripheral mononuclear cells from normal individuals and patients who are not undergoing an asthma attack has failed to induce mast cells[9]. Furthermore, human SCF induces the differentiation of human mast cells from bone marrow, peripheral blood mononuclear cells and fetal liver cells in long term culture[5,10]. One thing that is unclear in mast cell development is whether the two mast cell phenotypes derive from separate committed progenitors, or whether the local environment in which a single uncommitted precursor is deposited may influence the switching on of the genes that encode the proteases. Although by no means conclusive, the recent observation by Saito *et al.*[11] that a 10 week culture of CD34+ cord blood cells with SCF and IL-6 induced the differentiation of both MC_{TC} (83%) and MC_T (17%) mast cells would tend to support the hypothesis of discrete precursors.

HETEROGENEITY OF HUMAN MAST CELLS

Human mast cells are metachromatic as a result of their heparin proteoglycan, contain histamine[12], and bind IgE with high affinity to specific $Fc_\varepsilon RI$ receptors[13,14]. Although these features are common to all human mast cells, they have other features which distinguish subpopulations, particularly their protease content. In humans, granules with a grating/lattice structure are found in mast cells in which the granules contain tryptase, chymase, carboxypeptidase and a cathepsin G-like enzyme (MC_{TC}), while those rich in complete scrolls are found in mast cells which contain tryptase alone (MC_T)[15,16]. MC_T cells derived from lung contain 10 pg tryptase per cell, whereas MC_{TC} cells derived from foreskin contain 35 pg tryptase, 4.5 pg chymase, 16 pg carboxypeptidase and 12 pg cathepsin G per cell[17]. Tryptase, which is specific for mast cells, is located in secretory granules, is released in parallel with histamine during degranulation[18], and accounts for all of the substantial trypsin-like activity detected in human mast cells. Its biological role *in vivo* is uncertain, although *in vitro* studies show several potential activities in humans — for example fibrinogenolysis, C3a generation[19,20], high molecular weight kininogen destruction, and prostromelysin activation[21].

Heparin is present in all human mast cells and constitutes some 75% of the granular proteoglycan, the remainder being a mixture of chondroitin sulphates. The histamine content of MC_T in preparations of dispersed mast cells obtained from lung parenchyma ($17\,027 \pm 2072\,pmol/10^6$ mast cells) is significantly greater than that of MC_{TC} obtained from children's foreskin MC_{TC} ($4345 \pm 1002\,pmol/10^6$ mast cells)[22]. Although similar amounts of LTC_4 and PGD_2 are also produced by preparations of human mast cells, LTD_4/E_4 are also produced in dispersed lung cells, probably by extracellular metabolism of LTC_4[22].

Dispersed mast cell preparations obtained from various anatomical sites contain a variable mixture of MC_T and MC_{TC} cells, depending on the site examined, the pathological condition of the donor organ, and the methods of dispersion and purification. In addition, human mast cells from anatomical sites show functional heterogeneity that appears to be independent from their protease heterogeneity. For example, mast cells from the skin, but not the lung, adenoid, tonsil and intestinal mucosa, release histamine non-immunologically in response to agents such as substance P, vasoactive intestinal polypeptide (VIP), somatostatin and compound $48/80$[23–25]. Furthermore, human skin MC_{TC}, but not similar cells from the uterus, express on their cell membranes CD88, the receptor for C5a (P. Valent, personal communication), and may thus be stimulated to degranulate by this complement peptide[24].

The finding that sodium cromoglycate (SCG) and nedocromil sodium fail to inhibit IgE dependent histamine release from human skin mast cells clearly distinguishes human skin mast cells from those of the lung, tonsils, adenoid and intestine[26]. High concentrations of ketotifen alone induced histamine release from skin mast cells, but not from lung and tonsillar mast cells[27]. Furthermore, the responsiveness of tonsillar and adenoidal mast cells to SCG and nedocromil sodium is quite different[26]. Mast cell protease typing of the cell populations[16] showed the MC_T: MC_{TC} ratio of mast cells in lung, tonsils and skin to be 93:7, 40:60 and 0.3:99.7, respectively. Thus the majority of tonsillar mast cells are phenotypically more like those of the skin than those of the lung, and yet their responsiveness to ketotifen and SCG is similar to that of lung mast cells. These studies demonstrate that functional heterogeneity does not parallel the distribution of neutral protease content. Whether these functional differences reflect the influence of factors in the local tissue environment, or whether mast cell heterogeneity is more diverse than we realise at present, is still an unresolved question. In contrast, no heterogeneity in mast cell response is observed with the β-adrenoceptor agonists, procaterol and salbutamol[28]. β-Adrenoceptor stimulants are significantly more effective in inhibiting PGD_2 than in inhibiting histamine release[28]. No tachyphylaxis is seen with prolongation of the incubation time before challenge. Thus human mast cells appear to be heterogeneous with respect to modulation of mediator release by SCG, nedocromil sodium and H_1-antihistamines, but not β-adrenoceptor agonists.

INVOLVEMENT OF MAST CELLS IN DISEASES

Mast cells, in combination with eosinophils, have a role in many species to protect them against parasitic infection. The presence of a highly antigenic nematode at a mucosal surface stimulates the immune system to produce IgE antibody through the process of antigen recognition by members of the monocyte family. Subsequent interaction of parasite antigens with IgE stimulates the mast cells to degranulate and release their preformed and newly generated mediators into the local environment. The effect of these mediators is to cause a localised inflammatory response (Fig. 9.2) in order to create a hostile environment for the parasite. Secondary to this is the preferential recruitment of eosinophils, which are then activated by the antigen to release their cytotoxic mediators in an attempt to kill the parasite. These mediators also cause local tissue damage in the environment of their activation. Involvement of rodent mast cells in parasite infection has been suggested on the basis of the following observations: first, T lymphocyte dependent hyperplasia of mucosal mast cells[29-32] and second, an increased level of rat mast cell chymase II, a marker for the rat "mucosal" mast cell, in response to intestinal parasite infection[33]. However, the exact role for human mast cells in parasite infection is unclear.

Allergic reactions at all mucosal surfaces, including asthma, rhinitis, allergic conjunctivitis and intestinal allergies, may be considered to be inappropriate "antiparasitic" responses mounted against an allergen such as pollen or house-dust mite proteins. With some knowledge of the widely varying actions of

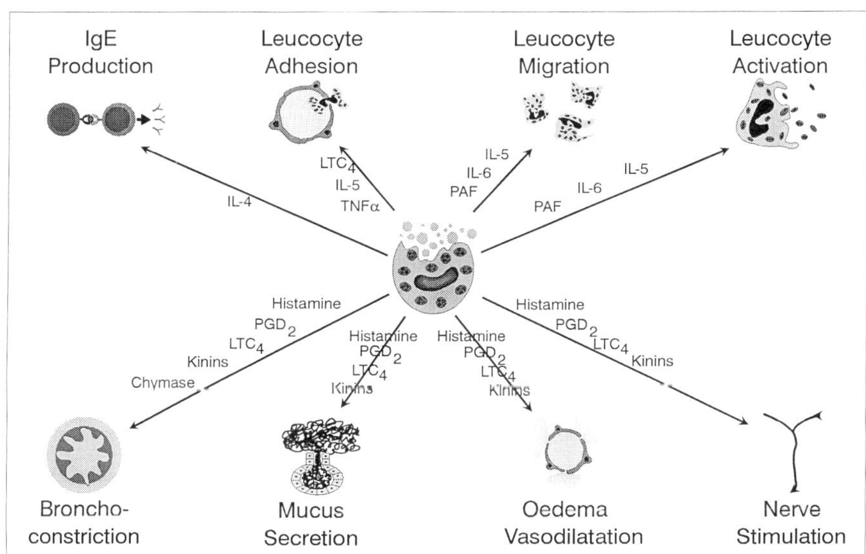

Figure 9.2. Immediate and cytokine actions of human mast cells. IL = Interleukin; LTC$_4$ = leukotriene C$_4$; TNFα = tumour necrosis factor α; PAF = platelet activating factor; PGD$_2$ = prostaglandin D$_2$

the major mast cell mediators, it is possible to account, at least partially, for the many pathophysiological features of the acute allergic reaction on the basis of these actions. Two features are apparent in the pathophysiology of bronchial asthma, namely hyperreactivity of the bronchi to specific or non-specific stimuli, and airway inflammation. Bronchial asthma is characterised by mucus hypersecretion, local eosinophilia of the airways, invasion of the airways by neutrophils and monocytes, epithelial damage or sloughing, thickening of airway basement membrane, smooth muscle hypertrophy and mucosal oedema[34]. Some of these events can be accounted for on the basis of mast cell mediator release and the subsequent secondary activation of other cells. Pulmonary mast cells have ready access to inhaled allergen. Human lung is a rich source of mast cells (0.01–0.1% of total cells) with more than 80% of these cells being in and around the airways[35]. Whilst many mast cells are located in the submucosa, it is those cells superficial to the basement membrane that assume particular importance in the response to allergen, as they come into direct contact with it. Activation of superficial mast cells, and later of cells lying within the epithelium, leads to the release of mediators which are capable of increasing bronchial mucus secretion, contracting airway smooth muscle both directly and indirectly by stimulation of vagal neuronal reflexes, and causing oedema of the airway mucosa. In man, bronchoconstrictory histamine receptor-H_1 receptors predominate over bronchodilatory histamine receptor-H_2 receptors on bronchial smooth muscle, and hence the major response to pulmonary mast cell histamine release is bronchoconstriction[36]. The role of the histamine receptor-H_3 receptor remains to be evaluated, although it has been reported that these receptors mediate inhibition of cholinergic neurotransmission in human airways[37]. The consequence of the release of mast cell proteases and exoglycosidases is damage to bronchial mucosa, thus promoting allergen contact with deeper lying mast cells. Release of chemotactic factors such as eosinophil chemotactic factor of anaphylaxis (ECF-A), neutrophil chemotactic factor of anaphylaxis (NCF-A) and LTB_4 would stimulate migration of inflammatory cells to the site of mast cell activation, aided by the increased vascular permeability and venodilatation caused by histamine, PGD_2 and LTC_4[38]. Moreover, both PGD_2 and LTC_4 produce bronchial hyperreactivity to stimuli such as histamine and methacholine in asthmatic patients, although it is only transient with the latter stimulus, unlike the two other slow reacting substances of anaphylaxis, LTD_4 and LTE_4, which produce prolonged hyperreactivity[39,40]. Eosinophils contribute their own spectrum of inflammatory mediators such as eosinophil major basic protein (MBP), which disrupts bronchial epithelium and LTB_4. By these mechanisms, the initial acute response to allergen by the mast cells can be prolonged to several hours.

In fibrotic lung diseases also, increased numbers of mast cells have been reported[41,42]. As described in the following section, mouse skin derived 3T3 fibroblasts prolong the survival of rat connective tissue mast cells[43] and human lung mast cells[44]. Consequently, the production of SCF by fibroblasts may explain, at least in part, mast cell growth and differentiation during fibrosis. Mast cell tryptase in turn enhances proliferation of fibroblasts, suggesting a two way interaction between mast cells and fibroblasts[45].

HUMAN MAST CELL CYTOKINE PRODUCTION

The interactions between immune and inflammatory cells are mediated in large part by cytokines which promote cell growth, differentiation, and functional activation. Cytokines represent the basis for complex networks of cell to cell signalling in more global physiological or pathological processes[46–49]. Recent technical developments in molecular biology and biochemical research have considerably extended our knowledge about allergic inflammation. *In vitro* experiments, particularly using cell lines, have provided information about some actions of cytokines relevant to allergic inflammation. For example, IL-1 stimulates the expression of the adhesion protein, endothelial leucocyte adhesion molecule (ELAM—now known as E-selectin)[50], IL-3 and IL-4 stimulate basophil growth and differentiation[51], IL-5 stimulates eosinophil differentiation and maturation[52–55], IL-4 switches B cell immunoglobulin production to IgE[56–59], and IL-6 activates T cells[60], induces the differentiation of B cells into high immunoglobulin secreting plasma cells[61] and potentiates IL-4 induced IgE synthesis by B cells[62]. Because of the association of cytokines with T lymphocytes, many workers have suggested that allergic inflammation is orchestrated by these cells[63]. However, mast cells may also participate significantly in cytokine production (Fig. 9.2). Murine mast cell lines have been shown to produce IL-1, IL-2, IL-3, IL-4, IL-5, IL-6, granulocyte macrophage colony stimulating factor (GM-CSF), interferon gamma (IFNγ), tumour necrosis factor α (TNFα), macrophage inflammatory protein -1α (MIP-1α), MIP-1β, T cell activation antigen 3 (TCA-3) and monocyte chemoattractant protein-1 (MCP-1) following activation by IgE- and calcium ionophore-dependent stimuli[64–69]. However, the murine mast cell lines used in these studies were derived from the same progenitor cells as Th2 lymphocytes, which have the same spectrum of cytokine production.

The pertinent question is whether or not human mast cells generate cytokines and, if so, which cytokines. Using the reverse transcriptase polymerase chain reaction (RT-PCR) we have demonstrated the presence within human lung mast cells of mRNA for IL-4, IL-5, IL-6, IL-8, IL-10, IL-13, GM-CSF and TNFα[70–72], thus illustrating their potential to produce a unique and wide spectrum of cytokines.

Using sequential 2 µm glycolmethycrylate embedded sections stained with antibodies to mast cell tryptase and the cytokine under investigation, IL-4, IL-5, IL-6 and TNFα, immunoreactivity has been localised to mast cells of the bronchial and nasal mucosal[73–75]. There was a significant increase in the number of TNFα positive cells in the mucosa in asthma, but not of cells staining for IL-5 or IL-6[74,75]. IL-4 positive mast cells were also increased in the nasal and bronchial mucosa of patients with rhinitis and asthma, respectively[74,75]. Using a sandwich technique in which consecutive biopsy sections were stained with antibodies to human mast cell tryptase, the cytokine in question and human mast cell chymase, IL-4 was found to be present in both MC$_{TC}$ and MC$_T$, whereas IL-5 and IL-6 were associated exclusively with the MC$_T$ subset, suggesting that mast cell heterogeneity exists with respect to both cytokine expression and protease production[76]. Furthermore, immunogold electron microscopy indicated that IL-4 was localised to the granules of mast cells[77], although it is not known whether it is bound ionically to heparin in an inactive form, or is available for release in an active form on mast cell degranulation.

Our isolated human lung mast cell studies with RT-PCR and *in situ* hybridisation analysis of mRNA and enzyme linked immunosorbent assay (ELISA) measurement of cytokine product have concentrated on IL-4, IL-5, IL-6 and TNFα. Cross linkage of high affinity Fc$_\varepsilon$ receptors (Fc$_\varepsilon$RI) with anti-IgE consistently induced expression of mRNA for IL-5 at 2–48 or 2–72 h after stimulation, whereas mRNA for IL-4 was detectable in only six of 13 experiments[78]. Densitometric analysis of gels of RT-PCR indicated that, at all concentrations tested, anti-IgE enhanced the intensity of the IL-5 mRNA signal, the optimum concentration being 1–10 μg·ml^{-1}. Constitutive expression of IL-6 and TNFα was seen in purified mast cells cultured for 16 h with 10 ng·ml^{-1} SCF together with 3 μg·ml^{-1} myeloma IgE. However, mast cell activation with anti-IgE led to an increase in intensity of TNFα mRNA expression, suggesting the regulation of this cytokine by both SCF and IgE dependent stimulation.

The use of sandwich ELISAs has shown the mast cells to produce large amounts of IL-5 (up to 1.5 ng·10^{-6} mast cells per 24 h) and TNFα (up to 150 pg·10^{-6} mast cells per 24 h). Interestingly, the major stimulus appears to be different for generation of each of these cytokines, Fc$_\varepsilon$RI–IgE dependent stimulation initiating IL-5 production and SCF initiating TNFα production, although production of the latter is enhanced by immunological stimulation. Time course studies showed the peak production time for IL-5 to be 4–12 h after challenge, whereas that of TNFα was more rapid, the cytokine being generated maximally 2–4 h after stimulation.

IL-5, the main cytokine responsible for eosinophil differentiation, migration and activation, is expressed only by a limited group of fully differentiated cells: eosinophils, mast cells and subsets of T cells[79,80]. Our preliminary studies showed that human lung mast cells produce large amounts of IL-5. In studies of human T cell clones grown from human airway[81], a small number of clones weakly expressed IL-5 after stimulation. If the IL-5 signalling pathway is different from that in T cells, the fact that IL-5 appears to activate a unique set of transduction molecules in human mast cells may mean that highly specific agents targeting the actions of these molecules could form the basis of advanced treatments for allergy and asthma.

The consequences of cytokine release from mast cells remains to be determined in detail. However, it has been reported that these cytokines can influence a broad spectrum of biological responses. After activation, cytokines such as TNFα, which mediate "proinflammatory" events, may be involved in the initial accumulation of inflammatory cells in antigen stimulated tissue[82]. Indeed, endothelial cells can be stimulated by TNFα to express adherence proteins such as ELAM-1 and vascular cell adhesion molecule-1[83]. In addition, Gauchat *et al.* have demonstrated that IgE synthesis can be induced by the interaction of B cells with human mast cells and basophils in the presence of IL-4 by the interaction of CD40 and its ligand[59]. Thus the ability of mast cells to release cytokines with proinflammatory properties would suggest a role for these cells in the initiation and maintenance of allergic inflammation. Later, cytokines such as IL-5 have an effect on the proliferation or function of mast cells and other inflammatory cells[82].

The release of cytokines from mast cells may have a bearing on the migration and development of mast cells themselves. The response to tissue injury in asthma and other inflammatory disease is generally accompanied by an infiltration of mast cells into the damaged tissues, particularly along the basement membrane[84]. In human uterine mast cells, there is expression of very late activating antigen-4 (VLA-4) (CD49d/29), VLA-5 (CD49e/29), and vitronectin receptor (CD51/61), but not VLA-2 or VLA-6[85]. The derivation of mast cells in either mucosal or connective tissue sites from a putative common progenitor in man is not yet clear, nor is the lineage interrelationship between the two subtypes of mast cell. The mechanisms by which mature or immature mast cells recognise their final tissue site is not known, but may well be influenced by the profile of cytokines released by mast cells.

CONCLUSION

The potential of mast cells to act as important effector cells in mucosal defence and allergic disease is now well established. These cells can rapidly release histamine, PGD_2 and other potent mediators of inflammation in response to a range of agonists. The demonstration that mast cells can also release inflammatory cytokines confers on this cell type a role in the induction and modulation of immune reactions. There is a need for further investigation of the contribution made by cytokines from mast cells to inflammatory responses. Improved understanding of the ability of mast cells to produce cytokines and other mediators will greatly advance our knowledge of the cellular basis of the link between the early and later phases of IgE dependent inflammation.

REFERENCES

1. Furitsu T, Saito H, Dvorak A M, *et al*. Development of human mast cells *in vitro*. *Proc Natl Acad Sci USA* 1989; **86:** 10039–10043.
2. Irani A A, Bradford T R, Kepley C L, *et al*. Detection of MC_T and MC_{TC} types of human mast cells by immunohistochemistry using new monoclonal anti-tryptase and anti-chymase antibodies. *J Histochem Cytochem* 1989; **37:** 1509–1515.
3. Irani A A, Schechter N M, Craig S S, *et al*. Two types of human mast cells that have distinct neutral protease compositions. *Proc Natl Acad Sci USA* 1986; **83:** 4464–4468.
4. Irani A A, Buckley R, Haynes B, *et al*. Selective depletion of T mast cells in intestinal mucosa of patients with defective lymphocyte function [Abstract]. *J Allergy Clin Immunol* 1987; **79:** 178.
5. Irani A M, Nilsson G, Miettinen U, *et al*. Recombinant human stem cell factor stimulates differentiation of mast cells from dispersed human fetal liver cells. *Blood* 1992; **80:** 3009–3021.
6. Kirshenbaum A S, Goff J P, Dreskin S C, *et al*. IL-3-dependent growth of basophil-like cells and mast-like cells from human bone marrow. *J Immunol* 1989; **142:** 2424–2429.
7. Kirshenbaum A S, Goff J P, Kessler S W, *et al*. Effect of IL-3 and stem cell factor on the appearance of human basophils and mast cells from CD34[+] pluripotent progenitor cells. *J Immunol* 1991; **148:** 772–777.
8. Craig S S, Schechter N M, Schwartz L B. Ultrastructural analysis of maturing human T and TC mast cells *in situ*. *Lab Invest* 1989; **60:** 147–157.
9. Saito H, Matsumoto K, Sakaguchi N, *et al*. Emergence of mast cell precursors in human peripheral blood [Abstract]. *Allergy* 1992; **47:** 222.

10. Valent P, Spanblochl E, Sperr W R, *et al.* Induction of differentiation of human mast cells from bone marrow and peripheral blood mononuclear cells by recombinant human stem cell factor/kit-ligand in long-term culture. *Blood* 1992; **80:** 2237–2245.

11. Saito H, Sakaguchi N, Matsumoto K, *et al.* Growth in methylcellulose of human mast cells in hematopoietic colonies stimulated by steel factor, a c-kit ligand. *Int Arch Allergy Immunol* 1994; **103:** 143–151.

12. Riley J F, West G B. Skin histamine: its location in the tissue mast cells. *Arch Dermatol* 1956; **74:** 471–478.

13. Ishizaka T, Tomioka H, Ishizaka K. Mechanisms of passive sensitization. I. Presence of IgE and IgG molecules on human leukocytes. *J Immunol* 1970; **105:** 1459–1467.

14. Tomioka H, Ishizaka K. Mechanisms of passive sensitization. II. Presence of receptors for IgE on monkey mast cells. *J Immunol* 1971; **107:** 971–978.

15. Bienenstock J, Austen K F, Galli S J. Nomenclature of mast cells and basophils (1989). In: Galli S J, Austen K F, eds. *Mast Cell and Basophil Differentiation and Function in Health and Disease.* New York: Raven Press, 1989; 329–331.

16. Irani A A, Schwartz L B. Neutral proteases as indicators of human mast cell heterogeneity. In: Schwartz L B, ed. *Neutral Proteases of Mast Cells.* Basel: Karger, 1990; 146–162.

17. Schwartz L B, Atkins P C, Bradford T R, *et al.* Release of tryptase together with histamine during immediate cutaneous response to allergen. *J Allergy Clin Immunol* 1987; **80:** 850–855.

18. Raud J, Sydbom A, Dahlen S-E, *et al.* Prostaglandin E2 prevents diclofenac-induced enhancement of histamine release and inflammation evoked by *in vivo* challenge with compound 48/80 in the hamster cheek pouch. *Agents Actions* 1989; **28:** 108–114.

19. Schwartz L B, Kawahara M S, Hugli T E, *et al.* Generation of C3a anaphylatoxin from human C3 by human mast cell tryptase. *J Immunol* 1983; **130:** 1891–1895.

20. Schwartz L B, Bradford T M, Littman B L, *et al.* The fibrinogenolytic activity of purified tryptase from human lung mast cells. *J Immunol* 1985; **135:** 2762–2767.

21. Schwartz L B, Maier M, Spragg J. Interaction of human low molecular weight kininogen with human mast cell tryptase. *Adv Exp Med Biol* 1986; **198A:** 105–111.

22. Church M K, Benyon R C, Rees P H, *et al.* Functional heterogeneity of human mast cells. In: Galli S J, Austen K F, eds. *Mast Cell and Basophil Differentiation and Function in Health and Disease.* New York: Raven Press, 1989; 161–170.

23. Lowman M A, Benyon R C, Church M K. Characterization of neuropeptide-induced histamine released from human dispersed skin mast cells. *Br J Pharmacol* 1988; **95:** 121–130.

24. El Lati S G, Dahinden C A, Church M K. Complement peptides C3a- and C5a-induced mediator release from dissociated human skin mast cells. *J Invest Dermatol* 1994; **102:** 803–806.

25. Lowman M A, Rees P H, Benyon R C, *et al.* Human mast cell heterogeneity: histamine release from mast cells dispersed from skin, lung, adenoids, tonsils and intestinal mucosa in response to IgE-dependent and non-immunological stimuli. *J Allergy Clin Immunol* 1988; **81:** 590–597.

26. Okayama Y, Benyon R C, Rees P H, *et al.* Inhibition profiles of sodium cromoglycate and nedocromil sodium on mediator release from mast cells of human skin, lung, tonsil, adenoid and intestine. *Clin Exp Allergy* 1992; **22:** 401–409.

27. Okayama Y, Church M K. Comparison of the modulatory effect of ketotifen, sodium cromoglycate, procaterol and salbutamol in human skin, lung and tonsil mast cells. *Int Arch Allergy Immunol* 1992; **97:** 216–225.

28. Okayama Y, Benyon R C, Lowman M A, *et al.* In vitro effects of H-1-antihistamines on histamine and PGD(2) release from mast cells of human lung, tonsil, and skin. *Allergy* 1994; **49:** 246–253.

29. Ruitenberg E J, Elgersma A. Absence of intestinal mast cell response in congenitally athymic mice during *Trichinella spiralis* infection. *Nature* 1976; **264:** 258–260.

30. Mayrhofer G. The nature of the thymus dependency of mucosal mast cells. I. An adaptive secondary response to challenge with *Nippostrongylus brasiliensis. Cell Immunol* 1979; **47:** 304–311.

31. Mayrhofer G. The nature of the thymus dependency of mucosal mast cells. II. The effect of thymectomy and of depleting circulating lymphocytes on the response to *Nippostrongylus brasiliensis. Cell Immunol* 1979; **47:** 312–322.

32. Mayrhofer G, Bazin H. The nature of the thymus dependency of mucosal mast cells. III. Mucosal mast cells in nude mice and nude rats, in B rats and in a child with the Di George syndrome. *Int Arch Allergy Appl Immunol* 1981; **64:** 320–331.

33. Woodbury R G, Miller H R P, Huntley J F, *et al.* Mucosal mast cells are functionally active during spontaneous expulsion of intestinal nematode infections in the rat. *Nature* 1984; **312:** 450–452.

34. Hogg J C. Pathologic abnormalities in asthma. In: Lichtenstein L M. Austen K F, eds. *Asthma: Physiology, and Treatment, Second International Symposium.* New York: Academic Press, 1977; 1–120.

35. Lamb D, Lumsden A. Intra-epithelial mast cells in human airway epithelium—evidence for smoking-induced changes in their frequency. *Thorax* 1982; **37:** 334–342.

36. Eiser N M. Histamine. In: Barnes P J, Rodger I W, Thompson N C, eds. *Asthma: Basic Mechanisms and Clinical Management,* 2nd Edn. London: Academic Press, 1992; 249–275.

37. Ichinose M, Barnes P J. Inhibitory histamine H3-receptors on cholinergic nerves in human airways. *Eur J Pharmacol* 1989; **163:** 383–386.

38. Raphael G D, Metcalfe D D. Mediators of airway inflammation. *Eur J Respir Dis* 1986; **69** (suppl 147): 44–57.

39. O'Byrne P M. Prostaglandins and thromboxanes. In: Barnes P J, Rodger I W, Thompson N C, eds. *Asthma: Basic Mechanisms and Clinical Management,* 2nd Edn. London: Academic Press, 1992; 225–234.

40. Drazen J M. Cysteinyl leukotrienes. In: Barnes P J, Rodger I W, Thompson N C, eds. *Asthma: Basic Mechanisms and Clinical Treatment,* 2nd Edn. London: Academic Press, 1992; 235–247.

41. Kawanami O, Ferrans V J, Fulmer J D, *et al.* Ultrastructure of pulmonary mast cells in patients with fibrotic lung disorders. *Lab Invest* 1985; **40:** 717–734.

42. Goto T, Befus D, Low R, *et al.* Mast cell heterogeneity and hyperplasia in bleomycin-induced pulmonary fibrosis of rats. *Am Rev Respir Dis* 1984; **130:** 797–802.

43. Levi-Schaffer F, Austen K F, Caulfield J P, *et al.* Fibroblasts maintain the phenotype and viability of the rat heparin-containing mast cell in vitro. *J Immunol* 1985; **135:** 3454–3462.

44. Levi-Schaffer F, Austen K F, Caulfield J P, *et al.* Co-culture of human lung-derived mast cells with mouse 3T3 fibroblasts: morphology and IgE-mediated release of histamine, prostaglandin D2 and leukotrienes. *J Immunol* 1987; **139:** 494–500.

45. Ruoss S J, Hartmann T, Caughey G H. Mast cell tryptase is a mitogen for cultured fibroblasts. *J Clin Invest* 1991; **88:** 493–499.

46. McNeil H P, Austen K F, Somerville L L, *et al.* Molecular cloning of the mouse mast cell protease-5 gene. A novel secretory granule protease expressed early in the differentiation of serosal mast cells. *J Biol Chem* 1991; **266:** 20316–20322.

47. Knapp H R, Sladek K, Fitzgerald G A. Increased excretion of leukotriene E_4 during aspirin-induced asthma. *J Lab Clin Med* 1992; **119:** 48–51.

48. Solway J, Leff A R. Sensory neuropeptides and airway function. *J Appl Physiol* 1991; **71:** 2077–2087.

49. Taylor M B, Easmon C S F. The neutrophil chemiluminescence response to *Pneumocystis carinii* is stimulated by GM-CSF and gamma interferon. *FEMS Microbiol Immunol* 1991; **89:** 41–44.

50. Mizel S B. Interleukin 1 Biology and molecular biology. In: Poste G, Crooke S T, eds. *Cellular and Molecular Aspects of Inflammation.* New York: Plenum, 1988; 75–96.

51. Ishizaka T, Saito H, Furitsu T, *et al.* Growth of human basophils and mast cells *in vitro.* In: Galli S J, Austen K F, eds. *Mast Cell and Basophil Differentiation and Function in Health and Disease.* New York: Raven Press, 1989; 39–47.

52. Clutterbuck E J, Hirst E M, Sanderson C J. Human interleukin-5 (IL-5) regulates the production of eosinophils in human bone marrow cultures: comparison and interaction with IL-1, IL-3, IL-6, and GMCSF. *Blood* 1989; **73:** 1504–1512.

53. Lopez A F, Sanderson C J, Gamble J R, *et al.* Recombinant human interleukin-5 is a selective activator of human eosinophil function. *J Exp Med* 1988; **167:** 219–224.

54. Wang J M, Rambaldi A, Biondi A, *et al.* Recombinant human interleukin 5 is a selective eosinophil chemoattractant. *Eur J Immunol* 1989; **19:** 701–705.

55. Sher A, Coffman R L, Hieny S, *et al*. Interleukin-5 is required for the blood and tissue eosinophilia but not granuloma formation induced by infection with *Schistosoma mansoni*. *Proc Natl Acad Sci USA* 1990; **87:** 61–65.

56. Paul W E, Ohara J. B-cell stimulatory factor-1/interleukin 4. *Annu Rev Immunol* 1987; **5:** 429–460.

57. Delespesse G, Safati H, Heusser C. IgE synthesis. *Curr Opin Immunol* 1990; **2:** 506–512.

58. Finkelman F D, Urbàn J F, Beckmann M P, *et al*. Regulation of murine *in vivo* IgG and IgE responses by monoclonal anti-IL-4 receptor antibody. *Int Immunol* 1991; **3:** 599–607.

59. Gauchat J-F, Henchoz S, Mazzei G, *et al*. Induction of human IgE synthesis in B cells by mast cells and basophils. *Nature* 1993; **365:** 340–343.

60. Tosato G, Pike S E. Interferon-beta 2/interleukin 6 is a co-stimulant for human T lymphocytes. *J Immunol* 1988; **141:** 1556–1562.

61. Muraguchi A, Hirano T, Tang B, *et al*. The essential role of B cell stimulatory factor (BSF-2/IL-6) for the terminal differentiation of B cells. *J Exp Med* 1988; **167:** 332–344.

62. Vercelli D, Jabara H H, Arai K, *et al*. Endogenous interleukin 6 plays an obligatory role in interleukin 4-dependent human IgE synthesis. *Eur J Immunol* 1989; **19:** 1419–1424.

63. Frew A J, Kay A B. The relationship between infiltrating CD4+ lymphocytes, activated eosinophils and the magnitude of the allergen-induced late phase cutaneous reaction in man. *J Immunol* 1988; **141:** 4158–4164.

64. Chung S W, Wong P M C, Shen-Ong G, *et al*. Production of granulocyte-macrophage colony-stimulating factor by Abelson virus-induced tumorigenic mast cell lines. *Blood* 1986; **68:** 1074–1081.

65. Brown M A, Pierce J H, Watson C J, *et al*. B cell stimulatory factor-1/interleukin-4 mRNA is expressed by normal and transformed mast cells. *Cell* 1987; **50:** 809–818.

66. Humphries R K, Abraham S, Krystal G, *et al*. Activation of multiple hemopoietic growth factors in Abelson virus transformed myeloid cells. *Exp Hematol* 1988; **16:** 774–781.

67. Young J D E, Liu C C, Butler G, *et al*. Identification, purification and characterization of a mast cell associated cytolytic factor related to tumor necrosis factor. *Proc Natl Acad Sci USA* 1987; **84:** 9175–9179.

68. Richards A L, Okuno T, Takagaki Y, *et al*. Natural cytotoxic cell-specific cytotoxic factor produced by IL-3-dependent basophilic/mast cells. *J Immunol* 1988; **141:** 3061–3066.

69. Wodnar-Filipowicz A, Heusser C H, Moroni C. Production of the haemopoietic growth factors GM-CSF and interleukin-3 by mast cells in response to IgE receptor-mediated activation. *Nature* 1989; **11:** 150–152.

70. Okayama Y, Quint D J, Hunt T C, *et al*. Expression of IL-4 mRNA in human dermal mast cells in response to Fc receptor cross-linkage in the presence of SCF [Abstract]. *J Allergy Clin Immunol* 1993; **91:** 256.

71. Okayama Y, Petit-Frère C, Kassel O, *et al*. Expression of mRNA for IL-4 and IL-5 in human skin and lung mast cells in response to Fcε receptor cross-linkage and the presence of stem cell factor [Abstract]. *Allergy Clin Immunol News* 1994; (suppl 2): 37.

72. Okayama Y, Bradding P, Tunon de Lara J M, *et al*. Cytokine production by human mast cells. In: Marone G, ed. *Human Basophils and Mast Cells in Health and Disease*. Basel: Karger, 1995; 114–134.

73. Bradding P, Feather I H, Howarth P H, *et al*. Interleukin 4 is localized to and released by human mast cells. *J Exp Med* 1992; **176:** 1381–1386.

74. Bradding P, Feather I H, Wilson S, *et al*. Immunolocalization of cytokines in the nasal mucosa of normal and perennial rhinitic subjects: the mast cell as a source of IL-4, IL-5 and IL-6 in human allergic mucosal inflammation. *J Immunol* 1993; **151:** 3853–3865.

75. Bradding P, Roberts J A, Britten K M, *et al*. Interleukin-4, -5, and -6 and tumor necrosis factor-alpha in normal and asthmatic airways: evidence for the human mast cell as a source of these cytokines. *Am J Respir Cell Mol Biol* 1994; **10:** 471–480.

76. Church M K, Okayama Y, Bradding P. Functional mast cell heterogeneity. In: Busse W W, Holgate S T, eds. *Asthma and Rhinitis*. Oxford: Blackwell Scientific, 1995; 209–220.

77. Wilson S, Bradding P, Heusser C, *et al*. The subcellular localisation of interleukin 4 in the respiratory mucosa using immunoelectron microscopy [Abstract]. *Clin Exp Allergy* 1994; **24:** 980.

78. Okayama Y, Petit-Frère C, Kassel O, *et al.* The IgE-dependent expression of mRNA for IL-4 and IL-5 in human lung mast cells. *J Immunol* 1995; **155:** 1796–1808.

79. Yokota T, Arai N, De Vries J, *et al.* Molecular biology of interleukin 4 and interleukin 5 genes and biology of their products which stimulate B cells, T cells and hemopoietic cells. *Immunol Rev* 1988; **102:** 137–187.

80. Desreumaux P, Janin A, Colombel J F, *et al.* Interleukin 5 messenger RNA expression by eosinophils in the intestinal mucosa of patients with coeliac disease. *J Exp Med* 1992; **175:** 293–296.

81. Bodey K, Semper A E, Madden J, Cytokine mRNA pattern in BAL T cell clones from asthmatic airways [Abstract]. *Clin Exp Allergy* 1994; **24:** 981.

82. Gordon J R, Burd P R, Galli S J. Mast cells as a source of multifunctional cytokines. *Immunol Today* 1990; **11:** 458–464.

83. Osborn L, Hession C, Tizard R, *et al.* Direct expression cloning of vascular cell adhesion molecule 1, a cytokine-induced endothelial protein that binds to lymphocytes. *Cell* 1989; **59:** 1203–1211.

84. Varsano S, Lazarus S C, Gold W M, *et al.* Selective adhesion of mast cells to tracheal epithelial cells *in vitro*. *J Immunol* 1988; **140:** 2184–2192.

85. Guo C-B, Kagey-Sobotka A, Lichtenstein L M, *et al.* Immunophenotyping and functional analysis of purified human uterine mast cells. *Blood* 1992; **79:** 708–712.

10

Epithelial Cells in Host Defense

S. I. RENNARD, W. W. WEST AND RICHARD A. ROBBINS*

University of Nebraska Medical Center, Omaha, USA

INTRODUCTION

The epithelial cells which line the luminal surface of the airways and the air spaces of the lung provide essential components of host defense by a variety of mechanisms. Included among these are the production and clearance of secretions, maintenance of an effective barrier, recruitment and regulation of inflammatory cells, regulation of airway smooth muscle and subepithelial vascular function, metabolism of inhaled toxicants, and mediation of repair responses following injury. This review will briefly describe the epithelial cells of the lung and then describe the functioning of airway epithelial cells in host defense.

LUNG EPITHELIAL CELLS

The epithelial cells of the lung originate from the embryonic foregut[1,2]. The lung bud develops from an interaction between epithelial cells of the embryonic foregut together with surrounding mesenchyme: both cell types proliferate to form the bud, which both enlarges and undergoes dichotomous branching. The proximal portion remains connected to the embryonic foregut and forms the trachea. The more distal portions continue to branch, forming the conducting airways. Proliferation is maximal at the branching tips. Differentiation occurs after proliferation is diminished and, therefore, proceeds in a proximal to distal fashion. The bronchial circulation develops concurrently with the branching lung bud. The final stages of lung development, the formation of alveoli, takes place only after the conducting airways have formed. There is considerable species

---

* Present address: Overton Brooks Medical Center, Shreveport, USA.

Pulmonary Defences. Edited by Robert A. Stockley.
© 1997 John Wiley & Sons Ltd.

variation in the timing of alveolar development. In man, alveoli continue to develop after birth.

Because all epithelial cells of the lung share a common developmental origin, it is not surprising that they share many similarities despite the marked differences in differentiated phenotype. Much of current knowledge regarding lung epithelial cell function is derived from *in vitro* studies. In these circumstances, it is possible that cells have "de-differentiated." While there are species differences, the proximal airways are lined with a pseudostratified columnar epithelium which consists largely of ciliated cells, basal cells and smaller numbers of goblet cells[3,4] (Fig. 10.1). Glands are relatively common proximally. In the more distal airways, the epithelium becomes progressively less multilayered, glands become less frequent and cells become less columnar. In the most distal airways, basal cells are generally absent, ciliated cells and goblet cells are more cuboidal in shape, and Clara cells occur with increasing frequency (Fig. 10.2). These cells then merge with type II and type I alveolar epithelial cells which line the surface of respiratory bronchioles and alveoli[5,6].

The epithelial cells which form the lining of the luminal surface are attached to their neighbors by a number of cell–cell junctions. Included among these are tight junctions, intermediate junctions, gap junctions and desmosomes[3]. Desmosomes are believed to mediate the mechanical adhesion of cells to their neighbors, thus preserving the mechanical integrity of the epithelium[7]. Basal cells not only have desmosomes with which they interact with columnar cells, but also hemidesmosomes which are present on the basal surface[3,7]. These structures appear to interact with type VII collagen-containing anchoring fibrils, and are believed to be crucial in preserving the mechanical adhesion of the entire epithelium to the basement membrane[8–10]. Gap junctions serve as a means of cell–cell communication[11]. These connections between cells permit the epithelium to function as an electrically integrated unit, and also allow small molecules to travel between airway epithelial cells[11]. Communication via gap junctions is believed to help maintain uniform beating of cilia[12,13] and transport through gap junctions may be a means for cells to provide their neighbors with defense molecules such as antioxidants[14]. The intermediate junction, or zonule adherens, contains several cell–cell adhesion molecules[15–17] and provides an anchor point for cytoskeletal elements[18]. The tight junctions which are present just below the luminal surface are complex structures which completely obliterate the intercellular space[3,19]. These structures thus form a barrier segregating both the luminal space from the interior of the pulmonary parenchyma and, simultaneously, the external surfaces of the apical and basolateral cell membrane[20–22]. This organization serves at least two functions crucial to host defense. First, the close apposition of adjacent cells creates an effective mechanical barrier[21]. Second, many surface proteins are segregated into the apical or basolateral surfaces[20]. This organization therefore allows for polarity in function and permits maintenance of an ionic gradient and forms the basis for directional secretion of many substances.

The epithelial barrier can be disrupted by a variety of injuries, including those caused by inhaled particles and toxins[23,24]. It is likely that barrier function can also be modulated by inflammatory mediators[25,26]. In this regard, an

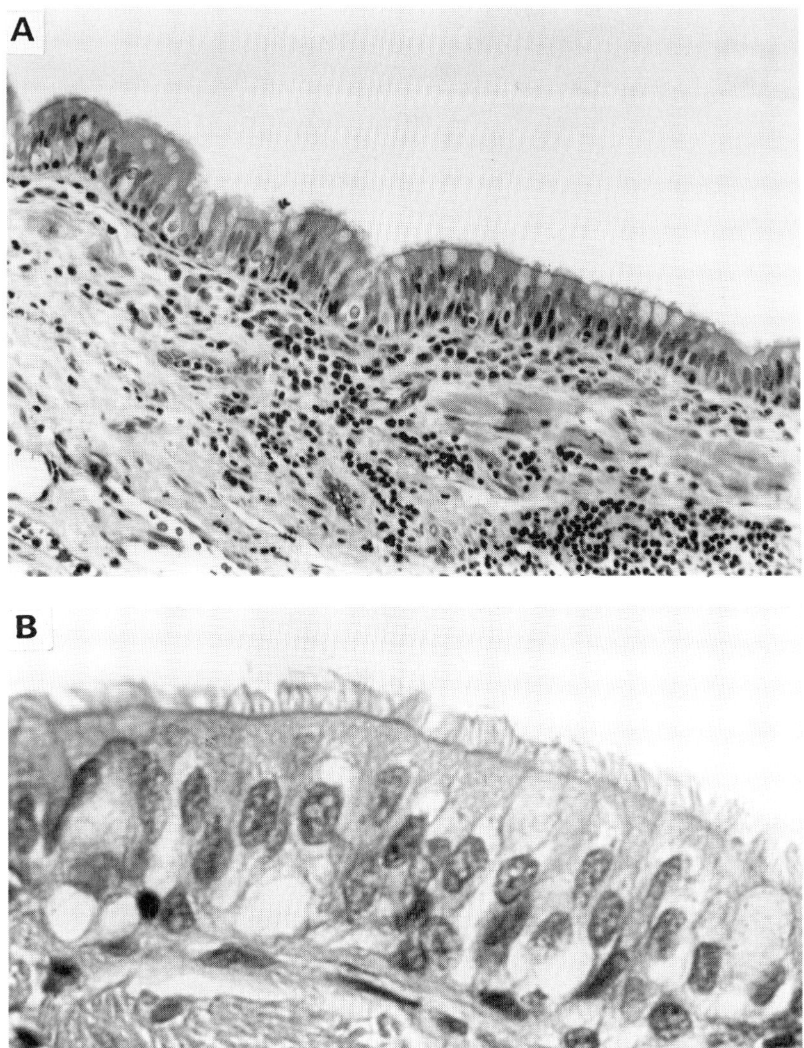

Figure 10.1. A: Proximal airway. Light microscopic view of the tall pseudostratified ciliated columnar epithelium overlying a thin basement membrane and a submucosa with scattered chronic inflammatory cells. **B:** Closer examination reveals a pseudostratified columnar mucosa that is predominantly composed of ciliated cells, with a smaller number of goblet cells and basal cells

increase in intracellular calcium and cAMP increases epithelial resistance[27,28], while activation of protein kinase C has the opposite effect[29]. Loss of barrier function probably plays an important pathogenetic part in many lung injuries. Conversely, maintenance and restoration of barrier function is likely to be an important aspect both of host defense and of repair following injury.

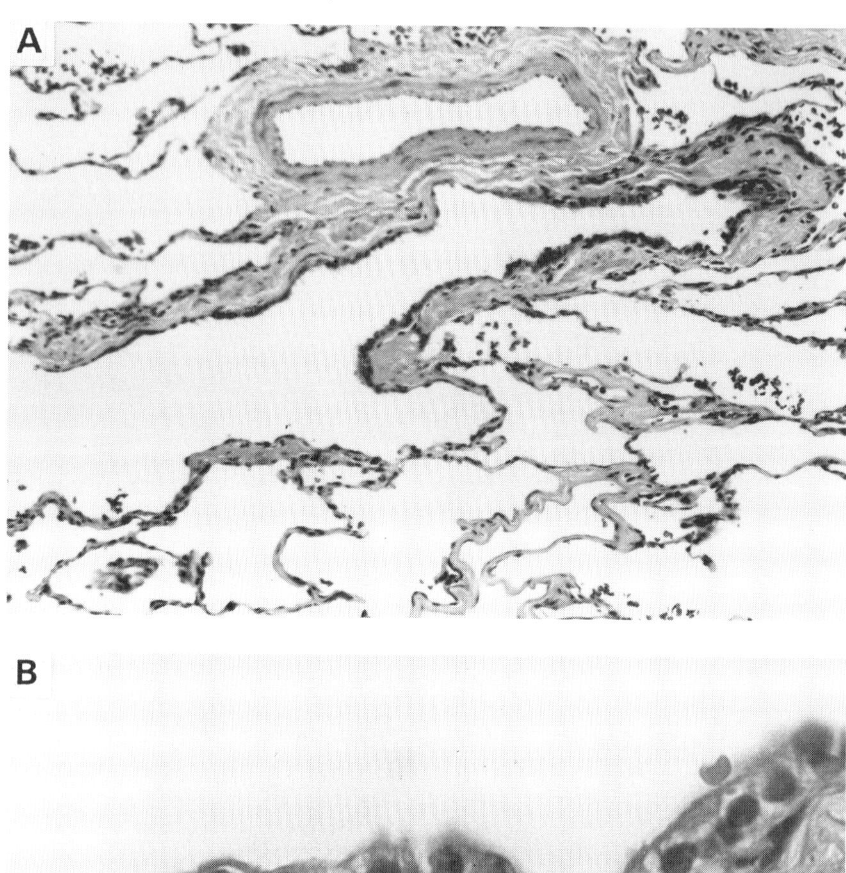

Figure 10.2. A: Distal airway at the level of the terminal bronchiole/respiratory bronchiole. Light microscopic view of the low columnar to cuboidal epithelium overlying a thin basement membrane and a thin fibromuscular submucosa. **B:** Closer examination reveals a simple mucosal lining with proportionately fewer ciliated cells and the relative absence of goblet cells. The epithelial cells become more cuboidal. Some of the cuboidal cells in this photo may represent Clara cells

AIRWAY EPITHELIAL CELLS IN HOST DEFENSE

MUCUS SECRETION AND MUCOCILIARY CLEARANCE

The luminal surface of the lung is lined by a fluid layer. Detailed reviews on the biochemistry, biology and production of the various components of airway secretion are available elsewhere[30-34]. This section will provide an overview of airway secretions in host defense.

The deepest layer of airway secretion is the "sol" layer. This is an aqueous solution, the volume and composition of which is determined by the activity of luminal secretory cells. The depth of the aqueous layer decreases from the proximal to the distal airways, but is generally believed to be sufficient for the cilia which line the apical surface of ciliated cells to just reach the "gel" layer which consists of a viscoelastic mixture of airway mucins, together with other secreted proteins.

Several transport mechanisms on airway epithelial cells have been described[31]. Importantly, the volume and composition of the aqueous airway secretions can be regulated through the activity of several ion transporters which, in turn, can be modulated by a variety of mediators acting through several signal transduction pathways. In this regard, the mutation in cystic fibrosis has been particularly well studied, and serves as a good example. The most common mutation in cystic fibrosis results in a defective cystic fibrosis transmembrane receptor protein which is responsible for mediating cyclic AMP induced increases in chloride secretion[35]. The resulting alterations in epithelial lining fluid composition, particularly at times of stress, are believed to lead to poor clearance of bacteria from the airway and, thus, to the recognized clinical syndrome. The recognition that alternate pathways for regulation of chloride secretion exist, however, has led to the suggestion that therapeutic strategies may be designed to bypass the defect in cystic fibrosis[36,37].

Airway mucins are produced primarily, but not exclusively, by glandular mucus cells and luminal goblet cells[33,34,38]. The relative volume of these two cells is believed to be approximately 40:1[39] and, as a result, glandular mucus cells are believed to contribute to the bulk of mucins in most conditions. However, both glandular hyperplasia and goblet cell metaplasia occur in many lung diseases. Serous cells are also present in glands, being located distally. These cells release a variety of molecules believed to have important roles in host defense, including antiproteases, antioxidants and substances with antibacterial activity[34,40]. These secretions mix with the mucous cell secretions during their course into the airway lumen. Their release can be regulated by a variety of neurogenic and inflammatory mediators, in addition to bacterial products[34,40].

The most superficial layer of the epithelial lining fluid is a thin layer of surfactant[32]. This layer consists of a mixture of phospholipids, primarily lecithin and sphingomyelin, together with several surfactant apoproteins. At least two airway epithelial cells, alveolar type II cells and Clara cells, produce surfactant components. One of the major functions of surfactant is to reduce the surface tension of the epithelial lining fluid layer. This function is believed to be crucial to prevent alveolar collapse, particularly in areas of poorly ventilated lung. Surfactant, however, has a number of other functions. It has antibacterial antioxidant activity[41,42], and may also aid the mechanical clearance of particles deposited in the lung, at least in part, by coating hydrophobic surfaces and by functioning as an opsonin[43]. Finally, by providing a separate phase, surfactant may help to segregate certain enzymes to the luminal surface[44].

The epithelial cell lining fluid of the lung, therefore, is literally the first line of lung defense. Inhaled particles initially encounter this fluid which possesses antibacterial, antioxidant and antiproteolytic activity. In the more proximal airways, large particles can be trapped in the relatively sticky mucus secretions and cleared by cough. Distal to the sixth or seventh division, cough is ineffective, and mucus clearance depends on ciliary transport[45]. In the most distal airways, the mechanisms for clearance of inhaled particles are less well understood. Phagocytosis of particles by both resident and recruited inflammatory cells and, perhaps, mechanical clearance resulting from interactions between lung motion during breathing and surfactant may have a role. The ability of epithelial cells to modulate the production, composition and clearance of these secretions is a key defense mechanism.

INFLAMMATION

Epithelial cells also participate in host defenses as active participants in inflammation. These cells are capable of both producing and responding to a variety of eicosinoids, cytokines and growth factors which form a complex network regulating inflammatory responses. In addition, they can express cell surface receptors that can interact directly with inflammatory cells. With current methods, airway epithelial cells are easier to produce and maintain *in vitro*, and have been more thoroughly studied. Much current knowledge regarding the abilities of epithelial cells to interact in inflammatory processes is consequently derived from *in vitro* studies. As a result, some caution is needed in interpretation of the findings. Nevertheless, epithelial cells from both airways and alveoli appear to be active in inflammatory processes, and a large number of inflammatory mediators have been described as potential products of epithelial cells in the lung (Table 10.1).

Inflammatory Mediators

The enzymatic basis for the generation of active eicosanoids by airway epithelial cells is being defined, and includes phospholipases A2, lipoxygenase and cyclo-oxygenase[46]. The phospholipases A2 are a family of enzymes that hydrolyze the SN-2-ester bond of phospholipids, generating free fatty acids and lysophospholipids. Both secreted and cytosolic phospholipase A2 (cPLA2) have been described[47]. The cytosolic form is believed to hydrolyze arachidonic acid-containing phospholipids selectively and, hence, to be crucially important in regulating the production of arachidonic acid-derived eicosanoids[48]. cPLA2 is a complex enzyme which can be regulated by phosphorylation. Its phosphorylation can be modulated, at least in some cells, by cytokines[49,50]. Human airway epithelial cells express cPLA2, and synthesis of this enzyme can be modulated by at least two cytokines: tumor necrosis factor α (TNFα) and interferon gamma (IFNγ)[51,52]. IFNγ, moreover, has been demonstrated to increase the activity of cPLA2 in response to ionophore stimulation[51].

After liberation of arachidonic acid, formation of eicosanoids requires the activity of either lipoxygenase or cyclo-oxygenase enzymes[46]. 15-Lipoxygenase inserts oxygen on the carbon-15 of the arachidonic acid molecule and generates biologically active 15-hydroxyeicosatetraenoic acid (15-HETE). 15-HETE is an active neutrophil chemoattractant, stimulates mitogenic activity, and can modulate immune cells and neural hypersensitivity[46]. 15-Lipoxygenase mRNA

Table 10.1. Inflammatory mediators produced by
lung epithelial cells

Lipids	Peptides
PGE$_2$	Chemokines
PGF$_{22}$	IL-8
15-HETE	*groα*
8, 15-diHETE	*groγ*
LTB$_4$	MCP-1
PAF	Chemoattractant factors
	LCF
Other	Colony stimulation factors
Nitric oxide	GM-CSF
	M-CSF
	G-CSF
	Other peptides
	IL-1, IL-6, IL-11
	TNFα
	TGFα, TGFβ1, TGFβ2
	Endothelin I
	Annexin I, annexin II
	Substance P
	Arginine-vasopressin
	Fibronectin

PG = Prostaglandin; HETE = hydroxyeicosatetraenoic acid; LT = leukotriene; PAF = platelet activating factor; IL = interleukin; MCP = monocyte chemoattractant protein; LCF = lymphocyte chemoattractant factor; GM-, M-, G-CSF = granulocyte macrophage, macrophage and granulocyte colony stimulating factors; TNF = tumor necrosis factor; TGF = transforming growth factor.

can be induced by interleukin-4 (IL-4) and, in some cells, this induction can be blocked by glucocorticoids and IFNγ[53]. Immunohistochemical studies suggest that 15-lipoxygenase is prominently expressed *in vivo* in the airway epithelium[46]. It remains controversial whether other lipoxygenases are expressed by normal airway epithelium. Five lipoxygenase products including, leukotriene B$_4$, (LTB$_4$), have been described in some species[54], but may be absent from man[46].

Cyclo-oxygenase catalyzes the oxygenation of arachidonic acid to yield prostaglandin H, from which prostaglandins, thromboxane and prostacyclin are derived[46]. Two forms of cyclo-oxygenase, cox 1 and cox 2, have been described. Cox 1 appears to be a constitutively expressed enzyme, whereas cox 2, at least in some cells, can be modulated by a variety of stimuli[55]. As prostaglandins, particularly prostaglandin E, appear to be major products of epithelial cells[46], regulation of cyclo-oxygenase enzymes is likely to play an important part in host defense.

Lung epithelial cells have also been described as sources of a large and increasing number of peptide mediators. Some of the mediators noted in Table 10.1 have been described only in *in vitro* studies, which may be subject to species variability and methodologic problems including purity of cell isolates and specificity of assay techniques. Nevertheless, it is clear that epithelial cells are potent sources of peptide mediators with a variety of functional capabilities. These studies have been paralleled by functional assays demonstrating the capability of epithelial cells to release mediators which can drive the chemotactic recruitment of neutrophils[56], monocytes[57], lymphocytes[58], eosinophils[59] and basophils[60]. It is likely that the chemotactic recruitment of any individual cell type can be mediated by several different factors. For example, airway epithelial cells are capable of releasing both peptide chemotactic factors, including IL-8[61,62], and eicosanoid chemotactic factors, including 15-HETE[46] and, in some species, LTB_4[54], which can drive the recruitment of neutrophils. A variety of stimuli have been demonstrated to induce the release of either neutrophil chemotactic activity or IL-8 from cultured lung epithelial cells. These include cigarette smoke[63], endotoxin[56] and other bacterial products[64], viral infection[61], neutrophil elastase[62], acetylcholine[65], neuropeptides[66] and a variety of cytokines, including IL-1, TNF and IFNγ[67,68]. The ability of epithelial cells to respond to such a diverse group of mediators by releasing a variety of chemotactic substances suggests these cells may have a crucial role in amplifying inflammatory responses. There is evidence to suggest, in addition, that epithelial cells can secrete IL-8 in a directional manner, with preferential secretion into the lumen[69]. Such polar secretion may function to drive inflammatory cells into the airway lumen, which can help to partition an inflammatory response, allowing the barrier function of the epithelium to protect the pulmonary parenchymal structures. In addition, it is likely that cytokines released by epithelial cells can modify the neighboring vascular structures both to increase capillary permeability[70] and to increase expression of endothelial cell adhesion molecules[71] — which are required for adherence of circulating inflammatory cells and their subsequent migration. The ability of epithelial cells to modulate the various aspects of the chemotactic recruitment of inflammatory cells suggests they not only amplify inflammatory signals, but also determine the specificity of cells recruited and direct these cells to their ultimate destination. In this regard, it is interesting to note that neutrophils migrating into the lumen of the airway appear to follow specific "channels" through the epithelial surface[72]. The structures involved and the mechanisms responsible for this level of control of inflammatory cell recruitment are unknown, but should serve to restrict "colateral" damage that ensues from inflammatory cell recruitment.

Epithelial cells not only recruit inflammatory cells, but release growth factors which can sustain these cells. In the absence of appropriate growth factors, most normal cells undergo apoptosis or a programmed cell death. Airway epithelial cells, for example, have been shown to release cytokines, among which GM-CSF appears to be particularly important and can sustain eosinophil survival[73]. Once inflammatory cells are recruited to a site of inflammation, their function is regulated through the interaction of various cell surface adhesion molecules. Epithelial cells in the lung are capable of upregulating the expression of the adhesion molecule, intercellular adhesion molecule-1 (ICAM-1) in response to proinflammatory stimuli[74,75]. ICAM-1 is a ligand for leukocyte integrins (cluster of differentiation (CD)11, CD18). By inducing the expression of this adhesion molecule, inflammatory stimuli can provoke the binding of neutrophils to epithelial cell surfaces[74,75]. Such a mechanism may both be important for regulating inflammatory cell activity, and lead to epithelial cell injury[74]. ICAM-1-independent cell adhesion mechanisms for neutrophils and monocytes have also been described. In addition, epithelial cells are capable of expressing antigens of the major histocompatibility complex (MHC)[76]. Both MHC-class I and class II antigens are expressed by epithelial cells, and MHC class II antigens are upregulated by cytokines, including IFNγ[77,78]. Consistent with their expression of MHC class II antigens, epithelial cells have some capacity to present antigen to lymphocytes and could, therefore, function to regulate antigen driven lymphocyte responses[78,79].

In addition to eicosanoid and peptide mediators, epithelial cells are also a source of nitric oxide[80,81]. Nitric oxide can be produced through the action of two enzymes, the constitutively expressed nitric oxide synthase (cNOS) and the inducible iNOS. Epithelial cells express both enzymes and a variety of cytokines, including IL-1, IFNγ and TNF can upregulate the expression of iNOS — an effect which can be blocked by glucocorticoids[82,83]. Nitric oxide produced by epithelial cells probably functions in a number of capacities. Cilia beat frequency, as noted above, can be regulated by a variety of mediators, all of which appear to act with nitric oxide as a final common pathway[81,82]. Rapidly acting stimuli appear to alter cilia beating through the activity of cNOS, and more slowly acting stimuli appear to regulate the beating through the induction of iNOS gene expression[81,84].

Nitric oxide is also capable of modulating inflammatory cell recruitment and adhesion, and it is likely that epithelial cell nitric oxide functions in this capacity[74,85]. Vasodilatation induced by nitric oxide produced by epithelial cells seems to be one mechanism for epithelial cell driven vascular control[86]. Nitric oxide could also function to relax airway smooth muscle. However, while epithelial cells clearly produce a bronchial smooth muscle relaxing activity, factors other than nitric oxide are likely to be involved.

Epithelial cells not only produce inflammatory mediators, but can degrade mediators present in the extracellular milieu. Epithelial cells, for example, express two surface proteases, neutral endopeptidase (NEP) and angiotensin converting enzyme (ACE), which are capable of cleaving kinins and neuropeptides[87]. ACE expression by epithelial cells can be upregulated by glucocorticoids[88]. NEP activity can be attenuated by a variety of injuries, for example viral infection[89]. Loss of NEP activity is associated with increased airways reactivity to substance P, as might be expected from loss of a degraded pathway[90]. In addition to degrading neuropeptides, epithelial cells are a source of histamine *N*-methyltransferase, which can degrade histamine and thus attenuate histamine mediated responses[91].

Epithelial cells do not produce immunoglobulins. However, in addition to recruiting lymphocytes, producing cytokines which can regulate lymphocyte activity, and expressing MHC receptors, epithelial cells, at least in the airway, can transport immunoglobulin A (IgA)[92]. Specifically, secretory component can be expressed on the basolateral surface of airway epithelial cells and bind IgA. The complex of IgA bound to secretory component is then internalized, transported to the apical surface and resecreted by the epithelial cells into the airway lumen. In this manner, relatively high levels of locally produced IgA can be achieved in the intraluminal space (see Chapter 3). The locally produced immunoglobulins are part of a systemic "mucosal" immunity[92]. That is, antigens exposed to one mucosal surface can be processed, leading to the recruitment of appropriate lymphocytes and the production of immune responses which, in turn lead to sensitization of mucosal surfaces throughout the body to those antigens. It is likely that epithelial cells have key roles in the regulation of this process as noted above.

Epithelial cells are capable not only of degrading endogenously produced mediators, but also of catabolizing inhaled foreign compounds. In this respect, inhaled xenobiotics can be either activated or inactivated by enzymes present in airway epithelial cells. These enzymes are differentially expressed along the length of the airway. For example, ethoxycoumarin *O*-deethylase is predominant in the nasal cavity and proximal airways[93], *P*-450 enzymes flavin monoxygenase and phenolsulphotransferase are present in increased concentrations distally[94,95], and Clara cells appear to have very high contents of both *P*-450 enzymes and other detoxifying enzymes, including aldehyde dehydrogenase[96]. It is likely that the aldehyde dehydrogenase, which can inactivate molecules such as acetaldehyde, accounts for the relative resistance of Clara cells to aldehyde mediated injury. In contrast, the increased concentration of *P*-450s may lead to activation of certain inhaled xenobiotics and may account for the relative sensitivity of Clara cells to xenobiotics such as 4-ipomeanol[93], carbon tetrachloride[97], naphthalene[98] and 1-1 dichloroethylene[99]. The ability of various stimuli to modulate the expression of these enzymes could alter the susceptibility of the lung to injury in a complex manner that would depend on the specific inhaled toxicants.

REPAIR PROCESSES

The lung possesses some capacity for repair after injury. Epithelial cells are active participants in this process. In experimental models of airway injury *in vivo*, epithelial cells are observed to migrate rapidly to cover a defect, following which they proliferate and redifferentiate[100–102]. In the alveolar structures, it appears that type I cells are uniquely susceptible to injury. These cells do not replicate, but rather type II cells are induced to proliferate and subsequently to migrate to restore alveolar integrity. Redifferentiation generally follows the period of active proliferation.

Epithelial cells are capable of migrating in response to a number of stimuli. Fibronectin, a multifunctional glycoprotein believed to have an important role in repair processes in general, appears to be particularly important as an epithelial cell chemoattractant[103]. Epithelial cells migrate towards fibronectin by crawling across a subjacent matrix[104], the nature of which appears to be an important variable determining the migratory capacity of the epithelial cells. Specifically, a matrix composed of basement membrane components allows adhesion of cells, but is less conducive to migration than a matrix composed of interstitial collagens. Teleologically, this would suggest that epithelial cells will close a defect more rapidly when basement membrane has been disrupted. The ability of epithelial cells to migrate appears to be modulated by cytokines. Transforming growth factor β(TGFβ), for example, increases the adhesion of epithelial cells to subjacent matrix, but decreases their migratory capacity[105]. In contrast, TNFα appears to increase epithelial cell migration for at least 24 h[106]. Epithelial cells are not only targets in the repair response, but can also produce mediators that can drive repair responses. In this capacity, epithelial cells can release fibronectin, which can function as a chemoattractant for neighboring epithelial cells[103]. The production of this fibronectin can be regulated by a number of cytokines and is dramatically increased by TGFβ[107,108], a cytokine also believed to participate in repair responses elsewhere. Furthermore, airway epithelial cells can produce and release TGFβ in its active form[109]. It is, therefore, reasonable to suggest that airway epithelial cells which remain at a site of injury can release TGFβ, which can function in an autocrine or paracrine manner to stimulate the release of fibronectin which, in turn, can subsequently recruit neighboring epithelial cells to help close an epithelial defect. Finally, epithelial cells are capable of releasing growth stimulating factors which can drive epithelial proliferation[110].

The mediators produced by epithelial cells can also drive the participation of fibroblasts in a repair response. Epithelial cell derived fibroblast chemotaxis can be mediated by fibronectin[111]. Epithelial cells are also capable of driving fibroblast proliferation[112]. In addition, TGFβ released by epithelial cells can increase fibroblast production of extracellular matrix macromolecules[113]. Finally, epithelial cell derived mediators can regulate fibroblast retraction of extracellular matrix[114]. Thus epithelial cells can not only participate in normal healing, but also drive all aspects of scar formation, including fibroblast recruitment, proliferation, matrix production and tissue disorganization.

Not only can epithelial cells drive repair responses, but they are also capable of releasing inhibitory factors. Prostaglandin E seems particularly important in this regard, as it is capable of attenuating fibroblast recruitment[115], proliferation[116,117], matrix production[118] and collagen gel retraction[119]. It is likely also that the activity of cells responding in the repair process is determined by mediators that are derived from a variety of cells. Epithelial cells, therefore, by virtue of their ability to recruit, activate and sustain mononuclear phagocytes, may also be important in regulating repair responses through indirect mechanisms.

SUMMARY

The cells which form the epithelial surface of the conducting airways and the pulmonary parenchyma are important participants in host defense. These cells function to form a complex barrier which includes secretions designed to trap and remove potentially dangerous substances and a relatively impermeable cell layer that prevents access of such substances to the "interior" of the body. The epithelial cells are active participants in the clearance of these trapped materials and are responsible for producing the complex secretions which line their surface. Finally, airway epithelial cells are capable of releasing a variety of regulatory molecules which can alter the behavior of both inflammatory and parenchymal cells in the lung. Through such mechanisms, lung epithelial cells are active participants in inflammatory and repair responses.

REFERENCES

1. Murray J F. Prenatal growth and development of the lung. In: *The Normal Lung*. Philadelphia: W B Saunders, 1976: 1–20.
2. Ten Have-Opbroek A A W. The development of the lung in mammals: an analysis of concepts and findings. *Am J Anat* 1981; **162:** 201–219.
3. Plopper C G, Mariassy A T, Wilson D W, *et al.* Comparison of nonciliated tracheal epithelial cells in six mammalian species: ultrastructure and population densities. *Exp Lung Res* 1983; **5:** 281–294.
4. Mercer R R, Russell M L, Roggli V L, *et al.* Cell number and distribution in human and rat airways. *Am J Respir Cell Mol Biol* 1994; **10:** 613–624.
5. Schneeberger E E. Alveolar type I cells. In: Crystal R G, West J B, eds. *The Lung: Scientific Foundations*. New York: Raven Press, 1991; **1:** 229–234.
6. Mason R J, Williams M C. Alveolar type II cells. In: Crystal R J, West J B, eds. *The Lung: Scientific Foundations*. New York: Raven Press, 1991; **1:** 235–247.
7. Evans M J, Plopper C G. The role of basal cells in adhesion of columnar epithelium to airway basement membrane. *Am Rev Respir Dis* 1988; **138:** 481–483.
8. Kawanami O, Ferrans V J, Crystal R G. Anchoring fibrils in the normal canine respiratory system. *Am Rev Respir Dis* 1979; **120:** 595–611.
9. Corwin P, Franke W W, Grand C, *et al.* The desmosome-intermediate filament complex. In: Edelman G, Thiery J, eds. *The Cell in Contact*. New York: John Wiley and Sons, 1985; 427–460.
10. Sakai L Y, Keene D R, Morris N P, *et al.* Type VII collagen is a major structural component of anchoring fibrils. *J Cell Biol* 1986; **103:** 1577–1586.
11. Revel J P, Nicholson B J, Yancey S B. Chemistry of gap junctions. *Ann Rev Physiol* 1985; **47:** 263–279.
12. Sanderson M J, Chow I, Dirksen E R. Intercellular communication between ciliated cells in culture. *Am J Physiol* 1988; **254:** C63–C74.
13. Sanderson M J, Charles A C, Boitano S, *et al.* Mechanisms and function of intercellular calcium signaling. *Mol Cell Endocrinol* 1994; **98:** 173–187.
14. Barhoumi R, Bowen J A, Stein L S, *et al.* Concurrent analysis of intracellular glutathione content and gap junctional intercellular communication. *Cytometry* 1993; **14:** 747–756.
15. Peyrieras N, Hyafil F, Louvard D, *et al.* Uvomorulin: a nonintegral membrane protein of early mouse embryo. *Proc Natl Acad Sci USA* 1983; **80:** 6274–6277.
16. Gallin W J, Edelman G M, Cunningham B A. Characterization of L-CAM, a major cell adhesion molecule from embryonic liver cells. *Proc Natl Acad Sci USA* 1983; **80:** 1038–1042.
17. Ogou S I, Yoshi-Noro C, Takeichi M. Calcium-dependent cell–cell adhesion molecules common to hepatocytes and teratocarcinoma stem cells. *J Cell Biol* 1983; **97:** 944–948.
18. Geiger B, Dutton A H, Tokuyasu K T, *et al.* Immunoelectron microscope studies of membrane–microfilament interactions: distributions of alpha-actinin, tropomyosin and vinculin in intestinal epithelial brush border and in chicken gizzard smooth muscle cell. *J Cell Biol* 1981; **91:** 614–628.
19. Schneeberger E E. Heterogeneity of tight junction morphology in extrapulmonary and intrapulmonary airways of the rat. *Anat Rec* 1980; **198:** 193–208.
20. Rodriguez-Boulan E, Nelson W J. Morphogenesis of the polarized epithelial cell phenotype. *Science* 1989; **245:** 718–725.
21. Claude P. Morphologic factors influencing transepithelial permeability: a model for the resistance of the zonula occludens. *J Membr Biol* 1978; **39:** 219–232.
22. Van Meer G, Simons K. The formation of tight junctions in maintaining differences in lipid composition between the apical and basolateral cell surface domains. *EMBO J* 1986; **5:** 1455–1464.
23. Gross T J, Cobb S M, Peterson M W. Asbestos exposure increases paracellular transport of fibrin degradation products across human airway epithelium. *Am J Physiol* 1994; **266:** L287–L295.
24. Kleeberger S R, Hudak B B. Acute ozone-induced change in airway permeability: role of infiltrating leukocytes. *J Appl Physiol* 1992; **72:** 670–676.

25. Heyman M, Darmon N, Dupont C, *et al*. Mononuclear cells from infants allergic to cow's milk secrete tumor necrosis factor alpha, altering intestinal function. *Gastroenterology* 1994; **106:** 1514–1523.
26. Yu X-Y, Schofield B H, Croxton T, *et al*. Physiologic modulation of bronchial epithelial cell barrier function by polycationic exposure. *Am J Respir Cell Mol Biol* 1994; **11:** 188–198.
27. Palant C E, Duffey M E, Mookerjee B K, *et al*. Ca++ regulation of tight junction permeability and structure in Necturus gallbladder. *Am J Physiol* 1983; **245:** C203–C212.
28. Duffey M E, Hainau B, Ho S, *et al*. Regulation of epithelial tight junction permeability by cyclic AMP. *Nature* 1981; **294:** 451–453.
29. Mullin J E, O'Brien T G. Effects of tumor promoters on LLC-PK, renal epithelial tight junctions and transepithelial fluxes. *Am J Physiol* 1986; **251:** C597–C602.
30. Noone P G, Olivier K N, Knowles M R. Modulation of the ionic milieu of the airway in health and disease. *Annu Rev Med* 1994; **45:** 421–434.
31. Basbaum C, Welsh M J. Mucus secretion and ion transport in airways. In: Murray J F, Nadel J A, eds. *Textbook of Respiratory Medicine*, Vol. 1. Philadelphia: W B Saunders, 1994; 323–344.
32. Hawgood S. Surfactant: composition, structure and metabolism. In: Crystal R G, West J B, eds. *The Lung: Scientific Foundations*, Vol. 1. New York: Raven Press, 1991; 247–261.
33. Jeffery P K. The origins of secretions in the lower respiratory tract. *Eur J Respir Dis Suppl* 1987; **153:** 34–42.
34. Basbaum C, Welsh M J. Defense mechanisms and immunology. In: Murray J F, Nadel J A, eds. *Textbook of Respiratory Medicine*, Vol. 1. Philadelphia: W B Saunders, 1994: 323–344.
35. Boat T F, Boucher R C. Cystic fibrosis. In: Murray J F, Nadel J A, eds. *Textbook of Respiratory Medicine*, Vol. 1. Philadelphia: W B Saunders, 1994: 1418–1450.
36. Stutts M J, Chinet T C, Mason S J, *et al*. Regulation of Cl⁻ channels in normal and cystic fibrosis airway epithelial cells by extracellular ATP. *Proc Natl Acad Sci USA* 1992; **89:** 1621–1625.
37. Parr C E, Sullivan D M, Paradiso A M, *et al*. Cloning and expression of a human P2U nucleotide receptor, a target for cystic fibrosis pharmacotherapy. *Proc Natl Acad Sci USA* 1994; **91:** 3275–3279.
38. Jeffery P K, Gaillard D, Moret S. Human airway secretory cells during development and in mature airway epithelium. *Eur Respir J* 1992; **5:** 93–104.
39. Reid L M. Measurement of bronchial mucous gland layer. A diagnostic yardstick in chronic bronchitis. *Thorax* 1960; **15:** 132–141.
40. Thompson A B, Schultz H D, Sisson J H, *et al*. Airway mucociliary clearance. In: Bone R C, ed. *Pulmonary and Critical Care Medicine*. New York: Mosby Yearbook, Inc., 1993; 1–12.
41. Katsura H, Kawada H, Konno K. Rat surfactant apoprotein A (SP-A) exhibits antioxidant effects on alveolar macrophages. *Am J Respir Cell Mol Biol* 1993; **9:** 520–525.
42. Matalon S, Holm B A, Baker R R, *et al*. Characterization of antioxidant activities of pulmonary surfactant mixtures. *Biochim Biophys Acta* 1990; **1035:** 121–127.
43. Pison U, Max M, Neuendank A, *et al*. Host defence capacities of pulmonary surfactant: evidence for "non-surfactant" functions of the surfactant system. *Eur J Clin Invest* 1994; **24:** 586–599.
44. Joyce-Brady M, Takahashi Y, Oakes S M, *et al*. Synthesis and release of amphipathic gamma-glutamyl transferase by the pulmonary alveolar type 2 cell. Its redistribution throughout the gas exchange portion of the lung indicates a new role for surfactant. *J Biol Chem* 1994; **269:** 14219–14226.
45. Lee R M K W, Forrest J B. Structure and function of cilia. In: Crystal R G, West J B, eds. *The Lung: Scientific Foundations*, Vol. 1. New York: Raven Press, 1991; 169–181.
46. Holtzman M J. Arachidonic acid metabolism in airway epithelial cells. *Ann Rev Physiol* 1992; **54:** 303–329.
47. Mukhrjee A B, Miele L, Patabiraman N. Phopholipase A2 enzymes: regulation and physiological role. *Biochem Pharmacol* 1994; **48:** 1–10.
48. Lin L L, Lin A Y, Knopf J L. Cytosolic phospholipase A2 is coupled to hormonally regulated release of arachidonic acid. *Proc Natl Acad Sci USA* 1992; **89:** 6147–6151.

49. Lin L L, Lin A Y, DeWitt D L. Interleukin-1a induces the accumulation of cytosolic phospholipase A2 and the release of prostaglandin E2 in human fibroblasts. *J Biol Chem* 1992; **267:** 23451–23454.

50. Hoeck W G, Ramesha C S, Chang D J, *et al.* Cytoplasmic phospholipase A2 activity and gene expression are stimulated by tumour necrosis factor: dexamethasone blocks the induced synthesis. *Proc Natl Acad Sci USA* 1993; **90:** 4475–4479.

51. Wu T, Levine S, Lawrence M G, *et al.* Interferon-gamma induces the synthesis and activation of cytosolic phospholipase A2. *J Clin Invest* 1994; **93:** 571–577.

52. Wu T, Angus C W, Shelhamer J H. Tumor necrosis factor induces cytosolic phospholipase A2 gene expression in airway epithelial cells through post-transcriptional regulation. *Am J Respir Crit Care Med* 1994; **149:** A1069.

53. Conrad D J, Kuh H, Mulkins M, *et al.* Specific inflammatory cytokines regulate the expression of human monocyte 15-lipoxygenase. *Proc Natl Acad Sci USA* 1992; **89:** 217–221.

54. Holtzman M J, Aizawa H, Nadel J A, *et al.* Selective generation of leukotriene B4 by tracheal epithelial cells from dogs. *Biochem Biophys Res Commun* 1983; **114:** 1071–1076.

55. Crofford L J, Wilder R L, Ristimaki A P, *et al.* Cyclooxygenase-1 and -2 expression in rheumatoid synovial tissues: effects of interleukin-1b, phorbol ester, and corticosteroids. *J Clin Invest* 1994; **93:** 1095–1101.

56. Koyama S, Rennard S I, Leikauf G, *et al.* Endotoxin stimulates bronchial epithelial cells to release chemotactic factors for neutrophils. *J Immunol* 1991; **147:** 4293–4301.

57. Koyama S, Rennard S I, Leikauf G D, *et al.* Bronchial epithelial cells release monocyte chemotactic activity in response to smoke and endotoxin. *J Immunol* 1991; **147:** 972–979.

58. Robbins R A, Shoji S, Linder J, *et al.* Bronchial epithelial cells release chemotactic activity for lymphocytes. *Am J Physiol* 1989; **257:** L109–L115.

59. Koyama S, Fujimoto K, Sato E, *et al.* Bradykinin stimulates bronchial epithelial cells to release eosinophil chemotactic activity. *Am Rev Respir Dis* 1993; **147:** A241.

60. Shoji S, Kitani S, Takizawa H, *et al.* Bronchial epithelial cells release a chemotactic activity for rat basophilic leukemia (RBL-2H3) cells [Abstract]. *Am Rev Respir Dis* 1993; **147:** A45.

61. Choi A M, Jacoby D B. Influenza virus A infection induces interleukin-8 gene expression in human airway epithelial cells. *FEBS Lett* 1992; **309:** 327–329.

62. Bedard M, McClure C D, Schiller N L, *et al.* Release of interleukin-8, interleukin-6 and colony-stimulating factors by upper airway epithelial cells: implications for cystic fibrosis. *Am J Respir Cell Mol Biol* 1993; **9:** 455–462.

63. Shoji S, Ertl R F, Koyama S, *et al.* Cigarette smoke stimulates release of neutrophil chemotactic activity from cultured bovine bronchial epithelial cells. *Clin Sci* 1995; **88:** 337–344.

64. Massion P P, Inoue H, Richman-Eisenstat J, *et al.* Novel pseudomonas product stimulates interleukin-8 production in airway epithelial cells *in vitro. J Clin Invest* 1994; **93:** 26–32.

65. Koyama S, Rennard S I, Robbins R A. Acetylcholine stimulates bronchial epithelial cells to release neutrophil and monocyte chemotactic activity. *Am J Physiol* 1992; **262:** L466–L471.

66. Von Essen S G, O'Neill D P, Mio T, *et al.* Challenge of human bronchial epithelial cells with substance P and CGRP causes IL-8 release. *Am J Respir Crit Care Med* 1995; **151:** A342.

67. Adler K B, Fischer B M, Wright D T, *et al.* Interactions between respiratory epithelial cells and cytokines: relationships to lung inflammation. *Ann NY Acad Sci* 1994; **725:** 128–145.

68. Kwon O J, Au T B, Collins P D, *et al.* Inhibition of interleukin-8 expression by dexamethasone in human cultured airway epithelial cells. *Immunology* 1994; **81:** 389–394.

69. Mio T, Adachi Y, Romberger D J, *et al.* Modulation of IL-8 release from human bronchial epithelial cells by tumor necrosis factor-alpha, endotoxin and cigarette smoke. *Am J Respir Crit Care Med* 1994; **149:** A1070.

70. Moncada S, Higgs E A. Endogenous nitric oxide: physiology, pathology and clinical relevance. *Eur J Clin Invest* 1991; **21:** 361–374.

71. Smith C W. Leukocyte–endothelial cell interactions. *Semin Hematol* 1993; **30:** 45–53.

72. Hulbert W C, Walker D C, Hogg J C. The site of leukocyte migration through the tracheal mucosa in the guinea pig. *Am Rev Respir Dis* 1981; **124:** 310–316.

73. Cox G, Vancheri C, Ohtoshi T, *et al.* Human bronchial epithelial cell-derived granulocyte-macrophage colony stimulating factor (GM-CSF) prolongs survival of human eosinophils. *J Allergy Clin Immunol* 1990; **85:** 233.

74. Robbins R A, Nelson K J, Gossman G L, *et al.* Modulation of neutrophil adhesion to bronchial epithelial cells by nitric oxide. *Am Rev Respir Dis* 1993; **147**: A435.

75. DeRose V, Robbins R A, Snider R M, *et al.* Substance P increases neutrophil adhesion to bronchial epithelial cells. *J Immunol* 1994; **152**: 1339–1346.

76. Glanville A R, Tazelaar H D, Theodore J, *et al.* The distribution of MHC class I and II antigens on bronchial epithelium. *Am Rev Respir Dis* 1989; **139**: 330–334.

77. Spurzem J R, Sacco O, Rossi G A, *et al.* MHC class II expression by bronchial epithelial cells is modulated by lymphokines and corticosteroids. *Am Rev Respir Dis* 1990; **141**: A681.

78. Rossi G A, Sacco O, Balbi B, *et al.* Human ciliated bronchial epithelial cells: expression of the HLA-DR antigens and of the HLA-DR alpha gene, modulation of the HLA-DR antigens by gamma-interferon and antigen-presenting function in the mixed leukocyte reaction. *Am J Respir Cell Mol Biol* 1990; **3**: 431–439.

79. Kalb T H, Chuang M T, Marom Z, *et al.* Evidence for accessory cell function by class II MHC antigen-expressing airway epithelial cells. *Am J Respir Cell Mol Biol* 1991; **4**: 320–329.

80. Robbins R A, Hamel F G, Floreani A A, *et al.* Bovine bronchial epithelial cells metabolize L-arginine to L-citrulline: possible role of nitric oxide synthase. *Life Sci* 1993; **52**: 709–716.

81. Jain B, Rubinstein I, Robbins R A, *et al.* Modulation of airway epithelial cell ciliary beat frequency by nitric oxide. *Biochem Biophys Res Commun* 1993; **191**: 83–88.

82. Robbins R A, Springall D R, Warren J B, *et al.* Inducible nitric oxide synthase is increased in murine lung epithelial cells by cytokine stimulation. *Biochem Biophys Res Commun* 1994; **198**: 835–843.

83. Robbins R A, Barnes P J, Springall D R, *et al.* Expression of inducible nitric oxide in human lung epithelial cells. *Biochem Biophys Res Commun* 1994; **203**: 209–218.

84. Jain B, Robbins R, Rubinstein I, *et al.* TNF-alpha and IL-1beta modulate airway epithelial ciliary activity by a nitric oxide-dependent mechanism. *Am J Physiol* 1995; **268**: L911–L917.

85. Belenky S N, Robbins R A, Gossman G L, *et al.* Inhibitors of nitric oxide synthase attenuate human neutrophil chemotaxis *in vitro*. *J Lab Clin Med* 1993; **122**: 388–394.

86. Alving K, Fornhem C, Wietzberg E, *et al.* Nitric oxide mediates cigarette-smoke-induced vasodilatory responses in the lung. *Acta Physiol Scand* 1992; **146**: 407–408.

87. Barnes P J. Regulatory peptides in the respiratory system. *Experentia Suppl* 1989; **56**: 317–333.

88. Muns G, Vishwanatha J K, Rubinstein I. Regulation of angiotensin I-converting enzyme in cultured bovine bronchial epithelial cells. *J Cell Biochem* 1993; **53**: 352–359.

89. Jacoby D B, Tamaoki J, Borson D B, *et al.* Influenza infection causes airway hyperresponsiveness by decreasing enkephalinase. *J Appl Physiol* 1988; **64** 6 : 2653–2658.

90. Sekizawa K, Tamaoki J, Nadel J A, *et al.* Enkephalinase inhibitor potentiates substance P- and electrically induced contraction in ferret trachea. *J Appl Physiol* 1987; **60**: 1401–1405.

91. Ohuri T, Yamauchi K, Sekizawa K, *et al.* Histamine *N*-methyltransferase controls the contractile response of guinea pig trachea to histamine. *J Pharmacol Exp Ther* 1992; **261**: 1268–1272.

92. Mestecky J, Lue C, Russell M W. Selective transport of IgA. Cellular and molecular aspects. *Gastroenterol Clin North Am* 1991; **20**: 441–471.

93. Bond J A, Dahl A R. Metabolism of xenobiotics in the respiratory tract. In: Hutson D H, Caldwell J, Paulson G D, eds. *Intermediary Xenobiotic Metabolism in Animals: Methodology, Mechanisms and Significance*. London: Taylor & Francis, 1990: 41–64.

94. Foster J R, Elcombe C R, Boobis A R, *et al.* Immunocytochemical localization of cytochrome P-450 in hepatic and extrahepatic tissues of the rat with a monoclonal antibody against cytochrome P-450. *Biochem Pharmacol* 1986; **35**: 4543–4554.

95. Plopper C G, Cranz D L, Kemp L, *et al.* Immunohistochemical demonstration of cytochrome P-450 monooxygenase in Clara cells throughout the tracheobronchial airways of the rabbit. *Exp Lung Res* 1987; **13**: 59–68.

96. Bogdanffy M S, Randall H W, Morgan K T. Histochemical localization of aldehyde dehydrogenase in the respiratory tract of the Fischer-344 rats. *Toxicol Appl Pharmacol* 1986; **82**: 560–567.

97. Boyd M R, Statham C N, Longo N S. The pulmonary Clara cell as a target for toxic chemicals requiring metabolic activation; studies with carbon tetrachloride. *J Pharmacol Exp Ther* 1980; **212**: 109–114.

98.   Mahvi D, Bank H, Harley R. Morphology of naphthalene-induced bronchiolar lesions. *Am J Pathol* 1977; **86:** 559–572.

99.   Forkert P G, Stringer V, Racz W J. Effects of administration of metabolic inducers and inhibitors on pulmonary toxicity and covalent binding by 1,1-dichloroethylene in CD-1 mice. *Exp Mol Pathol* 1986; **45:** 44–58.

100. Lane B P, Gordon R. Regeneration of rat tracheal epithelium after mechanical injury. I. *Proc Soc Exp Biol Med* 1974; **145:** 1139–1144.

101. McDowell E M, Ben T, Newkirk C, *et al.* Differentiation of tracheal mucociliary epithelium in primary cell culture recapitulates normal fetal development and regeneration following injury in hamsters. *Am J Pathol* 1987; **139:** 511–522.

102. Shimizu T, Nishihara M, Kawaguchi S, *et al.* Expression of phenotypic markers during regeneration of rat tracheal epithelium following mechanical injury. *Am J Respir Cell Mol Biol* 1994; **11:** 85–94.

103. Shoji S, Ertl R F, Linder J, *et al.* Bronchial epithelial cells produce chemotactic activity for bronchial epithelial cells: possible role for fibronectin in airway repair. *Am Rev Respir Dis* 1990; **141:** 218–225.

104. Rickard K A, Taylor J, Rennard S I, *et al.* Migration of bovine bronchial epithelial cells to extracellular matrix components. *Am J Respir Cell Mol Biol* 1993; **8:** 63–68.

105. Spurzem J R, Sacco O, Veys T, *et al.* TGF-beta increases expression of extracellular matrix receptors on cultured bovine bronchial epithelial cells. *Am Rev Respir Dis* 1992; **145:** A668.

106. Ito H, Romberger D J, Rennard S I, *et al.* TNF-alpha enhances bronchial epithelial cell migration and attachment to fibronectin. *Am Rev Respir Dis* 1993; **147:** A46.

107. Wang A, Cohen D S, Palmer E, *et al.* Polarized regulation of fibronectin secretion and alternative splicing by transforming growth factor. *J Biol Chem* 1991; **266:** 15598–15601.

108. Romberger D J, Beckmann J D, Claassen L, *et al.* Modulation of fibronectin production of bovine bronchial epithelial cells by transforming growth factor-beta. *Am J Respir Cell Mol Biol* 1992; **7:** 149–155.

109. Sacco O, Romberger D, Rizzino A, *et al.* Spontaneous production of transforming growth factor beta 2 by primary cultures of bronchial epithelial cells: effects on cell behavior *in vitro*. *J Clin Invest* 1992; **90:** 1379–1385.

110. Ferriola P C, Robertson A T, Rusnak D W, *et al.* Epidermal growth factor dependence and TGF alpha autocrine growth regulation in primary rat tracheal epithelial cells. *J Cell Physiol* 1992; **152:** 302–309.

111. Shoji S, Rickard K A, Ertl R F, *et al.* Bronchial epithelial cells produce lung fibroblast chemotactic factor: fibronectin. *Am J Respir Cell Mol Biol* 1989; **1:** 13–20.

112. Koizumi S, Ertl R, Rennard S. Bronchial epithelial cells stimulate fibroblast proliferation. *Am Rev Respir Dis* 1991; **143:** A526.

113. Kawamoto M, Nakamura Y, Tate L, *et al.* Modulation of fibroblast type I collagen and fibronectin production by bronchial epithelial cells. *Am Rev Respir Dis* 1992; **145:** A842.

114. Mio T, Striz I, Adachi Y, *et al.* Responses of human bronchial epithelial cells to acid injury. *Am J Respir Crit Care Med* 1995; **151:** A367.

115. Ertl R F, Valenti V, Spurzem J R, *et al.* Prostaglandin E inhibits fibroblast recruitment. *Am Rev Respir Dis* 1992; **145:** A19.

116. Bitterman P B, Wewers M D, Rennard S I, *et al.* Modulation of alveolar macrophage-driven fibroblast proliferation by alternative macrophage mediators. *J Clin Invest* 1986; **77:** 700–708.

117. Nakamura Y, Ertl R F, Kawamoto M, *et al.* Bronchial epithelial cells modulate fibroblast proliferation: role of prostaglandin E2. *Am Rev Respir Dis* 1992; **145:** A827.

118. Diaz A, Munoz E, Johnston R, *et al.* Regulation of human lung fibroblast alpha 1 procollagen gene expression by tumor necrosis factor alpha, interleukin-1 beta, and prostaglandin E2. *J Biol Chem* 1993; **268:** 10364–10371.

119. Ehrlich H P, Wyler D J. Fibroblast contraction of collagen lattices *in vitro:* inhibition by chronic inflammatory cell mediators. *J Cell Physiol* 1983; **116:** 345–351.

11

Antigen Processing and Presentation

R. J. MOOTS AND STEPHEN P. YOUNG

University of Birmingham, Birmingham, UK

INTRODUCTION

It is essential that the human organism can correctly recognise and respond to a continually changing environment. There are few places where this is as important as the immune system, which must quickly and efficiently detect and react selectively to the presence of invading micro-organisms. This is of great importance within the respiratory system, which is constantly exposed to pathogens within inhaled air. Once a pathogen has entered, there is the potential for it or its products to occupy diverse compartments that may be extracellular, or intracellular such as the cytoplasm or membrane bound endocytic vesicles. T lymphocytes are central to the specific immune response, and have evolved mechanisms to recognise and respond to foreign antigens in a highly selective manner. Activation of these cells may have drastic consequences, ranging from direct cytolysis of cells expressing an antigen, to chemokine secretion providing help for B lymphocytes in the production of antibodies.

In order for something to be recognised as "foreign", it must differ from the host in a recognisable manner. However, the differences may often be subtle, involving changes in only a few, or even a single amino acid. T lymphocytes have evolved to exploit this by recognising antigens after they have first been fragmented from proteins into short peptides and then stably bound to major histocompatibility complex (MHC) molecules. They may then be presented to the T cell antigen receptor (TCR), an antibody-like protein on the surface of T cells, and in the presence of appropriate accessory signals result in activation of the T cell. Such a requirement for processing of antigen and presentation by MHC molecules before recognition by the TCR, is an important difference between T and B lymphocyte function. As a consequence of this, T and B cells tend to interact with different regions of an antigen: B cell epitopes tend to be on the

Pulmonary Defences. Edited by Robert A. Stockley.
© 1997 John Wiley & Sons Ltd.

surface of antigens or cells and dependent on conformation, and T cell epitopes are more often within the core of the antigen or cell and more dependent upon the amino acid sequence of the protein rather than conformation.

These independent recognition pathways have allowed the evolution of an immunological surveillance system designed to recognise potential pathogens within a "soup" of only subtly different self antigens.

THE MAJOR HISTOCOMPATIBILITY COMPLEX

The MHC first attracted the attention of immunologists because "histocompatibility antigens" interfered with tissue grafting experiments[1]. It is now known to be a critical component in antigen presentation to T cells[2,3] and not present merely to confound organ transplantation. Although there has recently been an exponential increase in knowledge about the immunology of the MHC, there is still much more to learn about it.

The MHC is a complex genetic region coding for a highly polymorphic set of glycoproteins that act as antigen binders, transporters and presenters, and are ultimately expressed on the cell surface. In humans, the alleles are found on the short arm of chromosome 6 and are known as the human leucocyte antigen (HLA) system. There are analogous systems in other mammals—in the mouse, for example, which is often used as a model for studying the immune response, it is known as the H-2 system. The MHC is divided into three main groups: class I MHC, expressed on most nucleated cells; class II MHC, expressed primarily on B cells, macrophages, monocytes, dendritic cells and endothelium (except under the influence of interferon gamma (IFNγ), which induces class II expression

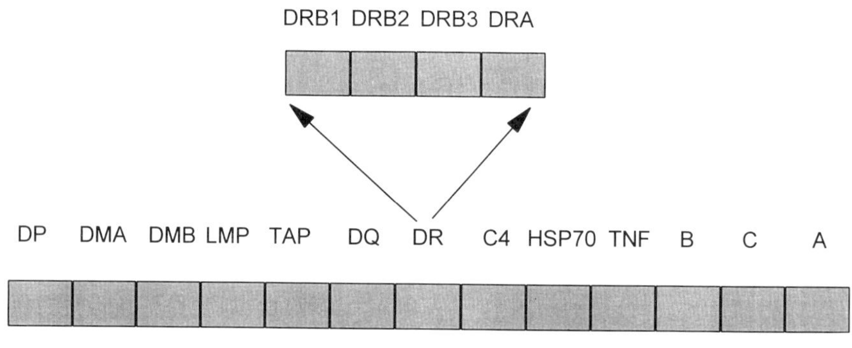

Figure 11.1. Simplified map of the HLA region of chromosome 6. The possible impact of genes other than those of the MHC molecules on the function of the MHC is emphasised by the close proximity of a number of other important genes in this region. Many of them are involved in antigen processing (TAP, DM, LMP and possibly HSP70), whereas others are important in the immune system (TNF and C4). Genetic associations of a variety of diseases may involve combinations of several of these genes

on diverse cell types); and the class III region, coding for various molecules in antigen transport, presentation and complement components. A simplified genetic map of the MHC in man is shown in Fig. 11.1.

STRUCTURE OF THE MHC

Structural analysis of MHC molecules has proved important in elucidating the mechanisms whereby they can fulfil their important role. The most helpful technique to date for determining the structure of the MHC has been that of x ray crystallography, which has allowed the structures of both class I and class II molecules to be resolved in detail. The first MHC molecule to be so characterised was the human class I molecule HLA-A0201[4,5] and since then many more class I molecules, both human and murine, have been crystallised and resolved. Class I MHC molecules have two immunoglobulin-like domains, corresponding to the highly conserved membrane proximal portion of the heavy chain and to the monomorphic light chain, β_2 microglobulin (β_2 m) (Fig. 11.2A). These support the highly polymorphic peptide binding site which is made up from two α-helical walls, lying on top of a floor formed by eight strands of a β-pleated sheet. One of the α helices is firmly attached to the floor of the groove by a disulphide bond (α_1 domain α helix), whilst the other is not so rigidly attached to the floor. The net result is to form a groove or cleft in the highly polymorphic region of this molecule where peptide can be bound, and a conserved area which acts as a support for this. The peptide binding groove is closed off at each end, limiting the potential length of peptide that can be bound (Fig. 11.3A).

Class II MHC molecules, unlike class I, are not composed of a heavy chain and light chain, but are formed as a heterodimer of α and β chains of similar molecular weight (Fig. 11.2B). The crystal structure of a class II molecule is, however, very similar to that of class I[6,7], with non-covalently associated α and β chains contributing equally to the final structure, including peptide binding groove and immunoglobulin-like membrane proximal part. The β chain α helix is disulphide bonded to the floor of the groove (like one α helix in class I), whilst the α chain α helix is not. Unlike class I MHC, the ends of the groove in class II MHC are open, and thus do not impose the same sort of restriction as class I MHC regarding the length of peptide that may bind (Fig. 11.3B). A constant feature of the MHC class II crystals studied to date is that they crystallise as tetramers, composed of dimers of the heterodimeric α chain and β chain complex[6–8]. As yet, it is not known whether this is a crystal artefact, or reflects the physiological state at the cell surface.

Both class I and II MHC molecules have to bind a potentially huge repertoire of peptides, but must do so in a way that allows a certain selectivity in the peptides so bound — one of the most intriguing paradoxes in immunology. This is achieved in part by two distinct and complementary mechanisms for binding peptide. For both MHC classes, a broad peptide binding capacity arises from molecular interactions, predominantly hydrogen bonding, between the peptide backbone and conserved residues in the groove of the MHC molecule. For class I MHC, there are conserved areas at either end of the groove, forming electrostatic depressions, or pockets, that bind the carboxyl (C) and amino (N) termini of

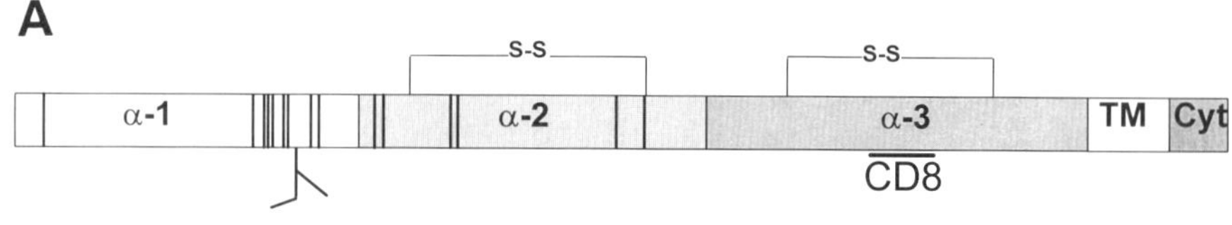

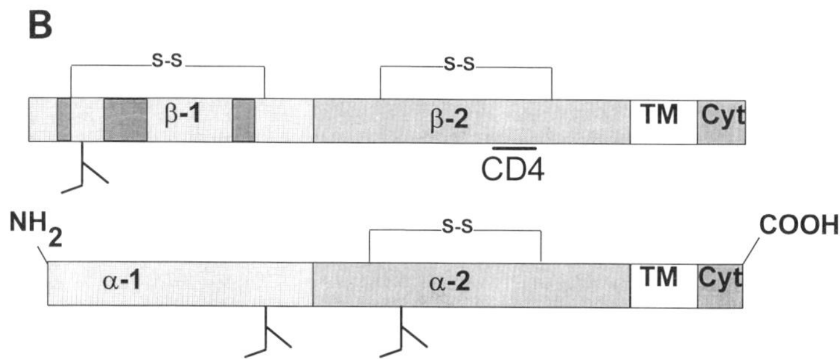

Figure 11.2. A: Structure of the heavy chain of human class I MHC. Hypervariable residues are found throughout the α-1 and α-2 regions. The α-3 region is not variable and contains the CD8 binding site. Note the small size of the cytoplasmic (Cyt) region. **B:** Structure of the α and β chains of the human class II DR molecule. The α chain is more heavily glycosylated and so appears to be heavier than the β when separated electrophoretically. The β chain contains all of the variable residues, largely confined to three regions of hypervariability, in addition to the CD4 binding site, in a position comparable to that of the CD8 site in class I. TM = Transmembrane domain

peptides[5,9,10]. The groove is closed at each end, fixing the peptide inside. Such constraints on N- and C-terminal binding, in the presence of a closed groove, ensure that class I MHC can bind only short peptides, of about eight to 10 amino acids. The differences in length are accommodated by a central bulge in the peptide which is greater in the slightly longer peptides (Fig. 11.3B).

The class I groove is also in the area of maximum polymorphism, and polymorphic amino acids also form pockets that are specific to a particular allele, generating "specificity pockets"[5,10–13]. These pockets, of sizes, shapes, and electrostatic charges appropriate to accommodate and bind the side chains of individual amino acids characterising a peptide, may confer specificity in binding. This is reflected when MHC molecules are affinity purified from the surface of cells in culture and the prebound peptides are eluted and sequenced. Sequences of peptides eluted from a particular MHC molecule may have an excess of one particular amino acid at certain positions (determined by pockets), known as anchor residues[14–16]. Most MHC molecules require peptides to contain a certain number of anchor residues at the correct positions, for binding to occur. The net result in class I is for peptide to bind with the termini buried at either end of the groove, some peptide amino acid side chains lying in specificity pockets, and the peptide forming a looped shape with a bulge in the middle, allowing the side chains of amino acids in the middle of the peptide to interact with the TCR.

A

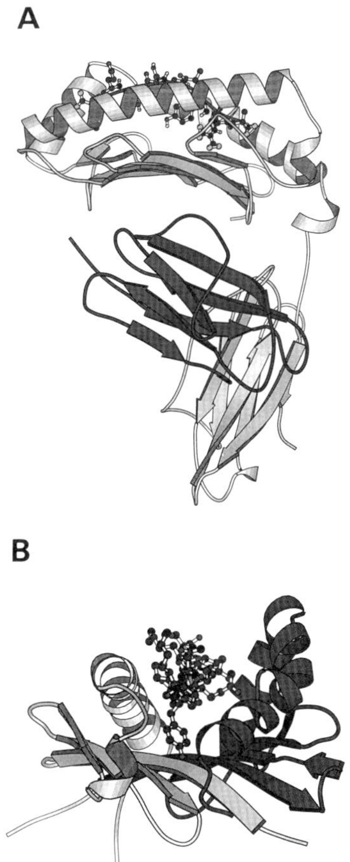

B

Figure 11.3. A: Crystal structure of HLA B27 complexed with a peptide.The peptide is held between the two α helices of the MHC heavy chain at the membrane distal part of the molecule. Note the bend in the peptide (shown on its own in **C**) and how one residue in particular, and arginine, points down into the protein. The small β_2-microglobulin subunit (darker print), non-covalently bound, is at the lower end of the complex nearest to you. Association of the β_2-microglobulin is believed to occur after the peptide has been bound by the MHC heavy chain. **B:** Crystal structure of human class II MHC DR1 with peptide. The overall configuration is very similar to class I. In this picture an end view of the peptide binding groove is shown, demonstrating that the peptide fills much of the space, creating an overall surface of peptide and MHC onto which the T cell antigen receptor docks. Note again how one residue, a tyrosine, is buried deeply in the protein. The peptide is, however, in a much more extended form than that bound to B27, as shown in C overleaf

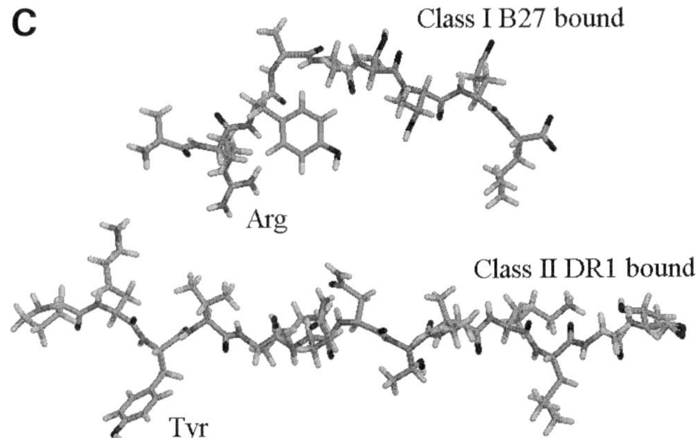

Figure 11.3. (*Continued*) C: Comparison of B27 and DR1 bound peptides. Peptides from the two complexes have been aligned in their original bound conformations to demonstrate the contrasts between them. The class I binds peptides largely by the ends, leaving the middle part to bulge out, whereas class II binds all the way along, keeping the peptide much more rigid and linear. The Arg of the B27 peptide and the Tyr of the DR1 peptide probably make the major contribution to defining the MHC restriction of these peptides

Although there are also specificity pockets at the polymorphic regions of class II, these do not appear to play as large a part in peptide binding as the analogous pockets in class I. This is consistent with reports that the sequences of peptides eluted from affinity purified class II MHC do not reveal the strong allele specific "anchor" residues observed with peptides eluted from class I. The main interaction between class II MHC molecules and peptide, in contrast, appears to be with main chain atoms of the peptide. In addition, the observation from structural studies that the groove in class II is not closed off, potentially allowing the peptide to extend at either end, may explain why there is not so stringent a requirement for peptide length (Fig. 11.3B). Indeed, it has been shown that peptides of up to 100 amino acids may bind to class II MHC in a manner still recognisable by T cells (E. Epstein and S.P. Young, unpublished observations).

MHC molecules have therefore sacrificed the ability to bind the broadest possible repertoire of peptides, in order to provide an effective yet selective display of peptides at the surface of the cell, in a form available for interaction with the TCR. The limitations of this are minimised by the highly polymorphic nature of the MHC and the simultaneous expression of multiple class I and class II alleles in both the individual and the species[17].

ANTIGEN PROCESSING

Given that MHC molecules are responsible for presenting peptide antigen to T lymphocytes, it is important to consider how the peptide–MHC complex arrives at the correct place, the cell surface, at the correct time. This starts with uptake of antigen, and is followed by binding of antigen by MHC and transport of the peptide–MHC complex to the cell surface. To ensure efficient surveillance for antigens, this process must work for peptides that arise from different cellular compartments. Two different pathways have therefore evolved, one to process cytoplasmic derived and the other, endosomal derived antigens. These processing pathways present peptide to two different types of T lymphocyte. The class II MHC restricted pathway presents peptide to cluster of differentiation (CD)4+ T helper (Th) cells, and the class I restricted pathway presents peptide to CD8+ cytotoxic T lymphocytes (CTL). These two types of lymphocyte appear to have different functions within an immune response. CTLs recognise peptide presented by the cytoplasmic pathway class I MHC route and lyse cells expressing appropriate antigen. Th cells are responsible for killing and clearance of pathogen—of special importance within the lungs. They work by recruitment of B lymphocytes and accessory cells, and respond to antigens processed by the endosomal, class II MHC route.

PROCESSING OF CYTOPLASMIC DERIVED (CLASS I MHC RESTRICTED) ANTIGENS

Generation of Peptides

It has been known for a while that MHC class I molecules present peptides derived from cytosolic antigens such as the influenza A nucleoprotein[18]. However, exactly how antigenic peptides arise, and the mechanism whereby they reach the correct compartment to combine with the class I MHC have been studied in detail only recently. Cytosolic antigens may either be synthesised by the antigen presenting cell, as in virus infection, or penetrate into the cytosol from the extracellular space, carried by invasive micro-organisms or experimentally by techniques such as osmotic lysis or electroporation[19,20]. This pathway is by no means exclusive because, in some cases, exogenous antigens with no known cytosolic penetration are presented by the class I MHC pathway[21−23]. The mechanisms for this remain unclear.

In vitro cytotoxicity[13], peptide elution[24,25] and x ray crystallographic studies[26−28] have revealed that class I MHC binds peptides approximately nine amino acids in length. These observations have prompted a concerted search for the cytosolic proteases that are responsible for breaking down proteins to generate the nonapeptides that bind to class I MHC. The discovery of mutant cell lines that are deficient in some aspect of antigen processing has allowed this search to begin. One such cell line was the murine line, RMA-S, which did not express class I MHC at $37°C$[29]. Genetic analysis of the regions of the chromosome to which the defects in the murine cells were mapped showed that one gene in the region between the K locus and the MHC class II coded for a proteasome subunit[30], and, since then, other similar proteasome genes have been reported[31]. Proteosomes are IFN_γ inducible non-lysosomal proteinase complexes abundantly present in the cytosol. They have several proteolytically active sites and are of high relative molecular mass (M_r about 600 000), consisting of about 20–30 subunits with M_r between 15 000 and 30 000. The deficient gene in RMA-S was, in turn, tightly linked to the HAM1 gene, believed to be required for translocating peptide fragments of endogenous antigens into the endoplasmic reticulum for association with MHC class I molecules (discussed later). Further analysis of the genomic organisation in this region of human chromosome 6 has identified two proteasome related genes (low molecular mass polypeptides (LMP) 2 and 7), believed to be involved in the proteolytic degradation of cytoplasmic antigens[30–35]. The subunits coded for by these genes are, however, not critical for antigen processing, because mutant cell lines lacking these genes can still process antigens for presentation by MHC class I[36,37], perhaps by other proteasomes containing alternative subunits.

Transport of Peptides to MHC Molecules

After cleavage to appropriate size in the cytosol, peptides need to cross to the endoplasmic reticulum, to the site of production of class I molecules. The mechanisms for this are now becoming clear, again using mutant cell lines that are deficient in some aspect of antigen processing. Experiments using the mouse line RMA-S[29] revealed that association between class I MHC and β_2 m, and transport of this complex in physiological amounts to the cell surface, were dependent on the presence of peptide, which appeared to have a rate limiting and vital role in the final folding of the MHC complex before its surface expression[38]. A similar defect has also been found in a human mutant cell line, mapped to within chromosome 6. These cell lines were found to be defective in genes that code for peptide transporters. Two transporter genes (TAP1 and TAP2), believed to code for proteins that pump the degraded peptides across the endoplasmic reticulum membrane have been isolated in various species, including man, mice and rats[33,39–46]. Discovery of these genes now provides an explanation for the defect in the RMA-S cell, which contains only one copy of the TAP2 gene[40], that in turn contains a point mutation resulting in a premature stop codon: as the peptide transporter protein is absent from RMA-S cells, class I fails to assemble and is not transported to the cell surface.

Direct evidence of the peptide transporting properties of the TAP products came from Levy *et al.*[48], who studied peptide uptake by microsomes, which was found to be very rapid, allowing assembly of class I MHC within 1 min[48]. The same group of investigators found that this assembly process requires ATP[48], but that the translocation of peptide across the endoplasmic reticulum membrane did not require ATP. They therefore suggested that ATP is required in the lumen of the endoplasmic reticulum for efficient assembly to occur. However, more recent work by Shepherd *et al.* suggested that the peptide translocation may not be ATP dependent[49], leaving the exact role for the ATP open. That study also showed some discrimination by the transporter amongst peptides[49], which was also found by Androlewicz *et al.*[50] who showed that the transport of short peptides (eight to 10 amino acids) was more effective than that of longer peptides. In this last work it was also found that transport occurred, albeit inefficiently, even in the absence of the specific transporter, in an ATP independent manner[50]. Presentation of Sendai virus by the RMA-S cell can also take place inefficiently[51], in spite of its lack of peptide transporter. Similarly, peptides can be transported into the endoplasmic reticulum for presentation by peptide transporter deficient T2 cells. In one case, a peptide with three charged residues was presented poorly unless the peptide was preceded by an endoplasmic reticulum translocation signal sequence, normally found on proteins destined for secretion. However, this signal sequence was not always required for presentation to occur, and the hydrophobicity of the peptide does not appear to be a major determinant in selecting peptides for this alternate pathway[52]. This suggests a certain degeneracy in the processing pathway for class I MHC presentation, and may also be the case for the proteolytic steps, as proteasome subunits are not generally required for the processing of peptides bound by class I MHC[37].

Allelic variation in the peptide transporters has been described[42], although there is limited genetic variability. Four different nucleotide substitutions have been found in the TAP2 gene, and attempts to evaluate whether TAP2 variants are associated with MHC related conditions such as insulin dependent diabetes mellitus or reactive arthritis have been largely unsuccessful. However, the transporters may be important in other non-genetic diseases, as cytomegalovirus can prevent antigen presentation by blocking the transport of peptide loaded MHC class I molecules into the Golgi compartment[53], and other viruses may use this strategy to avoid immune surveillance.

Transport to the Cell Surface

After binding of peptides and β_2 m to MHC heavy chains to form trimolecular complexes, MHC molecules undergo a conformational change that results in an increased thermostability, detectable by conformation dependent monoclonal antibodies. The MHC are released by chaperonin-like molecules that bind

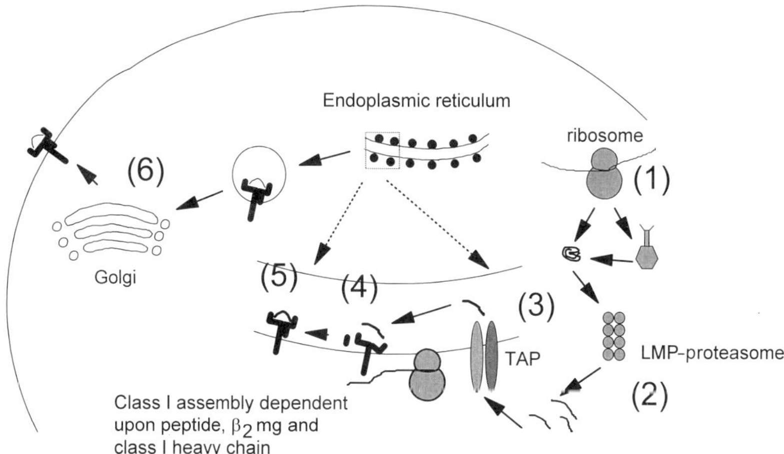

Figure 11.4. Antigen processing for class I MHC. Viral or self proteins produced within the cell on ribosomes (1) are captured and partially degraded, a process perhaps involving the LMP–proteasome complex (2). Peptides are selectively transported into the lumen of the endoplasmic reticulum via the TAP complex (3), where they bind to the nascent class I heavy chain (4) inducing it to fold. β_2-Microglobulin then binds (5), locking the complex in a stable conformation. It is then exported to the cell surface, via the Golgi (6), where glycosylation takes place

unassembled MHC class I heavy chains in the endoplasmic reticulum[54]. Transport of the peptide–MHC class I complex to the cell surface is blocked by brefeldin A, which blocks movement of membrane proteins from the endoplasmic reticulum to the Golgi, and it appears that the MHC follows constitutive biosynthetic/secretory pathways, with sorting in the *trans*-Golgi reticulum. At this point, the pathways of classes I and II MHC appear to diverge (see below)[55]. The class I restricted antigen processing pathway is illustrated in Fig. 11.4, p. 187.

PROCESSING OF ENDOSOMAL DERIVED (CLASS II MHC RESTRICTED) ANTIGENS

Generation of Peptides

Many microbial antigens do not reach the cytoplasm. They may instead reach a compartment inside the cell by mechanisms such as pinocytosis, finally locating in endosomes. Such antigens are presented to T cells by class II MHC. The fine specificity of the pathway of antigen processing by the class II pathway is also not fully understood. The mechanism of antigen uptake may vary depending on circumstances. Class II MHC expressing antigen presenting cells such as B lymphocytes are able to endocytose immunoglobulin bound antigen or take in antigen by pinocytosis. After uptake, protein enters early endosomal compartments which fuse with other similar compartments, ultimately forming a larger, late endosomal complex. Subsequently, the contents of the late endosome may fuse with lysosomal compartments, which are considered the terminal stage of the endocytic route[56]. The early and late endosomal compartments are at pH 6–6.5 and 5.5, respectively, and probably represent a continuum of increasing proteolytic potential proportional to the degree of acidity[56]. The lysosome contains a greater concentration of proteases which are at maximum levels of activation within the low pH environment[57].

Recent evidence favours the lysosome, or possibly the late endosome, as the key organelle involved in denaturation and proteolysis of protein. This is supported by many studies that included isolation of intracellular compartments after pulsing with a synthetic protein, demonstrating the lysosome to be the only organelle in which denaturation of this protein occurred[58]. Furthermore, encapsulation of protein within liposomes, with varied compositions, such that the protein was released into the different intracellular compartments, also suggested the lysosome, or possibly the late endosome, to be the main organelle involved in processing[59,60]. These data, however, are questioned by other studies showing that the endosome is of key importance in processing, thus highlighting that the issue is far from resolved. The factors that dictate the particular intracellular compartment in which protein is processed may depend on a complex interplay of accessibility of proteolytic cleavage sites within the protein and variations of the concentration of proteases within the endocytic pathway between cell types.

The studies suggesting that endosomal compartments are of importance in processing do not make the distinction between early and late endosomes. The evidence that the early endosomal compartments, in isolation, are able to process antigen rests on the isolation of cathepsins B and D within this compartment; however, it is not known if this is sufficient for antigen processing.

The possible importance of the prelysosomal and lysosomal compartments as the main organelles involved in processing required the development of a theory to explain how the antigen fragment can withstand the degradative potential of these organelles. It appears possible that the groove of class II MHC is able to provide protection against proteolysis. This is confirmed, in part, by a cell free system demonstrating that class II MHC is able to protect peptides against degradation from cathepsin D and offer partial protection against pronase[61]. In fact, MHC class II can bind directly to partially unfolded proteins[62] and protect regions against proteolysis and, as the naturally processed fragments are of at least 13–17 amino acids[16], longer than the MHC class II groove[7], this supports the idea of MHC playing an active part in determining which peptides survive.

The Invariant Chain and MHC Trafficking

MHC class II molecules are assembled in the endoplasmic reticulum as a stoichiometric complex of α chains, β chains and a monomorphic, non-MHC encoded polypeptide chain termed the invariant chain (Ii), for which various functions have been proposed[63,64]. Peptide is unable to associate with class II MHC until Ii has been cleaved from the class II MHC molecule, suggesting that Ii deters association of cellular peptides en route to the endocytic pathway. It is also believed that class II MHC is targeted to the endocytic pathway from the endoplasmic reticulum by Ii. Cells that are deficient in Ii show a marked decrease in the ability to process class II restricted antigens[65], decreased ability to assemble α and β chains, and inefficient transport of the chains to the cell surface as stable dimers[66,67]. The few class II dimers that reach the cell surface do not appear to present antigen, as if their binding regions were empty. There is an obvious parallel here with mutant cell lines possessing deficiencies in the class I antigen processing pathway: Ii provides for class II MHC the functions that fully processed peptides provide for class I MHC.

An explanation for this observation may come from consideration of the biochemistry of ligand binding by class II molecules. Class II MHC associated Ii might regulate binding of digested peptides to the antigen binding site of class II MHC proteins by directly or allosterically blocking that site until cleavage and release of Ii from MHC α and β chains at the time of peptide charging. Indeed, cathepsin B may be the main protease for cleaving off Ii. This protease has been shown to colocalise with class II MHC molecules in intracellular compartments, to generate antigenic peptide fragments, and to cleave off Ii[68].

Because Ii appears to block peptide loading, it has been suggested that it must interact with the class II peptide binding groove and, indeed, Ii peptides are among those eluted from class II[69]. The precise mechanism whereby Ii blocks peptide loading by class II MHC is not known. Although Ii peptides occupy the groove, there also appears to be an allosteric effect from part of the Ii that is not inside the groove[70]. If this is the case, then Ii may prevent peptide loading of class II MHC not by directly blocking the peptide binding site, but rather by inducing an allosteric change in the protein such that it cannot bind the peptides.

190 *R. J. Moots and Stephen P. Young*

Truncation of the cytoplasmic domain of Ii results in the failure of Ii to dissociate from the class II MHC and leads to stable expression of class II MHC α chain, β chain–Ii complexes on the cell surface which are very inefficient in their ability to present peptides. The cytoplasmic domain of Ii may therefore be important in endosomal targeting of the class II MHC[63].

When a mouse model that does not express invariant chain is created by genetic manipulation, there are defects in MHC class II assembly, transport, peptide acquisition, and CD4+ T cell selection[67]. Cells from these "Ii chain knockout" mice showed a dramatic reduction in surface class II MHC, resulting from both defective association of MHC class II α and β chains and markedly decreased post-Golgi transport. The few class II MHC α–β heterodimers reaching the cell surface behave as if empty or occupied by an easily displaced peptide, and display a distinct structure. Mutant spleen cells are defective in their ability to present intact protein antigens, but stimulate enhanced responses in the presence of peptides. Class II MHC restricted processing is illustrated in Fig. 11.5.

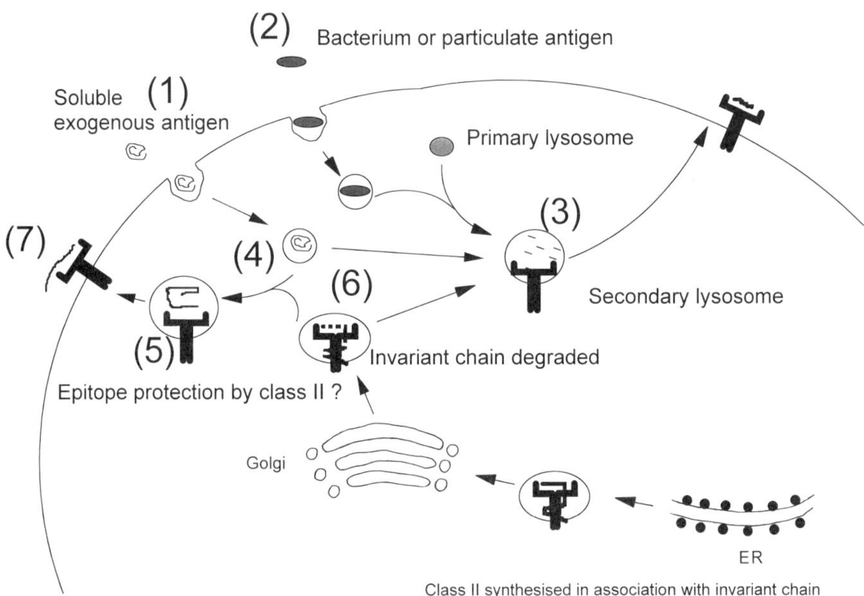

Figure 11.5. Antigen processing for class II MHC. In contrast to class I, antigen for class II presentation comes largely from exogenous sources, in the form of soluble proteins (1) or phagocytosed bacteria, viruses and immune complexes (2). Some antigens such as bacteria or particulates, require vigorous processing by lysosome (3), while others require little degradation, which can take place in non-lysosomal acidic vesicles (4). Class II MHC may be present in these vesicles and may have an active role in protecting regions of antigens against degradation (5). Before binding, however, class II MHC α–β heterodimers are released from the invariant chain by the action of cathepsins (6). The class II MHC–antigen complex probably undergoes a conformational change to produce a stable complex and is then exported to the surface (7)

ACCESSORY MOLECULES IN ANTIGEN PRESENTATION

Presentation of peptide antigen by MHC is not on its own sufficient for optimal T cell activation. This idea is supported by the observation that purified T cells do not produce interleukin-2 in response to mitogenic lectins or monoclonal antibodies to TCR in the absence of viable accessory cells, even though signalling has occurred through the TCR[71,72]. Furthermore, there is a great difference in the capacity of B cells to stimulate T cells to produce cytokines under conditions in which the B cells should be presenting the same number of peptide–MHC complexes to the T cell for recognition[73]. These data suggest that antigen presenting cells do more than just present peptide to the TCR: they must also provide "costimulatory" signals.

Costimulatory signals may be defined as those that: (i) require cell–cell contact (and therefore are not attributable to cytokines); (ii) do not require MHC compatibility between presenting and responding cells; (iii) are provided most efficiently by dendritic cells, less effectively by macrophages and activated B cells, poorly by resting B cells and not at all by resting T cells; (iv) are not mediated by increases in intracellular calcium or inositol phosphate metabolism[71]. Several receptor–coreceptor pairs providing such costimulatory signals have now been characterised. The best known of these is the CD28–CD80 (B7) receptor–ligand pair.

CD28 is a cell surface glycoprotein composed of two identical disulphide linked 44 kDa subunits that are coded for by an Ig-like gene[74]. It is expressed on all human (and murine) CD4+ cells and 50% of CD8+ T cells. The CD28 ligand, CD80 (also known as B7 or BB-1), is a heavily glycosylated integral membrane protein of about 50 kDa, also of the Ig superfamily. CD80 is constitutively expressed on splenic and blood dendritic cells, inducible on B cells and monocytes, and not expressed on resting T cells[75]. Interference with the signals transduced through this pathway *in vitro* can block T cell proliferation despite TCR activation[76,77].

Other receptor–ligand pairs (reviewed elsewhere[78]), including lymphocyte function associated antigen (LFA)-1–intercellular adhesion molecule (ICAM)-1 or ICAM-2, CD2–LFA-3 and very late activation antigen-4–vascular cell adhesion molecule-1, also enhance T cell activation. These molecules probably act both by transducing activation signals in the T cell and by promoting adhesion between antigen presenting cells and T cells, allowing the cells to come into contact in a greater proximity and possibly for a longer period. This may in turn allow other signalling molecules such as the TCR and CD28 to interact more efficiently with their ligands.

Normal activation of the T lymphocyte occurs as a consequence of two signals occurring together: signal 1, produced by the T cell–antigen receptor complex, and signal 2, produced by accessory molecule interaction (e.g. CD28–CD80) (Fig. 11.6). Data have emerged that suggest that if signal 1 occurs in the absence of signal 2, this may result in a state of anergy, in which the responding T cell is rendered unable to be activated[79]. This phenomenon may have implications in understanding and possibly treating autoimmune pulmonary disorders, such as

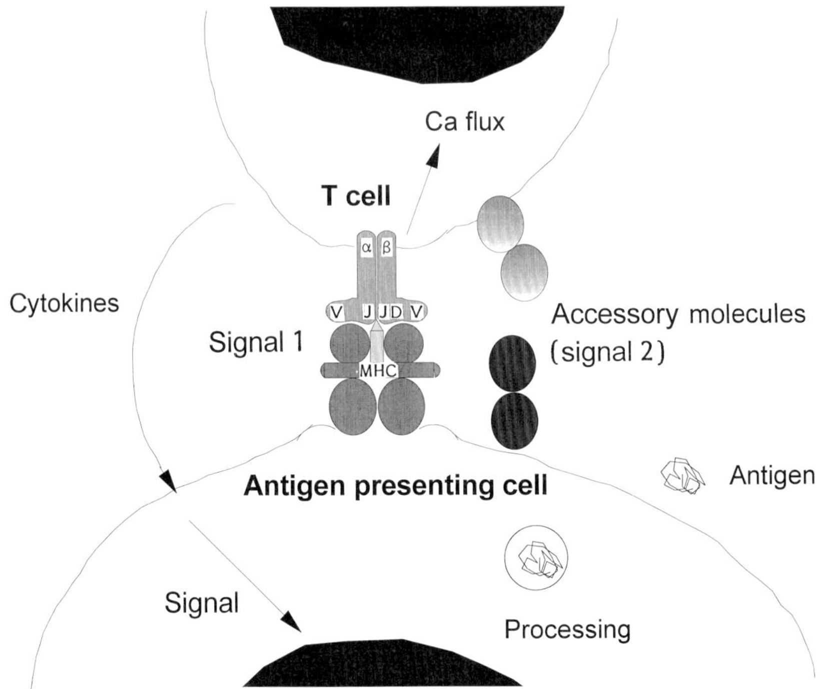

Figure 11.6. Important accessory signalling is involved in antigen presentation. While the peptide–MHC complex is primarily responsible for the specificity of a cellular immune response, many other interactions determine the final outcome. Without the interaction of a variety of accessory molecules (see text) the T cell may become unresponsive, and without the feedback of cytokines from the T cell, the presenting cell may not respond adequately for sufficient time to enable a full immune response to occur

cryptogenic pulmonary fibrosis, in which normal anergy appears to have been broken, and an autoimmune state has resulted.

CONCLUSIONS

MHC molecules are critical to the specific immune system, serving as peptide receptors with a number of purposes. They function first as peptide binders, protecting the peptides from further degradation. Second, they transport the peptides to the cell surface. Finally, they serve as a platform for the display of peptides to the TCR, also comprising part of the determinant recognised by the TCR. The different pathways of peptide processing that have evolved allow the immune system to survey both intra- and extracellular compartments. Cyto-plasm derived peptides are transported into the endoplasmic reticulum, where they bind to nascent MHC class I molecules, which are then transported to the surface membrane along the constitutive biosynthetic/secretory pathway. MHC class II molecules, in contrast, diverge at the trans-Golgi region, and target with the invariant chain to late endocytic compartments where peptide–MHC binding occurs. In each case, the targeting patterns of the MHC molecules determine the source of peptides to be presented to the immune system.

REFERENCES

1. Counce S, Smith P, Barth R, *et al.* Strong and weak histocompatibility gene differences in mice and their role in the rejection of homografts of tumor and skin. *Ann Surg* 1956; **144**: 198–204.
2. Bennacerraf B, McDevitt H O. Histocompatibility-linked immune response genes. *Science* 1972; **175**: 273–279.
3. Schwartz R H. T-lymphocyte recognition of antigen in association with gene products of the major histocompatibility complex. *Annu Rev Immunol* 1985; **3**: 237–261.
4. Bjorkman P J, Saper M A, Samraoui B, *et al.* Structure of the human class I major histocompatibility antigen HLA-A2. *Nature* 1987; **329**: 506–512.
5. Madden D R, Gorga J C, Strominger J L, *et al.* The three-dimensional structure of HLA-B27 at 2.1 Å resolution suggests a general mechanism for tight peptide binding to MHC. *Cell* 1992; **70**: 1035–1048.
6. Stern L J, Brown J H, Jardetzky T S, *et al.* Crystal structure of the human class II MHC protein HLA-DR1 complexed with an influenza virus peptide. *Nature* 1994; **368**: 215–221.
7. Brown J H, Jardetzky T S, Gorga J C, *et al.* Three-dimensional structure of the human class II histocompatibility antigen HLA-DR1. *Nature* 1993; **364**: 33–39.
8. Jardetzky T S, Brown J H, Gorga J C, *et al.* Three-dimensional structure of a human class II histocompatibility molecule complexed with superantigen. *Nature* 1994; **368**: 711–718.
9. Latron F, Pazmany L, Moots R J, *et al.* A critical role for conserved residues in the cleft of HLA-A2 in presentation of a nonapeptide to T cells. *Science* 1992; **257**: 964–967.
10. Matsumura M, Fremont D H, Peterson P A, *et al.* Emerging principles for the recognition of peptide antigens by MHC class I molecules [see comments]. *Science* 1992; **257**:927–934.
11. Brown E L, Wooters J L, Ferenz C R, *et al.* Peptide binding to the murine MHC class-I h-2kk allele. *J Cell Biochem Suppl* 1993; **17C**: 54.
12. Moots R J, Matsui M, Pazmany L, *et al.* A cluster of mutations in HLA-A2 a-helix abolishes peptide recognition by T cells. *Immunogenetics* 1991; **34**: 141–148.
13. Morrison J, Latron F, Moots R J, *et al.* Identification of the nonamer peptide from influenza A matrix protein and the role of pockets of HLA-A2 in its recognition by cytotoxic T lymphocytes. *Eur J Immunol* 1992; **22**: 903–907.
14. Falk K, Rotzschke O, Stevanovic S, *et al.* Allele-specific motifs revealed by sequencing of self-peptides eluted from MHC molecules. *Nature* 1991; **351**: 290–296.
15. Jardetzky T S, Lane W S, Robinson R A, *et al.* Identification of self peptides bound to purified HLA-B27. *Nature* 1991; **353**: 326–329.
16. Rudensky A Y, Preston Hurlburt P, Hong S C, *et al.* Sequence analysis of peptides bound to MHC class II molecules [see comments]. *Nature* 1991; **353**: 622–627.
17. Germain R N. MHC-dependent antigen processing and peptide presentation: providing ligands for T lymphocyte activation. *Cell* 1994; **76**: 287–299.
18. Townsend A R M, Gotch F M, Davey J, Cytotoxic T cells recognize fragments of the influenza nucleoprotein. *Cell* 1985; **42**: 457–467.
19. Moore M W, Carbone F R, Bevan M J. Introduction of soluble protein into the class I pathway of antigen processing and presentation. *Cell* 1988; **54**: 777–785.
20. Harding C V. Electroporation of exogenous antigen into the cytosol for antigen processing and class I major histocompatibility complex (MHC) presentation: weak base amines and hypothermia (18 degrees C) inhibit the class I MHC processing pathway. *Eur J Immunol* 1992; **22**: 1865–1869.
21. Grant E P, Rock K I. MHC class I-restricted presentation of exogenous antigen by thymic antigen presenting cells. *J Immunol* 1992; **148**: 13–18.
22. Pfeifer J D, Wick M J, Roberts R I, *et al.* Phagocytic processing of bacterial antigens for class I MHC presentation to T cells. *Nature* 1993; **361**: 359–362.

23. Carbone F R, Bevan M J. Class I-restricted processing and presentation of exogenous cell-associated antigen *in vivo*. *J Exp Med* 1990; **171:** 377–387.

24. Rotzschke O, Falk K, Deres K, *et al*. Isolation and analysis of naturally processed viral peptides as recognized by cytotoxic T cells. *Nature* 1990; **348:** 252–254.

25. Falk K, Rotzschke O, Rammensee H. Cellular peptide composition governed by major histocompatibility complex class I molecules. *Nature* 1990; **348:** 248–251.

26. Madden D R, Gorga J C, Strominger J L, *et al*. The structure of HLA-B27 reveals nonamer self-peptides bound in an extended conformation. *Nature* 1991; **353:** 321–325.

27. Saper M A, Bjorkman P J, Wiley D C. Refined structure of the human histocompatibility antigen HLA-A2 at 2.6 Å resolution. *J Mol Biol* 1991; **219:** 277–319.

28. Fremont D H, Matsumura M, Stura E A, *et al*. Crystal structures of two viral peptides in complex with murine MHC class I H-2Kb [see comments]. *Science* 1992; **257:** 919–927.

29. Ljunggren H G, Stam N J, Ohlen C, *et al*. Empty MHC class-I molecules come out in the cold. *Nature* 1990; **346:** 476–480.

30. Ortiz Navarrete V, Seelig A, Gernold M, *et al*. Subunit of the '20S' proteasome (multicatalytic proteinase) encoded by the major histocompatibility complex. *Nature* 1991; **353:** 662–664.

31. Martinez C K, Monaco J J. Homology of proteasome subunits to a major histocompatibility complex-linked LMP gene. *Nature* 1991; **353:** 664–667.

32. Driscoll J, Brown M G, Finley D, *et al*. MHC-linked *LMP* gene products specifically alter peptidase activities of the proteasome. *Nature* 1993; **365:** 262–264.

33. Kelly A, Powis S H, Glynne R, *et al*. Second proteasome-related gene in the human MHC class II region. *Nature* 1991; **353:** 667–668.

34. Glynne R, Powis S H, Beck S, *et al*. A proteasome-related gene between the two ABC transporter loci in the class II region of the human MHC [see comments]. *Nature* 1991; **353:** 357–360.

35. Brown M G, Driscoll J, Monaco J J. Structural and serological similarity of MHC-linked LMP and proteasome (multicatalytic proteinase) complexes [see comments]. *Nature* 1991; **353:** 355–357.

36. Yewdell J, Lapham C, Bacik I, *et al*. MHC-encoded proteasome subunits LMP2 and LMP7 are not required for efficient antigen presentation. *J Immunol* 1994; **152:** 1163–1170.

37. Arnold D, Driscoll J, Androlewicz M, *et al*. Proteasome subunits encoded in the MHC are not generally required for the processing of peptides bound by MHC class-I molecules. *Nature* 1992; **360:** 171–174.

38. Townsend A, Ohlen C, Bastin J, *et al*. Association of class I major histocompatibility complex heavy and light chains induced by viral peptide. *Nature* 1989; **340:** 443–448.

39. Bahram S, Arnold D, Bresnahan M, *et al*. Two putative subunits of a peptide pump encoded in the human major histocompatibility complex class II region. *Proc Natl Acad Sci USA* 1991; **88:** 10094–10098.

40. Yang Y, Fruh K, Chambers J, *et al*. Major histocompatibility complex (MHC)-encoded HAM2 is necessary for antigenic peptide loading onto class I MHC molecules. *J Biol Chem* 1992; **267:** 11669–11672.

41. Monaco J J. Genes in the MHC that may affect antigen processing. *Curr Opin Immunol* 1992; **4:** 70–73.

42. Spies T, Cerundolo V, Colonna M, *et al*. Presentation of viral antigen by MHC class I molecules is dependent on a putative peptide transporter heterodimer. *Nature* 1992; **355:** 644–646.

43. Monaco J J, Cho S, Attaya M. Transport protein genes in the murine MHC: possible implications for antigen processing. *Science* 1990; **250:** 1723–1726.

44. Yewdell J W, Esquivel F, Arnold D, *et al*. Presentation of numerous viral peptides to mouse major histocompatibility complex (MHC) class I-restricted T lymphocytes is mediated by the human MHC-encoded transporter or by a hybrid mouse–human transporter. *J Exp Med* 1993; **177:** 1785–1790.

45. Spies T, Bresnahan M, Bahram S, *et al*. A gene in the human major histocompatibility complex class II region controlling the class I antigen presentation pathway [see comments]. *Nature* 1990; **348:** 744–747.

46. De la Salle H, Hanau D, Fricker D, *et al*. Homozygous human TAP peptide transporter mutation in HLA class I deficiency. *Science* 1994; **265:** 237–241.

47. Levy F, Larsson R, Kvist S. Translocation of peptides through microsomal membranes is a rapid process and promotes assembly of HLA-B27 heavy chain and beta 2-microglobulin translated *in vitro*. *J Cell Biol* 1991; **115:** 959–970.

48. Levy F, Gabathuler R, Larsson R, *et al.* ATP is required for *in vitro* assembly of MHC class I antigens but not for transfer of peptides across the ER membrane. *Cell* 1991; **67:** 265–274.

49. Shepherd J C, Schumacher T N, Ashton Rickardt P G, *et al.* TAP1-dependent peptide translocation *in vitro* is ATP dependent and peptide selective. *Cell* 1993; **74:** 577–584.

50. Androlewicz M J, Anderson K S, Cresswell P. Evidence that transporters associated with antigen processing translocate a major histocompatibility complex class I-binding peptide into the endoplasmic reticulum in an ATP-dependent manner. *Proc Natl Acad Sci USA* 1993; **90:** 9130–9134.

51. Zhou X, Glas R, Momburg F, *et al.* TAP2-defective RMA-S cells present Sendai virus antigen to cytotoxic T lymphocytes. *Eur J Immunol* 1993; **23:**1796–1801.

52. Zweerink H J, Gammon M C, Utz U, *et al.* Presentation of endogenous peptides to MHC class I-restricted cytotoxic T lymphocytes in transport deletion mutant T2 cells. *J Immunol* 1993; **150:** 1763–1765.

53. Del Val M, Hengel H, Hacker H, *et al.* Cytomegalovirus prevents antigen presentation by blocking the transport of peptide-loaded major histocompatibility complex class I molecules into the medial-Golgi compartment. *J Exp Med* 1992; **176:** 729–738.

54. Degen E, Williams D B. Participation of a novel 88kD protein in the biogenesis of murine class I histocompatibility molecules. *J Biol Chem* 1991; **112:** 1099–1115.

55. Peters P J, Neefjes J J, Oorschot V, *et al.* Segregation of MHC class-II molecules from MHC class-I molecules in the golgi-complex for transport to lysosomal compartments. *Nature* 1991; **349:** 669–676.

56. Brodsky F M, Guagliardi L E. The cell biology of antigen processing and presentation. *Annu Rev Immunol* 1991; **9:** 707–744.

57. Jensen P E. Enhanced binding of peptide antigen to purified class II major histocompatibility glycoproteins at acidic pH. *J Exp Med* 1991; **174:** 1111–1120.

58. Collins D S, Unanue E R, Harding C V. Reduction of disulfide bonds within lysosomes is a key step in antigen processing. *J Immunol* 1991; **147:** 4054–4059.

59. Harding C V. Pathways of antigen processing. *Curr Opin Immunol* 1991; **3:** 3–9.

60. Harding C V, Collins D S, Kanagawa O, *et al.* Liposome-encapsulated antigens engender lysosomal processing for class-II MHC presentation and cytosolic processing for class-I presentation. *J Immunol* 1991; **147:** 2860–2863.

61. Mouritsen S, Meldal M, Werdelin O, *et al.* MHC molecules protect T cell epitopes against proteolytic destruction. *J Immunol* 1992; **149:** 1987–1993.

62. Sette A, Adorini L, Colon S M, *et al.* Capacity of intact proteins to bind to MHC class II molecules. *J Immunol* 1989; **143:** 1265–1267.

63. Roche P A, Teletski C L, Karp D R, *et al.* Stable surface expression of invariant chain prevents peptide presentation by HLA-DR. *EMBO J* 1992; **11:** 2841–2847.

64. Cresswell P. Assembly, transport, and function of MHC class II molecules. *Annu Rev Immunol* 1994; **12:** 259–293.

65. Layet C, Germain R N. Invariant chain promotes egress of poorly expressed, haplotype-mismatched class II major histocompatibility complex A alpha A beta dimers from the endoplasmic reticulum/cis-Golgi compartment. *Proc Natl Acad Sci USA* 1991; **88:** 2346–2350.

66. Viville S, Neefjes J, Lotteau V, *et al.* Mice lacking the MIIC class II associated invariant chain. *Cell* 1993; **72:** 635–648.

67. Bikoff E K, Huang L Y, Episkopou V, *et al.* Defective major histocompatibility complex class II assembly, transport, peptide acquisition, and CD4+ T cell selection in mice lacking invariant chain expression. *J Exp Med* 1993; **177:** 1699–1712.

68. Reyes V E, Lu S, Humphreys R E. Cathepsin B cleavage of Ii from class II MHC alpha-and beta-chains. *J Immunol* 1991; **146:** 3877–3880.

69. Chicz R M, Urban R G, Gorga J C, *et al.* Specificity and promiscuity among naturally processed peptides bound to HLA-DR alleles. *J Exp Med* 1993; **178:** 27–47.

70. Freisewinkel I N, Schenck K, Koch N. The segment of invariant chain that is critical for association with major histocompatibility complex class II molecules contains the sequence of a peptide eluted from class II polypeptides. *Proc Natl Acad Sci USA* 1993; **90:** 9703–9706.

71. Schwartz R H. Costimulation of T lymphocytes: the role of CD28, CTLA-4, and B7/BB1 in IL-2 production and immunotherapy. *Cell* 1992; **71:** 1065–1068.
72. Mueller D L, Jenkins M K, Schwartz R H. Clonal expansion versus functional clonal inactivation: a costimulatory signalling pathway determines the outcome of T cell antigen receptor occupancy. *Annu Rev Immunol* 1989; **7:** 445–480.
73. Jenkins M K, Burrell E, Ashwell J D. Antigen presentation by resting B cells. Effectiveness at inducing T cell proliferation is determined by costimulatory signals, not T cell receptor occupancy. *J Immunol* 1990; **144:** 1585–1590.
74. June C H, Ledbetter J A, Linsley P S, *et al.* Role of the CD28 receptor in T cell activation. *Immunology Today* 1990; **11:** 211–216.
75. Jenkins M K, Johnson J G. Molecules involved in T-cell costimulation. *Curr Opin Immunol* 1993; **5:** 361–367.
76. Young J W, Koulova L, Soergel S A, *et al.* The B7/BB1 antigen provides one of several costimulatory signals for the activation of CD4+ T lymphocytes by human blood dendritic cells *in vitro. J Clin Invest* 1992; **90:** 229–237.
77. Koulova L, Clark E A, Shu G, *et al.* The CD28 ligand B7/BB-1 provides a costimulatory signal for alloactivation of CD4+ T cells. *J Exp Med* 1991; **173:** 759–762.
78. Liu Y, Linsley P S. Costimulation of T cell growth. *Curr Opin Immunol* 1992; **4:** 265–270.
79. Lenschow D J, Bluestone J A. T cell co-stimulation and *in vivo* tolerance. *Curr Opin Immunol* 1993; **5:** 747–752.

12

Animal Models of Immune Defenses

GALEN B. TOEWS

University of Michigan Medical Center, Ann Arbor, USA

INTRODUCTION

The lung is an important interface between the host and an environment that contains numerous species of potentially harmful microbes. While the airways and the alveoli are regularly exposed to infectious agents (normal ventilation, aerosols, aspiration) infection occurs only relatively rarely. Microbes deposited in the lung encounter a variety of efficient defenses that are capable of eliminating micro-organisms before their multiplication has a deleterious effect on the internal milieu of the host. This complex array of defense mechanisms is spread throughout the entire respiratory tract from the nares to the alveolar surface. It includes mechanical, neural, and immune mechanisms. Mechanical barriers include filtration, sedimentation, and impaction followed by mucociliary clearance. Neural reflexes are involved in cough and bronchoconstriction. Immune mechanisms provide innate immune defenses, inflammatory responses and antigen specific antibody and cell mediated immune responses[1-6].

The immune system exists, first and foremost, to protect the host from infection. The evolutionary history of the immune system has been shaped largely by microbial challenge. Pulmonary immune responses are critical for the defense of the lung; the absence of components of the immune system almost invariably manifests itself by an increased susceptibility to infection. For effective protection, all components of the immune system must function in an integrated fashion. *In vivo* animal models of infection have had a key role in determining the importance of individual components of host defense against microbes.

Pulmonary Defences. Edited by Robert A. Stockley.
© 1997 John Wiley & Sons Ltd.

MECHANICAL DEFENSES

Animal Models

The roles of mechanical barriers and innate immune defenses have been studied in experimental animals, utilizing aerosolization of microbes which deposits them widely and uniformly in the respiratory tract. Variation in the size of the aerosolized particulate matter allows preferential deposition of particles in airways or in the lower respiratory tract. An aerosol exposure can deposit a large number of microbes in the lung, but the microbial burden in any given anatomic focus is small. The ratio of infectious agents to resident phagocytes is low after aerosol deposition. Aerosol deposition of microbes is a physiologic analog of droplet infection[7].

Expression of Mechanical Defenses in the Lung

The epithelial surface of the respiratory tract serves as an efficient barrier to most micro-organisms (Fig. 12.1). The nose and conducting airways are lined by ciliated epithelium[8], and mucociliary clearance has been shown to be of importance for microbes that are deposited in the airways of mice[9]. Effective mucociliary clearance depends not only on the effective function of ciliated epithelial cells, but also on normal tracheobronchial secretions. The latter are composed of goblet cell and bronchial gland mucus fluid mixed with Clara cell secretions and electrolytes[10]. Malfunctions of mucociliary clearance in man may result from inherited or acquired defects in ciliary motion, loss of ciliated epithelium and

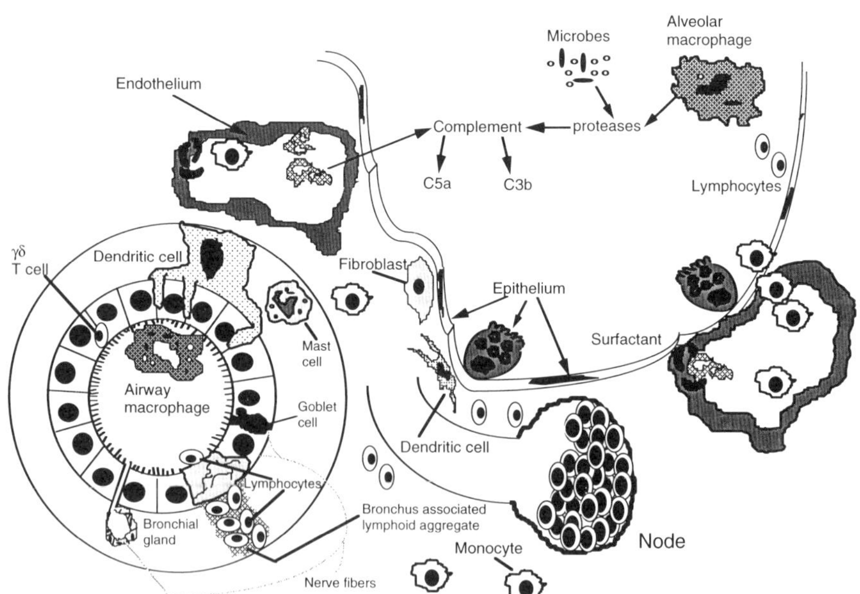

Figure 12.1. Resident defenses of the lung (see text for details)

excessive or abnormal mucus production[11-17]. Sneezing and coughing probably enhance the clearance of microbes deposited within the airways.

Microbes that evade upper respiratory tract mechanical or mucociliary defenses, or those that are deposited in the alveoli, encounter a different group of host defenses. The alveolar epithelium is more than a mere physical barrier to microbial invasion. Bacteria which reach the lower respiratory tract replicate rapidly on the surface of the alveolar epithelium, and microbes which enter the alveolar space encounter alveolar epithelial cell derived substances that might inactivate them. Surfactant (secreted by type II pneumocytes) obtained from rat lung has antibacterial activity against staphylococci, rough colony strains of Gram negative bacteria and some fungi[18-19].

INNATE IMMUNE DEFENSES

All vertebrates counter invasion by microbes with innate immune defenses that exist in the respiratory tract of all individuals. These defenses are not antigen specific, do not require a prolonged period for induction, and begin functioning within minutes of infection. Only when these innate immune defenses are overwhelmed is an inflammatory response or an antigen specific immune response required.

Expression of Innate Immune Defenses in the Lower Respiratory Tract

Innate immune defenses composed entirely of humoral and cellular factors have evolved to defend the lower respiratory tract against microbial invasion (Fig. 12.1). The alternative pathway of complement activation is an important first line of defense against many extracellular microbes[20], and bronchoalveolar lavage fluids contain a functional alternative complement pathway[21]. C3b–Bb complexes formed on the surface of a micro-organism function as active C3/C5 convertases. Complement regulatory proteins are not present on bacterial surfaces; this favors binding of properdin which stabilizes the C3b–Bb convertase activity. This convertase initiates the conversion of large amounts of free C3 molecule to C3b, which coats the surface of the microbe. The membrane bound complex binds C5, induces its cleavage, and initiates the lytic pathway. Inflammatory peptides, C3a and C5a, are also released[22]. Murine studies have confirmed that products of the alternate complement pathway are involved in pulmonary bacterial defenses by contributing opsonic and chemotactic fragments[23].

The alveolar macrophage is the only phagocytic cell normally present within the lower respiratory tract. Accordingly, the alveolar macrophage is the first line of phagocytic cellular defense against microbes[24]. These cells are derived from blood monocytes[25] and have a life span of months and perhaps years[25,26]. The resident alveolar macrophage population is maintained by movement of blood monocytes into the lung and by local proliferation[27], but the mechanisms which regulate monocyte traffic to the normal lung are unknown.

Alveolar macrophages avidly phagocytose inert particles, but ingest viable bacteria considerably less efficiently[4]. Encapsulated microbes resist phagocytosis by means of their polysaccharide capsule[28]. The ability of macrophages to interact with microbes is mediated by surface receptors capable of binding specific ligands including toxins, polysaccharides, lipopolysaccharides, complement proteins and immunoglobulins[29,30]. The ability to recognize surface lectins on microbes is crucial to innate immune defenses. The mannose receptor, a 162 kDa membrane glycoprotein that binds mannose and fucose bovine serum albumin with high affinity, is present on murine alveolar macrophages and inflammatory macrophages[31–33]. All cells transfected with cDNA for the mannose receptor acquire the capacity to ingest yeast, zymosan particles and *Pneumocystis carinii*, indicating that this receptor mediates phagocytosis[34,35]. Complement receptor III (CR3) can directly bind *Histoplasma capsulatum* in the absence of antibody or complement[36]. The capacity of CR3 to bind directly to microbes in the absence of an opsonin may represent another mechanism whereby macrophages recognize potential pathogens before the onset of immunity[37]. While the interaction between C3bi and CR3 mediates binding of complement coated particles, macrophages must be appropriately activated before ligand–CR3 interactions mediate phagocytosis[38,39]. Ligation of CR3 does not mediate release of arachidonic acid metabolites and does not promote secretion of hydrogen peroxide by macrophages[40,41].

Murine studies have shown that alveolar macrophages are capable of clearing small pulmonary inocula of *Staphylococcus aureus* ($<10^5$); however, larger inocula of *Staph. aureus* or Gram negative organisms lead to the generation of an inflammatory response. While small inocula of bacteria can be successfully ingested and killed by alveolar macrophages, larger inocula overwhelm resident alveolar macrophages. Both bacterial virulence and bacteria–phagocyte ratio may be crucial factors in determining whether resident alveolar macrophages are sufficient to clear the microbial challenge[42].

Animal models have been utilized to study the effects of altering resident host defenses on microbial clearance. Environmental manipulations, including exposure to cigarette smoke, pollutants, and noxious gases, alter host defenses. Alveolar hypoxemia, acidosis, ethanol ingestion, acidemia, and pulmonary edema have also been shown to decrease net bacterial clearance[43].

ALVEOLAR INFLAMMATORY RESPONSE

Animal Models

The instillation of microbes directly into a localized area of lung overwhelms innate immune defenses and leads to the generation of an inflammatory response, a specific immune response or both[44]. Microbes are inoculated through an endo-bronchial tube in lightly anesthetized animals and a high ratio of microbes to phagocytes can be achieved by manipulation of the inoculum size of the microbe. This technique mimics the aspiration of pharyngeal microbes into the lower respiratory tract. The importance of various components of the inflammatory response has been demonstrated utilizing animals selectively depleted of polymorphonuclear leukocytes and animals with specific genetic deficiencies[45–47].

Expression of Inflammatory Responses

The generation of an inflammatory response is crucial to the effective clearance of most microbes. The importance of polymorphonuclear neutrophils (PMN) in early bacterial clearance has been shown in experimental animals selectively depleted of PMNs. Animals depleted of neutrophils were unable to clear inocula of *Pseudomonas aeruginosa, Klebsiella pneumoniae*, and *Haemophilus influenzae* as efficiently as normal animals[45,47]. While alveolar macrophages can clear small inocula of some microbes, the recruitment of granulocytes is required to clear most extracellular pulmonary pathogens effectively.

Alveolar macrophages have an important role in the recruitment of additional phagocytic cells and effector molecules to the site of pulmonary infections, through the release of monokines including tumor necrosis factor α (TNFα), interleukin-1 (IL-1), interleukin-6 (IL-6), and interleukin-12 (IL-12)[48]. The synthesis of all of these monokines is stimulated when macrophages recognize microbial constituents; lipopolysaccharide (LPS) is a particularly potent stimulus for the synthesis of these monokines. TNFα increases the vascular diameter of local blood vessels, leading to increased local blood flow and increased vascular permeability, which in turn leads to the local accumulation of immunoglobulins, complement and other blood proteins. The expression of adhesion molecules on the surface of the endothelium that bind to ligands on the surface of circulating polymorphonuclear leukocytes is induced by TNFα and greatly enhances the rate at which phagocytic cells migrate across blood vessel walls into the lung[49].

The migration of leukocytes into the lung has been extensively studied in animal models. Leukocyte migration is believed to occur in four steps[50–52]. The *initial step* involves the weak binding of PMNs to the vascular endothelium through interactions between carbohydrate ligands on the PMNs and selectins on the endothelium. TNFα rapidly induces the expression of P-selectin on endothelial cells and induces the expression of E-selectin within a few hours. These selectins recognize the sialyl Lewis X moiety on the surface of PMNs. While this weak binding does not anchor cells against the shear forces generated by the flow of blood, it does cause PMNs to roll along the endothelium as a result of continually making and losing contact with the endothelium. The *second step* in leukocyte migration is dependent on the interaction between intercellular adhesion molecule-1 (ICAM-1) on endothelial cells and the leukocyte function antigen-1 (LFA-1) on the surface of the PMN. TNFα is importantly involved in the induction of ICAM-1 on endothelial cells. Tight binding between LFA-1 and ICAM-1 arrests the rolling leukocyte and allows it to attach firmly to the endothelium. The *third step* involves the migration of the leukocyte between the endothelial cells. The extravasation of leukocytes involves LFA-1 and platelet endothelial cell adhension molecule (PECAM; cluster of differentiation (CD) 31), which is expressed both on the leukocyte and at the junction of endothelial cells. The *fourth step* is the migration of leukocytes through the tissues under the influence of a chemotactic gradient.

Chemotaxins are present in bronchoalveolar lavage fluid after bacterial challenge and the number of granulocytes present correlates positively with the amount of chemotactic activity present[47,53–56]. The C5 molecule and its fragments have been shown to be important chemotaxins in the lung during an inflammatory response to *Staph. aureus*, *Streptococcus pneumoniae*, *H. influenza*, and *P. aeruginosa*. Bacteria might generate these chemotactic fragments by activating the alternative pathway. C5 might also be cleaved by proteases derived from alveolar macrophages. Non-complement-derived chemotactic factors are also involved in PMN recruitment after bacterial challenges. Alveolar macrophages generate products of arachidonic acid such as 5- or 11-monohydroxyeicosatetraenoic acid and leukotriene B_4[57,58]. Chemokines, small polypeptides belonging to a family of closely related proteins, are also critically involved in granulocyte recruitment to the lung. This group of cytokines are related by primary structural similarities and by the conservation of a 4-cysteine motif. Members of the chemokine family fall into two broad groups, classified according to the position of the first two cysteines in the conserved motif: the C-X-C branch, which includes IL-8 and epithelial neutrophil activating peptide-78 (ENA-78), is characterized by the separation of the first two cysteines by an intervening amino acid, whereas in the C-C branch, which contains monocyte chemoattractant protein-1 (MCP-1), macrophage inflammatory protein-1 (MIP-1) and RANTES (rapid on activation normal T cell expressed and secreted chemokine), these two cysteines are directly adjacent. C-X-C molecules promote the migration of neutrophils, whereas C-C cytokines promote the migration of monocytes[59–61]. All of the receptors for chemokines are similar in structure; all are integral membrane proteins that have seven membrane spanning helices. This structure is characteristic of receptors that are coupled to G proteins. The binding of chemokines to the receptors activates G proteins.

Chemokines are synthesized by a wide array of immune and non-immune parenchymal cells in the lung: macrophages, endothelial cells, epithelial cells, fibroblasts, and smooth muscle cells[62–69]. Stimulus specificity for the elaboration of these chemokines has been demonstrated *in vitro*. Mononuclear phagocytes, endothelial cells and epithelial cells have the ability to generate chemokines in response to microbial products such as LPS. In contrast, endogenous host derived stimuli such as TNFα or IL-1 are required for the production of fibroblast or smooth muscle derived chemokines. TNFα and IL-1 markedly increase gene expression for chemokines in endothelial cells, fibroblasts and epithelial cells. Chemokines bind to proteoglycan molecules both in the extracellular matrix and on parenchymal cells. Chemokines are thus displayed on a solid substrate along which leukocytes might migrate. Chemokines also activate recruited phagocytes for microbicidal activity.

The generation of an inflammatory response following the entry of microbes into the lower respiratory tract requires a complex series of events (Fig. 12.2). The arrival of microbes in the lower respiratory tract activates the alternative complement pathway. Complement activation generates C3bi on the surface of microbes, thereby enhancing the likelihood that microbes will bind to alveolar macrophages, and also generates the important early chemotaxin, C5a. Alveolar macrophages are anatomically positioned to provide a communication link between the microbe and the parenchyma of the lung. They recognize microbes via the binding of microbial products to receptors that are either non-clonal or of very limited diversity. Microbial products such as LPS induce the synthesis of a broad array of monokines which act in a paracrine fashion to induce the synthesis

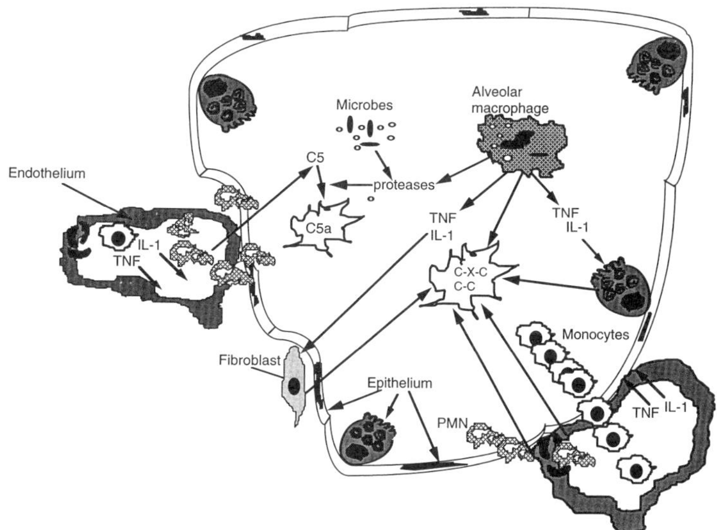

Figure 12.2. Initiation of alveolar inflammatory responses (see text for details). TNF = Tumor necrosis factor; IL-1 = interleukin-1; C5 = fifth component of complement; C-X-C = C-X-C chemokine family; C-C = C-C chemokine family; PMN = polymorphonuclear neutrophil

of chemokines by cells of the alveolar wall. The migration of leukocytes from the vasculature and the generation of a chemotactic gradient is the result of a complex cytokine mediated cell–cell communication network.

ANTIGEN SPECIFIC IMMUNE RESPONSES

Antigen specific immune responses are triggered by microbial infections which elude the innate defense mechanisms and the inflammatory response and generate a threshold dose of antigen. Such responses are effective only after 7–10 days; this time is required for the proliferation and differentiation of antigen specific T cells and B cells into effector cells. During the period during which immune responses develop, the pathogen may continue to grow in the host, being held in check by innate and inflammatory mechanisms.

INITIATION OF SPECIFIC LYMPHOCYTE RESPONSES TO PULMONARY ANTIGENS

Specific pulmonary immune responses are essential for the elimination of virulent encapsulated bacteria, viruses and intracellular organisms that survive in normal phagocytic cells. Activation of T lymphocytes is an early event in all immune responses; it occurs in the draining lymphoid organs. Extensive studies in experimental animals support the following sequence of events for the generation of cell

G. B. Toews

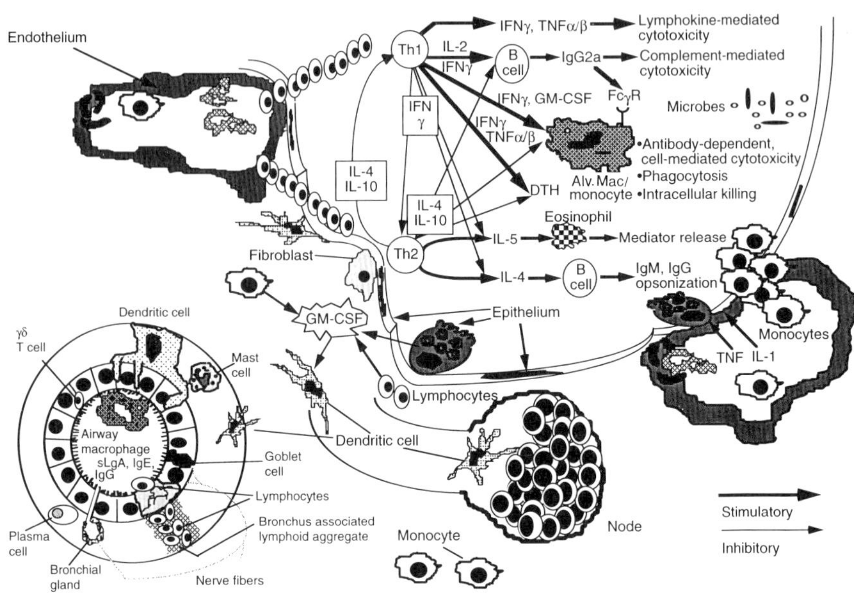

Figure 12.3. Initiation, regulation and expression of specific immune responses in the lung. Dendritic cells (DC) function as sentinel cells in the initiation of immune responses. In the non-perturbed state, DC are located in the interstium of the lung and in the airway epithelium in close contact with pulmonary parenchymal cells. After exposure to antigens, DC differentiation occurs as a result of (i) the action of cytokines produced by cells of the innate immune system (macrophages) in response to interaction with microbes or microbial products, or (ii) the action of cytokines produced as a result of microenvironmental injury to pulmonary epithelial cells. After differentiation, DC migrate to local lymph nodes and present antigen to naive T lymphocytes. After T cell activation, T cells migrate to the pulmonary parenchyma. The control of T cell subset differentiation and their effector functions occurs via complex, cross regulatory interaction mediated by lymphokines. See text for details. Alv. Mac/monocyte = Alveolar macrophage/monocyte; DTH = delayed type hypersensitivity reaction; $Fc_\gamma R$ = Fc_γ receptor; GM − CSF = granulocyte macrophage colony stimulating factor; IFN = interferon; IL = interleukin; sIgA = secretory IgA; TNF = tumor necrosis factor

mediated immune responses to antigens deposited in the lower respiratory tract (Fig. 12.3). Activation of T cells requires the participation of "antigen presenting cells"(APC) that recognize and process antigen, display antigen on their surface in association with major histocompatibility complex (MHC) molecules, and deliver crucial costimulatory signals to responding lymphocytes[70]. An effective APC is present in the lung parenchyma[71]; rapidly accumulating evidence from experimental animals suggests that pulmonary dendritic cells are the major APC in the lung[71−76]. Dendritic cells are found in the interstitium of the lung and are dispersed throughout the columnar epithelium of bronchi. Thus dendritic cells are ideally distributed to interact with antigens that penetrate the bronchial or alveolar epithelial barriers[77]. Antigens which breech the epithelial barrier would be transported by dendritic cells to the regional and hilar lymph node complex via lymphatics. Initiation of a primary immune response probably requires maturation of dendritic cells from antigen recognition and processing cells to potent antigen presenting, immunostimulatory cells. Granulocyte macrophage colony stimulating factor (GM-CSF), TNFα, IL-1, and IL-4 are required for this differentiative step[78]. The source of these differentiation inducing cytokines within the lung might include interstitial macrophages and epithelial cells[78,79]. The secretion of these cytokines might be generated via antigen induced injury to parenchymal cells. Following migration to draining hilar nodes, immunostimulatory dendritic cells would interact with and activate antigen reactive lymphocytes, resulting in expansion of specific clones of T and B lymphocytes.

T CELL MEDIATED IMMUNE RESPONSES IN THE LOWER RESPIRATORY TRACT

The effective clearance of intracellular microbes requires T cell mediated immune responses. Intracellular microbes can be subdivided into two categories: microbes which replicate in the cytosol, such as viruses and certain bacteria (chlamydia), and those that replicate in cellular vesicles, such as mycobacteria and fungi. Antigens from microbes which replicate in the cytosol are presented by MHC class I molecules which are recognized by CD8 $\alpha\beta$ T cells. Antigens from microbes which replicate in the vesicular compartment are presented by class II MHC molecules which are recognized by CD4 $\alpha\beta$ T cells.

Lymphocyte Recruitment to the Lower Respiratory Tract

Activated effector T lymphocytes must travel from lymph nodes to sites of infection to be involved in host defense[50−52]. The activation of naive T cells is accompanied by changes in cell surface adhesion molecules that are involved in this trafficking to sites of infection in the peripheral tissues. Activated effector T lymphocytes lose the L-selectin molecule that mediates homing of naive cells to the lymph node. The expression of other adhesion molecules, including very late activating antigen-4 (VLA-4), is markedly increased. VLA-4 binds to vascular cell adhesion molecule-1 (VCAM-1). TNFα generated during the innate immune response induces the expression of VCAM-1 on endothelial cells at sites of infection in the lung.

A separate means of "traffic control" may be involved for infections that do not trigger innate immune responses. Effector T cells appear to enter all tissues in very small numbers. This traffic is believed to be mediated by the binding of LFA-1 to ICAM-2 which is constitutively expressed on all endothelial cells. If circulating effector T cells recognize specific antigen in the tissue they enter, the effector cells are believed to produce cytokines, including TNFα, that activate endothelial cells to express selectins, ICAM-1, and VCAM-1. The increased levels of ICAM-1 and VCAM-1 would then bind LFA-1 and VLA-4 receptors, respectively, on other activated T cells. The net result would be the recruitment of additional activated T lymphocytes. This interaction could also serve to recruit more monocytes to the lung by adhesion to E-selectin.

Expression of T Cell Mediated Immune Responses in the Lower Respiratory Tract

Animal Models

Intracellular microbes represent an extremely heterogeneous group of pathogens. Animal models exist of *Mycobacterium tuberculosis, M. bovis, Legionella pneumophila, Hist. capsulatum, Cryptococcus neoformans* and influenza[80-85].

T Cell Subpopulations

The kinetics of T cell mediated immune responses in the lung parenchyma and the lymphocyte subsets involved in pulmonary host defenses have been defined almost exclusively from serial studies of experimental models of mycobacterial, fungal, and viral infections. T cells are critical to host defenses against each of these infections.

T cells can be separated into subsets according to their use of accessory molecules and T cell receptors which interact with the MHC gene product[86]. CD4 $\alpha\beta$ T cells recognize antigens presented by class II molecules and CD8 $\alpha\beta$ T cells recognize antigens presented by MHC class I molecules, but γ^δ T cells utilize different molecules (γ and δ chains) to construct the T cell receptor and lack both CD4 and CD8 molecules. CD4 cells can be further separated into two subsets according to their pattern of secretion of lymphokines[87-89]. Th1 cells produce interferon gamma (IFNγ) and IL-2, and Th2 cells produce IL-4, IL-5, and IL-10, whereas both subsets produce IL-3, GM-CSF and TNF$_\alpha$. Th1 cells mediate delayed type hypersensitivity reactions, activate macrophages for microbicidal function, and induce IgG2a; Th2 cells provide help for antibody responses and induce IgG1, IgA, and IgE. The two subsets are mutually inhibitory. IFNγ inhibits the proliferation of Th2 cells, IL-4 inhibits the expression of IL-2 receptors and IFNγ by Th1 cells, and IL-10 inhibits cytokine secretion by Th1 cells. A Th0 subset of cells produces cytokines characteristic of both Th1 and Th2 subsets of cells; Th0 cells are considered to be a precursor from which the Th1 and Th2 phenotype can differentiate[90] (Fig. 12.3).

CD4 T lymphocytes play a central part in host defense against mycobacteria and fungi[82,91-95]. Antigen specific CD4 T cells isolated from *M. tuberculosis* infected mice produce IL-2 and IFNγ and hence are of a Th1 type. Small amounts of IL-4 have been detected in mice immunized with mycobacteria, raising the possibility that Th0 cells also have a role in host defenses against this microbe.

CD8 T cells also participate in host defenses against mycobacterial and fungal pathogens[96-100]. They are present in the outer mantle of granulomatous lesions, and are necessary during the challenge and immunizing phases and for the expression of delayed type hypersensitivity to intact *C. neoformans*[99].

The relative roles of lymphocyte subsets in host defenses against microbes can be investigated by *in vivo* elimination of T cells by treatment with monoclonal antibodies and by adoptive transfer of T cells. These two approaches have revealed important roles for both CD4 and CD8 T cells in murine tuberculosis and fungal infections[91-100]. Mice depleted of CD4 T cells have earlier dissemination of *C. neoformans* from the lung and the burden of the organism is greater in extrapulmonary organs. The survival of mice depleted of CD4 lymphocytes is reduced, while mice depleted of CD8 T cells have both reduced survival and impaired pulmonary clearance.

Recruitment of macrophages and neutrophils to the lungs following *C. neoformans* infection is absolutely T cell dependent[94,95,101]. Cellular recruitment to the lungs is significantly reduced in both CD4 and CD8 T cell deficient mice and depletion of both CD4 and CD8 T cells ablates inflammation. A CD4 deficiency had a more profound effect on the total number of inflammatory cells recruited to the lung than a CD8 deficiency. Recruitment of CD8 T cells occurs independently of CD4 cells, but CD4 T cell recruitment to the lungs was significantly reduced in CD8 deficient mice, suggesting a role for CD8 cells in optimal CD4 T cell recruitment.

Role of Cytokines in Antimicrobial Defense

The cytokines produced during these infections have also been defined. CD4 T cells from *M. tuberculosis* infected mice produce IL-2 and IFNγ[91,102]. Using sensitive detection assays, IL-4 has also been detected in mice immunized with mycobacteria. Thus Th0 and Th1 cells appear to be importantly involved in pulmonary host responses to *M. tuberculosis*. T cells isolated from *C. neoformans* infected mice also produced both Th1 and Th2 cytokines[95]. CD4 depletion resulted in marked decreases in production of IL-4, IL-5, and IL-10. The remaining CD8 T cells secreted IL-2 and IFNγ, although IFNγ secretion was at a lower level than in intact mice. CD8 depleted mice secreted the same or greater levels of IL-4, IL-5, and IL-10 compared with intact mice, whereas IFNγ production was reduced by a CD8 deficiency. Thus a combination of Th1 and Th2 T cells, or Th0 T cells, or all three, are present in the lung during protective immune responses to *C. neoformans*.

The role of individual cytokines in cell mediated immune responses against microbes in the lung has been studied in animal models; both administration of recombinant cytokines and the neutralization of individual cytokines with specific monoclonal antibodies have been utilized. TNFα has been identified as an important mediator of granuloma formation. Administration of TNFα to severe combined immunodeficiency disease mice allows granuloma formation to occur, and neutralization of TNFα results in decreased granuloma formation[103,104]. Blockade of TNFα function inhibits ICAM-1 expression in forming granulomas[105]. ICAM-1 is required for leukocyte recruitment and T lymphocyte activation. TNFα also regulates cell mediated immunity by controlling the induction of chemokine gene expression[106,107]. It induces pulmonary fibroblasts and epithelial cells to express MCP-1 mRNA[64,108]. Both MCP-1 and MIP-1α have crucial roles in leukocyte accumulation and granuloma development in the lung.

Both Th1 and Th2 cytokines have important effector roles in pulmonary defenses. IFNγ, produced by CD4 T cells, CD8 T cells, γδ cells and natural killer cells, has a central role in microbicidal activity against most intracellular microbes. Recombinant IFNγ protects mice against lethal *M. tuberculosis* infection, whereas neutralization with IFNγ antibodies markedly exacerbates the disease[109]. The use of mutant mice with specific, targeted gene disruptions (knock-out mice) has allowed the identification of vital elements in host defenses.

Studies with IFNγ deletion (IFNγ-/-) and IFNγ receptor deletion (IFNγR-/-) mutants have underlined the central role of this cytokine in immunity to tuberculosis in mice. Knockout mice were more severely infected than control mice. *M. tuberculosis* infected IFNγ-/- mice developed granulomas with caseous necrosis and widespread tissue destruction, and widespread dissemination of the infection occurred. Both IFNγ-/- and IFNγR-/- animals failed to produce reactive nitrogen intermediates which are essential for antimicrobial killing[110−113]. IFNγ is a potent stimulator of *in vitro* tuberculostasis and fungistasis in murine mononuclear phagocytes[114−116]. IFNγ and TNFα are synergistic in activating the tuberculostatic capacities of murine phagocytes[114]. GM-CSF is produced by Th0, Th1, and Th2 subsets. It activates macrophages for killing of *Candida albicans* and *C. neoformans*[117−119]. GM-CSF and IFNγ have cooperative activities for the induction of anticryptococcal killing, but are not effective as an activation scheme in mycobacterial systems. GM-CSF primes macrophages for enhanced TNFα production after stimulation by other cytokines, thus participating in an autocrine cytokine loop to activate macrophages[120].

Th2 lymphokines also have important roles in certain granulomatous diseases. Leukocyte accumulation is diminished by neutralization of IL-4 during acute granulomatous responses to schistosomes[121]. IL-4 induces tuberculostatic activity in murine mononuclear phagocytes[122] and is capable of reducing mycobacterial growth even when given after infection of the animal.

Cell mediated cytotoxic responses are important in defense against pulmonary viral infections. Antigen specific CD8 cytotoxic T lymphocytes appear in the lung parenchyma within 1 week after pulmonary viral infections[85]. Viral pathogens replicate in the cytosol. Viral antigens are presented on the surface of infected cells in conjunction with MHC class I molecules. Eradication of viral infections is accomplished when cytotoxic CD8 cells recognize these MHC class I associated viral antigens on the surface of infected cells and lyse them.

B CELL MEDIATED IMMUNE RESPONSES IN LUNG PARENCHYMA

Animal Models

Studies of experimental animals after the instillation of T cell dependent particulate antigens have defined the mechanisms of accumulation of antibody forming cells in the lung[123−126]. Humoral immune responses to protein antigen cannot occur until after antigen specific helper CD4 T cells have been generated, because B cells specific for protein antigens cannot be activated until they encounter an activated helper CD4 T cell specific for one of the peptides derived from the antigen.

Accumulation of Antibody forming Cells in the Lung

The initial phase of B cell proliferation occurs in T cell areas of lymphoid tissues. Primary foci of B cell clonal expansion appear approximately 5 days after primary immunization; this time course correlates with the time required for helper CD4 T cell activation and development. B cells then migrate to the follicle, where they undergo further proliferation, somatic hypermutation, and selection. Some

B cells remain in the medullary cords of lymph nodes and the spleen. Other activated lymphocytes leave the lymph node via efferent lymphatics. Some migrate to bone marrow to complete their differentiation into plasma cells; other B cells migrate to the lung after the instillation of antigens in the lung. Approximately 90% of all antibody produced *in vivo* is produced by bone marrow plasma cells. CD4 T cells enter the interstitium and alveoli initially, followed by B cells and CD8 cells[126]. Lymphocytes are attracted to the lung by spontaneous migration[127], persistence of antigen[123,125,126] or by inflammatory mediators[128]. A pulmonary immune response ensues, with progressive accumulation of antibody forming B cells in the lung parenchyma[125,126]. The pulmonary immune response is accelerated and augmented in primed animals, presumably because of memory cells available for early recruitment into the lung[129].

Expression of B Cell Mediated Immune Responses in the Lower Respiratory Tract

The availability of specific antibody is an important ingredient in host defenses against extracellular microbes. Most extracellular bacteria possess polysaccharide capsules which allow them to evade phagocytic cells. Antibodies have three protective functions: (i) they neutralize pathogens or their toxins by binding to microbes or their products, thereby preventing injury to cells; (ii) they serve as opsonins which allow macrophages to recognize and ingest phagocytes via the involvement of Fc receptors; and (iii) they activate complement which enhances opsonization and can directly lyse some bacteria. Particles recognized by antibodies will be ingested by phagocytic cells.

Immunization can clearly enhance antibacterial defenses in the lower respiratory tract in animal models of bacterial infection. Immunization enhanced the clearance of aerosols of *P. aeruginosa* and *Proteus mirabilis*[130]. Systemic immunization also enhanced pulmonary clearance of bolus inoculated *P. aeruginosa* and *H. influenzae*[131−134]. Mice systemically immunized by parenteral injection of whole non-typable *H. influenzae, H. influenzae* type b, or a cell surface antigen complex consisting of the porin protein (P2) and a lipo-oligosaccharide exhibited an enhanced ability to clear a subsequent pulmonary bolus inoculation of these organisms. This enhanced clearance correlated with the appearance of antibodies in serum and bronchoalveolar lavage fluid which were directed against the organisms. Western blot analysis revealed that the antigenic specificities of the serum antibodies were identical with those of antibodies in lavage fluid. The antibodies obtained from serum were functional, exhibiting bactericidal and opsonic activity against non-typable *H. influenzae*[132,133].

It is difficult to determine the relative contributions of serum antibody and locally produced antibody to the enhanced clearance. Serum IgG antibody can, clearly, directly enhance bacterial clearance from the lower respiratory tract, as intravenous injection of a murine IgG monoclonal antibody specific for a cell surface exposed epitope of non-typable *H. influenzae* lipo-oligosaccharide resulted in enhanced pulmonary clearance[134,135]. IgG antibody accumulated in the alveolar spaces even in the absence of an inflammatory response. Thus serum IgG directly enters the alveolar spaces of the lung. Accordingly, direct airway immunization is not required to obtain protective antibodies in the lung. Immune enhancement of clearance from the lung may be augmented by the exudation of opsonic and bactericidal antibodies from the serum into the alveoli in response to an inflammatory challenge[132,133].

CONCLUSION

The ability of the host to defend itself against pulmonary pathogens that endanger its integrity depends on the coordinated response of many different cells. Animal models of pulmonary infectious diseases have enabled the characterization of the involved cells using criteria such as cell surface markers and the production of secretory products. While animal models which evaluate the interaction of microbes in the host are invariably complex, important information concerning the way in which cells of the immune system communicate, both through direct cell–cell interactions and through the release of cytokines, has been generated. Through the use of animal models, we have come to understand that extraordinary plasticity and adaptability are required to deal successfully with invasive, viable antigens. The complex web of cytokine regulation of immune cell function is gradually being untangled and immunotherapy aimed at manipulating these regulatory signals has already shown some success. Deeper understanding of host defense mechanisms will provide rational strategies for vaccination and immunotherapy.

REFERENCES

1. Newhouse M, Sanchis J, Bienenstock J. Lung defense mechanisms. *N Engl J Med* 1976; **295:** 990–998, 1045–1052.
2. Green G M, Jakab G J, Low R B, *et al.* Defense mechanisms of the respiratory membrane. *Am Rev Respir Dis* 1977; **115:** 479–519.
3. Reynolds H Y. Respiratory infections may reflect deficiencies in host defense mechanisms. *Dis Mon* 1985; **31:** 1–98.
4. Sibille Y, Reynolds H Y. Macrophages and polymorphonuclear neutrophils in lung defense and injury: state of the art. *Am Rev Respir Dis* 1990; **141:** 471–501.
5. Toews G B. Pulmonary clearance of infectious agents. In: Pennington J E, ed. *Respiratory Infections: Diagnosis and Management.* New York: Raven Press, 1994; 43–53.
6. Reynolds H Y. Normal and defective respiratory host defenses. In: Pennington J E, ed. *Respiratory Infections: Diagnosis and Management.* New York: Raven Press, 1994; 1–34.
7. Jay S J, Johanson W G Jr, Pierce A K, *et al.* Determinants of lung bacterial clearance in normal mice. *J Clin Invest* 1976; **57:** 811–817.
8. Reynolds H Y. Pulmonary host defense state of the art. *Chest* 1989; **95:** 2235–2305.
9. Laurenzi G A, Berman L, First M, *et al.* A quantitative study of the deposition and clearance of bacteria in the murine lung. *J Clin Invest* 1964; **43:** 759–768.
10. Reynolds H Y, Newball H H. Analysis of proteins and respiratory cells obtained from human lungs by bronchial lavage. *J Lab Clin Med* 1974; **84:** 559–573.
11. Afzelius B A. A human syndrome caused by immotile cilia. *Science* 1976; **193:** 317–319.
12. Afzelius B A. Immotile-cilia syndrome and ciliary abnormalities induced by infection and injury. *Am Rev Respir Dis* 1981; **124:** 107–109.
13. Fernald G W, Clyde W A Jr. Pulmonary immune mechanisms in *Mycoplasma pneumonia* disease. In: Kirkpatrick C H, Reynolds H Y, eds. *Immunologic and Infectious Reactions in the Lung.* New York: Marcel Dekker, 1976; 101–130.

14. Rubin B K, Ramirez O, Zayas J G, *et al.* Respiratory mucus from asymptomatic smokers is better hydrated and more easily cleared by mucociliary action. *Am Rev Respir Dis* 1992; **145:** 545–547.

15. Seybold Z V, Abraham W M, Gazeroglu H, *et al.* Impairment of airway mucociliary transport by *Pseudomonas aeruginosa* products. *Am Rev Respir Dis* 1992; **146:** 1173–1176.

16. Rutland J, de Iongh R U. Random ciliary orientation — a cause of respiratory tract disease. *N Eng J Med* 1990; **323:** 1681–1684.

17. Rutland J, Griffin W M, Cole P J. Human ciliary beat frequency in epithelium from intrathoracic and extrathoracic airways. *Am Rev Respir Dis* 1982; **125:** 100–105.

18. Coonrod J D. The role of extracellular bactericidal factors in pulmonary host defense. *Semin Respir Infect* 1986; **1:** 118–129.

19. Coonrod J D, Lester R L, Hsu L C. Characterization of the extracellular bactericidal factors of rat alveolar lung material. *J Clin Invest* 1984; **74:** 1269–1279.

20. Gross G N, Rehm S R, Pierce A K. The effect of complement depletion on lung clearance of bacteria. *J Clin Invest* 1978; **62:** 373–378.

21. Robertson J, Coldwell J R, Castle J R, *et al.* Evidence for the presence of components of the alternative (properdin) pathway of complement activation in respiratory secretions. *J Immunol* 1976; **117:** 900–903.

22. Pangburn M K. The alternative pathway In: Ross G D, ed. *Immunobiology of the Complement System.* Orlando: Academic Press, 1986; 45–62.

23. Heidbrink P J, Toews G B, Gross G N, *et al.* Mechanisms of complement-mediated clearance of bacteria from the murine lung. *Am Rev Respir Dis* 1982; **124:** 517–520.

24. Goldstein E, Lippert W, Warshauer D. Pulmonary alveolar macrophage: defender against bacterial infection of the lung. *J Clin Invest* 1974; **54:** 519–528.

25. Thomas E D, Rambergh R E, Sale G E, *et al.* Direct evidence for bone marrow origin of the alveolar macrophage in man. *Science* 1976; **192:** 1016–1018.

26. Winston D J, Territo M C, Ho W G, *et al.* Alveolar macrophage dysfunction in human bone marrow transplant recipients. *Am J Med* 1982; **73:** 859–866.

27. Bitterman P B, Saltzman L E, Adelberg S, *et al.* Alveolar macrophage replication: one mechanism for the expansion of the mononuclear phagocyte population in the chronically inflamed lung. *J Clin Invest* 1984; **74:** 460–469.

28. Gaskel J F. Pathology of the lung. *Lancet* 1927; **2:** 951–957.

29. Ulevitch R J, Tobias P S. Recognition of endotoxin by cells leading to transmembrane signaling. *Curr Opin Immunol* 1994; **6:** 125–128.

30. Wright S D, Ramos T A, Tobias P S, *et al.* CD14, a receptor for complexes of lipopolysaccharide (LPS) and LPS-binding protein. *Science* 1990; **249:** 1431–1433.

31. Ezekowitz R A B. The mannose receptor and phagocytosis. In: van Furth R, ed. *Mononuclear Phagocytes: Biology of Monocytes and Macrophages.* Dordrecht: Kluwer, 1992; 208–213.

32. Taylor M E, Conary J T, Lennartz M R, *et al.* Primary structure of the mannose receptor contains multiple motifs resembling carbohydrate-recognition domains. *J Biol Chem* 1990; **265:** 12156–12162.

33. Shepherd V L, Campbell E J, Senior R M, *et al.* Characterization of the mannose/fucose receptor on human mononuclear phagocytes. *J Reticuloendothel Soc* 1982; **32:** 423–431.

34. Ezekowitz R A, Williams D J, Koziel H, *et al.* Uptake of *Pneumocystis carinii* mediated by the macrophage mannose receptor. *Nature* 1991; **351:** 155–158.

35. Ezekowitz R A, Sastry K, Bailly P, *et al.* Molecular characterization of the human macrophage mannose receptor: demonstration of multiple carbohydrate recognition-like domains and phagocytosis of yeasts in Cos-1 cells. *J Exp Med* 1990; **172:** 1785–1794.

36. Bullock W E, Wright S D. The role of adherence-promoting receptors, CR3, LFA-1, and p150.95 in binding of *Histoplasma capsulatum* by human macrophages. *J Exp Med* 1987; **165:** 195–210.

37. Ehlenberger A G, Nussenzweig V. The role of membrane receptors for C3b and C3d in phagocytosis. *J Exp Med* 1977; **145:** 357–371.

38. Brown E J. Complement receptors and phagocytosis. *Curr Opin Immunol* 1991; **3:** 76–82.

39. Rosen H, Law S K A. The leukocyte cell surface receptor(s) for the iC3b product of complement. *Curr Top Microbiol Immunol* 1990; **153:** 99–122.

40. Yamamoto K, Johnson R B Jr. Dissociation of phagocytosis from stimulation of the oxidative metabolic burst in macrophages. *J Exp Med* 1984; **159:** 405–416.

41. Aderem A A, Wright S D, Silverstein S C, *et al.* Ligated complement receptors do not activate the arachidonic acid cascade in resident peritoneal macrophages. *J Exp Med* 1985; **161:** 617–622.

42. Toews G B, Gross G N, Pierce A K. The relationship of inoculum size to lung bacterial clearance and phagocytic cell response in mice. *Am Rev Respir Dis* 1979; **120:** 559–566.

43. Kass E H, Green G M, Goldstein E. Mechanisms of antibacterial action in the respiratory system. *Bacterial Rev* 1966; **30:** 488–497.

44. Onofrio J M, Toews G B, Lipscomb M F, *et al.* Granulocyte-alveolar macrophage interactions in the pulmonary clearance of *Staphylococcus aureus*. *Am Rev Respir Dis* 1983; **127:** 335–341.

45. Rehm S R, Gross G N, Pierce A K. Early bacterial clearance from murine lungs: species-dependent phagocyte response. *J Clin Invest* 1980; **66:** 194–199.

46. Koller B H, Smithies O. Allergy genes in animals by gene targeting. *Annu Rev Immunol* 1992; **10:** 705–730.

47. Larsen G L, Mitchell B C, Harper T B, *et al.* The pulmonary response of C5 sufficient and deficient mice to *Pseudomonas aeruginosa*. *Am Rev Respir Dis* 1982; **126:** 306–311.

48. Adams D O, Hamilton T A. Macrophages as destructive cells. In: Gallin J I, Goldstein I M, Snyderman R, eds. *Host Defenses in Inflammation: Basic Principles and Clinical Correllates*, 2nd edn. New York: Raven Press, 1992; 637–662.

49. Vassalli P. The pathophysiology of tumor necrosis factors. *Annu Rev Immunol* 1992; **10:** 411–452.

50. Berman J S, Beer D J, Theodore A C, *et al.* Lymphocyte recruitment to the lung. *Am Rev Respir Dis* 1990; **142:** 238–257.

51. Albelda S M, Smith C W, Ward P A. Adhesion molecules and inflammatory injury. *FASEB J* 1994; **8:** 504–512.

52. Springer T A. Adhesion receptors of the immune system. *Nature* 1990; **346:** 425–434.

53. Toews G B, Pierce A K. The fifth component of complement is not required for the clearance of *Staphylococcus aureus*. *Am Rev Respir Dis* 1984; **129:** 597–601.

54. Toews G B, Vial W C. The role of C5 in polymorphonuclear leukocyte recruitment in response to *Streptococcus pneumoniae*. *Am Rev Respir Dis* 1984; **129:** 82–86.

55. Toews G B, Vial W C, Hansen E J. Role of C5 and recruited neutrophils in early clearance of nontypable *Haemophilus influenzae* from murine lungs. *Infect Immun* 1985; **50:** 207–212.

56. Vial W C, Toews G B, Pierce A K. Early pulmonary granulocyte recruitment in response to *Streptococcus pneumoniae*. *Am Rev Respir Dis* 1984; **129:** 87–91.

57. Fels A O S, Pawlowski N A, Cramer E G, *et al.* Human alveolar macrophages produce leukotriene B_4. *Proc Natl Acad Sci USA* 1982; **79:** 7866–7870.

58. Valone F H, Franklin M, Sun G G, *et al.* Alveolar macrophage lipoxygenase products of arachidonic acid: isolation and recognition as the predominant constituents of the neutrophil chemotactic activity elaborated by alveolar macrophages. *Cell Immunol* 1985; **54:** 390–401.

59. Baggiolini M, Dewald B, Walz A. Interleukin-8 and related chemotactic cytokines. In: Galli J I, Goldstein I M, Snyderman R, eds. *Inflammation—Basic Principles and Clinical Correllates*. New York: Raven Press, 1992; 247–263.

60. Miller M P, Krangel M S. Biology and biochemistry of the chemokines: a family of chemotactic and inflammatory cytokines. *Crit Rev Immunol* 1992; **12:** 17–46.

61. Oppenheim J J, Zachariae L O L, Mukaida N, *et al.* Properties of the novel pro-inflammatory supergene intercrine cytokine family. *Annu Rev Immunol* 1993; **8:** 817–848.

62. Colotta F, Borre A, Ming Wamg J, *et al.* Expression of a monocyte chemotactic cytokine by human mononuclear phagocytes. *J Immunol* 1992; **148:** 760–765.

63. Matsusshima K, Oppenheim J J. Interleukin 8 and MCAF: novel inflammatory cytokines inducible by IL-1 and TNF. *Cytokine* 1989; **1:** 2–13.

64. Rolfe M W, Kunkel S L, Standiford T J, *et al.* Expression and regulation of human pulmonary fibroblast-derived monocyte chemotactic peptide (MCP-1). *Am J Physiol* 1992; **263:** L536–L545.

65. Standiford T J, Kunkel S L, Basha M A, *et al.* Interleukin-8 gene expression by a pulmonary epithelial cell line: a model for cytokine networks in the lung. *J Clin Invest* 1990; **86:** 1945–1953.

66. Standiford T J, Kunkel S L, Phan S H, *et al.* Alveolar macrophage-derived cytokines induce monocyte chemoattractant protein-1 expression from human pulmonary type II like epithelial cells. *J Biol Chem* 1991; **266:** 9912–9918.

67. Strieter R M, Chensue S W, Basha M A, *et al.* Human alveolar macrophage gene expression of interleukin-8 by TNF-α, LPS and IL-1β. *Am J Respir Cell Mol Biol* 1990; **2:** 321–326.

68. Strieter R M, Kunkel S L, Showell H, *et al.* Endothelial cell gene expression of a neutrophil chemotactic factor by TNF-α, LPS, and IL-1β. *Science* 1989; **243:** 1467–1469.

69. Strieter R M, Phan S H, Showell H J, *et al.* Monokine-induced neutrophil chemotactic factor gene expression in human fibroblasts. *J Biol Chem* 1989; **264:** 10621–10626.

70. Hance A J. Accessory cell lymphocyte interactions. In: Crystal R G, West J B, eds. *The Lung: Scientific Foundations.* New York: Raven Press, 1991; 483–498.

71. Weissler J C, Lyons C R, Lipscomb M F, *et al.* Human pulmonary macrophages: functional comparison of cells obtained from whole lung and by bronchoalveolar lavage. *Am Rev Respir Dis* 1986; **133:** 473–477.

72. Sertl K, Takemura T, Tschachler E, *et al.* Dendritic cells with antigen-presenting capability reside in airway epithelium, lung parenchyma, and visceral pleura. *J Exp Med* 1986; **163:** 436–51.

73. Holt P G, Schon-Hegrad M A. Localization of T cells, macrophages and dendritic cells in rat respiratory tract tissue: implications for immune function studies. *Immunology* 1987; **62:** 349–356.

74. Holt P G, Schon-Hegrad M A, Oliver J. MHC class II antigen-bearing dendritic cells in pulmonary tissues of the rat. *J Exp Med* 1988; **167:** 262–274.

75. Nicod L P, Lipscomb M F, Weissler J C, *et al.* Mononuclear cells in human lung parenchyma: characterization of a potent accessory cell not obtained by bronchoalveolar lavage. *Am Rev Respir Dis* 1987; **136:** 818–823.

76. Pollard A M, Lipscomb M F. Characterization of murine lung dendritic cells: similarities to langerhans cells and thymic dendritic cells. *J Exp Med* 1990; **172:** 159–167.

77. Toews G B. Pulmonary dendritic cells: sentinels of lung-associated lymphoid tissues. *Am J Respir Cell Mol Biol* 1991; **4:** 204–205.

78. Armstrong L R, Christensen P J, Paine R III, *et al.* Regulation of the immunostimulatory activity of rat pulmonary interstitial dendritic cells by cell–cell interactions and cytokines. *Am J Respir Cell Mol Biol* 1994; **11:** 682–691.

79. Christensen P J, Armstrong L R, Chen G-H, *et al.* Modulation of rat pulmonary dendritic cell function by alveolar epithelial cells *in vitro. Am J Respir Cell Mol Biol* 1995; **13:** 426–433.

80. Kaufmann S H E. Immunity to intracellular bacteria. Annu Rev Immunol 1992; **11:** 129–163.

81. Eisenstein B I, Engleberg N L. Genetics and molecular pathogenesis of *Legionella pneumophila*, an intracellular parasite of macrophages. *Mol Biol Med* 1989; **6:** 409–424.

82. Gomez A M, Bullock W E, Taylor C L, *et al.* Role of L3T4⁺ T cells in host defense against *Histoplasma capsulatum. Infect Immun* 1988; **56:** 1685–1691.

83. Lipscomb M F, Alvarellos T, Toews G B, *et al.* Role of natural killer cells in resistance to *Cryptococcus neoformans* infections in mice. *Am J Pathol* 1987; **128:** 354–361.

84. Mody C H, Toews G B, Lipscomb M F. Cyclosporin A inhibits the growth of *Cryptococcus neoformans* in a murine model. *Infect Immun* 1988; **56:** 7–12.

85. Wyde P R, Cate T R. Cellular changes in lungs of mice infected with influenza virus: characterization of the cytotoxic responses. *Infect Immun* 1978; **22:** 423–429.

86. Janeway C A. The T cell receptor as a multicomponent signaling machine: CD4/CD8 coreceptors and CD45 in T cell activation. *Annu Rev Immunol* 1992; **10:** 645–674.

87. Mosmann T R, Coffman R L. TH1 and TH2 cells: different patterns of lymphokine secretion lead to different functional properties. *Annu Rev Immunol* 1989; **7:** 145–173.

88. Mosmann T F, Coffman R L. Heterogeneity of cytokine secretion patterns and functions of helper T cells. *Adv Immunol* 1989; **46:** 111–147.

89. Powrie F, Coffman R L. Cytokine regulation of T-cell function: potential for therapeutic intervention. *Immunol Today* 1993; **14:** 270–274.

90. Firestein G S, Roeder W D, Laxer J A, *et al.* A new murine CD4$^+$ cell subset with an unrestricted cytokine profile. *J Immunol* 1989; **143:** 518–525.

91. Kaufmann S H E, Fleach I. Function and antigen recognition pattern of L3T4$^+$ T cell clones from *Mycobacterium tuberculosis*-immune mice. *Infect Immun* 1986; **54:** 291–296.

92. Mody C H, Lipscomb M F, Street N E, *et al.* Depletion of CD4+ [L3T4$^+$] lymphocytes *in vivo* impairs murine host defense to *Cryptococcus neoformans. J Immunol* 1990; **144:** 1472–1477.

93. Huffnagle G B, Yates J L, Lipscomb M F. T cell-mediated immunity in the lung: a *Cryptococcus neoformans* pulmonary infection model using SCID and athymic nude mice. *Infect Immun* 1991; **59:** 1423–1432.

94. Huffnagle G B, Yates J L, Lipscomb M F. Immunity to a pulmonary *Cryptococcus neoformans* infection requires both CD4+ and CD8+ T cells. *J Exp Med* 1991; **173:** 793–800.

95. Huffnagle G B, Lipscomb M F, Lovchik J L, *et al.* The role of CD4+ and CD8+ cells in the protective response to a pulmonary cryptococcal infection. *J Leukoc Biol* 1994; **55:** 35–42.

96. DeLibero G, Flesch I, Kaufmann S H E. Mycobacteria reactive Lyt2+ cell lines. *Eur J Immunol* 1988; **18:** 59–66.

97. Rees A D M, Scoging A, Mehlert A, *et al.* Specificity of proliferative response of human CD8 clones to mycobacterial antigens. *Eur J Immunol* 1988; **18:** 1881–1887.

98. Mody C H, Chen G-H, Jackson C, *et al.* Depletion of murine CD8+ T cells *in vivo* decreases pulmonary clearance of a moderately virulent strain of *Cryptococcus neoformans. J Lab Clin Med* 1993; **121:** 765–773.

99. Mody C H, Paine R III, Jackson C, *et al.* CD8 cells play a critical role in delayed type hypersensitivity to intact *Cryptococcus neoformans. J Immunol* 1994; **152:** 3870–3879.

100. Mody C H, Chen G-H, Jackson C, *et al.* Depletion of murine CD8 lymphocytes *in vivo* impairs survival following infection with a virulent strain of *Cryptococcus neoformans. Mycopathologica* 1994; **125:** 7–17.

101. Curtis J L, Chen G-H, Warnock M L, *et al.* Experimental pulmonary cryptococcosis: differences in pulmonary inflammation and lymphocyte recruitment induced by two strains of *C. neoformans. Lab Invest* 1994; **71:** 113–126.

102. Kelso A, Gough N M. Coexpression of granulocyte-macrophage colony-stimulating factor, γ interferon, and interleukin 3 and 4 is random in murine alloreactive T-lymphocyte clones. *Proc Natl Acad Sci USA* 1988; **85:** 9189–9193.

103. Amiri P, Locksley R M, Parslow T G, *et al.* Tumor necrosis factor α restores granulomas and induces parasite egg laying schistosome-infected SCID mice. *Nature* 1992; **356:** 604–607.

104. Joseph A L, Boros D L. TNF plays a role in *Schistosoma mansoni* egg-induced granulomatous inflammation. *J Immunol* 1993; **151:** 5461–5471.

105. Lukacs N W, Chensue S W, Strieter R M, *et al.* Inflammatory granuloma formation is mediated by TNFα-induced intercellular adhesion molecule-I. *J Immunol* 1994; **152:** 5883–5889.

106. van Seventer G A, Shimona Y, Horgan K J,*et al.* The lymphocyte function associated antigen I ligand intracellular adhesion molecule-1 provides an important costimulatory signal for T cell receptor-mediated activation of resting T cells. *J Immunol* 1990; **144:** 4579–4586.

107. Christensen P J, Rolfe M W, Standiford T J, *et al.* Characterization of the production of monocyte chemoattractant protein-1 and IL-8 in an allogenic immune response. *J Immunol* 1993; **151:** 1205–1213.

108. Paine R III, Rolfe M W, Standiford T J, *et al.* MCP-1 expression by rat type II alveolar epithelial cells in primary culture. *J Immunol* 1993; **150:** 4561–4570.

109. Denis M. Involvement of cytokines in determining resistance and acquired immunity in murine tuberculosis. *J Leukoc Biol* 1991; **50:** 495–501.

110. Huang S, Hendriks W, Athage A, *et al.* Immune responses in mice that lack the interferon-γ receptor. *Science* 1993; **259:** 1742–1745.

111. Dalton D K, Pitts-Meer S, Keshav S, *et al.* Multiple defects of immune cell function in mice with disrupted interferon-γ genes. *Science* 1993; **259:** 1739–1742.

112. Cooper A M, Dalton D K, Stewart T A, *et al.* Disseminated tuberculosis in interferon-γ gene disrupted mice. *J Exp Med* 1993; **178:** 2243–2247.

113. Flynn J L, Chan J, Triebold K J, *et al.* An essential role for interferon-γ in resistance to mycobacterium tuberculosis infection. *J Exp Med* 1993; **178:** 2249–2254.

114. Flesch I, Kaufmann S H E. Mycobacterial growth inhibition by interferon-γ-activated bone marrow macrophages and differential susceptibility among strains of *Mycobacterium tuberculosis. J Immunol* 1987; **138:** 4408–4413.

115. Denis M. Interferon-γ-treated murine macrophages inhibit growth of tubercle bacilli via the generation of reactive nitrogen intermediates. *Cell Immunol* 1991; **132:** 150–157.

116. Mody C H, Tyler C L, Sitrin R G, *et al.* Interferon-γ activates rat alveolar macrophages for anti-cryptococcal activity. *Am J Resp Cell Mol Biol* 1991; **5:** 19–26.

117. Wang M, Friedman H, Djeu J Y. Enhancement of human monocyte function against *Candida albicans* by the colony stimulating factors (CSF): IL-3 granulocyte-macrophage CSF and macrophage-CSF. *J Immunol* 1989; **143:** 671–677.

118. Chen G-H, Curtis J L, Mody C H, *et al.* Effect of granulocyte-macrophage colony-stimulating factor (GM-CSF) on rat alveolar macrophage anti-cryptococcal activity *in vitro. J Immunol* 1994; **152:** 724–734.

119. Levitz S M. Activation of human peripheral blood mononuclear cells by interleukin-2 and granulocyte-macrophage colony-stimulating factor to inhibit *Cryptococcus neoformans. Infect Immun* 1991; **59:** 3393–3397.

120. Heidenreich S, Gong J-H, Schmidt A, *et al.* Macrophage activation by granulocyte/macrophage colony-stimulating factor: priming for enhanced release of tumor necrosis factor alpha and prostaglandin E$_2$. *J Immunol* 1989; **143:** 1198–1205.

121. Chensue S W, Terebuh P D, Warmington K S, *et al.* Role of IL-4 and IFN-γ in *Schistosoma mansoni* egg-induced hypersensitivity granuloma formation. Orchestration, relative contribution, and relationship to macrophage function. *J Immunol* 1992; **148:** 900–906.

122. Flesch I E A, Kaufmann S H E. Activation of tuberculostatic macrophage functions by interferon-γ, interleukin 4 and tumor necrosis factor. *Infect Immun* 1990; **58:** 2675–2677.

123. Kaltreider H B, Byrd P K, Daughety T W, *et al.* The mechanism of appearance of specific antibody-forming cells in lungs of inbred mice after intratracheal immunization with sheep erythrocytes. *Am Rev Respir Dis* 1983; **127:** 316–321.

124. Bice D E, Shopp G M. Antibody responses after lung immunization. *Exp Lung Res* 1988; **14:** 133–155.

125. Kaltreider H B, Curtis J L, Arraj S M. The mechanism of appearance of specific antibody-forming cells in lungs of inbred mice after immunization with sheep erythrocytes intratracheally II. *Am Rev Respir Dis* 1987; **135:** 87–92.

126. Curtis J L, Kaltreider H B. Characterization of bronchoalveolar lymphocytes during a specific antibody-forming cell response in the lungs of mice. *Am Rev Respir Dis* 1989; **139:** 393–400.

127. Kaltreider H B, Barth E, Pellegrini C. The effect of splenectomy on the appearance of specific antibody-forming cells in lungs of dogs after intravenous immunization with sheep erythrocytes. *Exp Lung Res* 1981; **2:** 231–238.

128. Bice D E, Degen M A, Harris D L, *et al.* Recruitment of antibody-forming cells in the lung after local immunization is nonspecific. *Am Rev Respir Dis* 1982; **126:** 635–639.

129. Bice D E, Muggenburg B A. Localized immune memory in the lung. *Am Rev Respir Dis* 1988; **138:** 565–571.

130. Jakab G J. Factors influencing the immune enhancement of intrapulmonary bactericidal mechanisms. *Infect Immun* 1976; **14:** 389–398.

131. Dunn M M, Toews G B, Hart D, *et al.* The effects of systemic immunization on pulmonary clearance of *Pseudomonas aeruginosa. Am Rev Respir Dis* 1985; **131:** 426–431.

132. Hansen E J, Hart D A, McGehee J L, *et al.* Immune enhancement of pulmonary clearance of nontypable *Haemophilus influenzae. Infect Immun* 1988; **56:** 182–190.

133. Pennington J E, Hickey W F, Blackwood L O, *et al.* Active immunization with lipopolysaccharide Pseudomonas antigen for chronic Pseudomonas bronchopneumonia in guinea pigs. *J Clin Invest* 1981; **68:** 1140–1148.

134. Toews G B, Hart D A, Hansen E J. Effect of systemic immunization on pulmonary clearance of *Haemophilus influenzae* type b. *Infect Immun* 1985; **48:** 343–349.

135. McGehee J L, Radolf J R, Toews G B, *et al.* Effect of primary immunization on pulmonary clearance of non-typable *Haemophilus influenzae. Am J Respir Cell Mol Biol* 1989; **1:** 201–210.

13

Inhibition of Cell Migration

RICHARD A. ROBBINS*

University of Nebraska Medical Center, Omaha, USA

ROBERT G. TOWNLEY

Creighton University, Omaha, USA

INTRODUCTION

Directed cell migration, or chemotaxis, is a tightly regulated process. Much attention has focused on the migration of the blood leukocytes. This is not surprising, because the importance of the early migration of leukocytes into infected tissue sites for host defense has been long appreciated[1]. However, only recently has the concept that inflammatory cells themselves can cause tissue destruction been appreciated, emphasizing the importance for tight regulation of inflammatory cell migration[2]. Many other non-inflammatory cells can also migrate and their migration is becoming increasingly recognized as important in structure–function relationships and tissue repair[3,4]. Although inflammatory cell migration has been more extensively studied, many of the mechanisms and principles of cell migration derived from studies of inflammatory cells may also apply to non-inflammatory cells. It seems likely that future investigations will elucidate important similarities, in addition to differences, in the migration of inflammatory and non-inflammatory cells.

MECHANISMS OF CELL MIGRATION

The migration of cells is still incompletely understood, even in the neutrophil, which has been most extensively studied. Chemotaxis can be separated into at least three events: (i) release of a chemotactic factor from a cellular source or generation of a chemotactic factor from humoral factors; (ii) binding of

---

*Present address: Overton Brooks Medical Center, Shreveport, USA.

Pulmonary Defences. Edited by Robert A. Stockley.
© 1997 John Wiley & Sons Ltd.

the chemotactic factor to an appropriate receptor; (iii) activation of a complex series of events which initiate cell movement toward the chemotactic stimulus (Fig. 13.1). One extensively studied chemotactic factor is the bacterial peptide, *N*-formyl-methionyl-leucyl-phenylalanine (fMLP). fMLP binding to its receptor on the neutrophil results in the activation of a pertussis toxin sensitive G-protein[5]. Activation of the G-protein results in a large number of events, including cleavage of phophatidylinositol, release of calcium from intracellular stores, splitting of diacylglycerol, activation of protein kinase C, and an increase in arachidonate. This is followed by the phosphorylation and activation of many proteins and enzymes, including glycogen phosphorylase, phospholipase A2, and various ion pumps and channels[6]. The end result is the formation of lamellae, or pseudopods, which extend from the cell in the direction of migration, attach to the surface

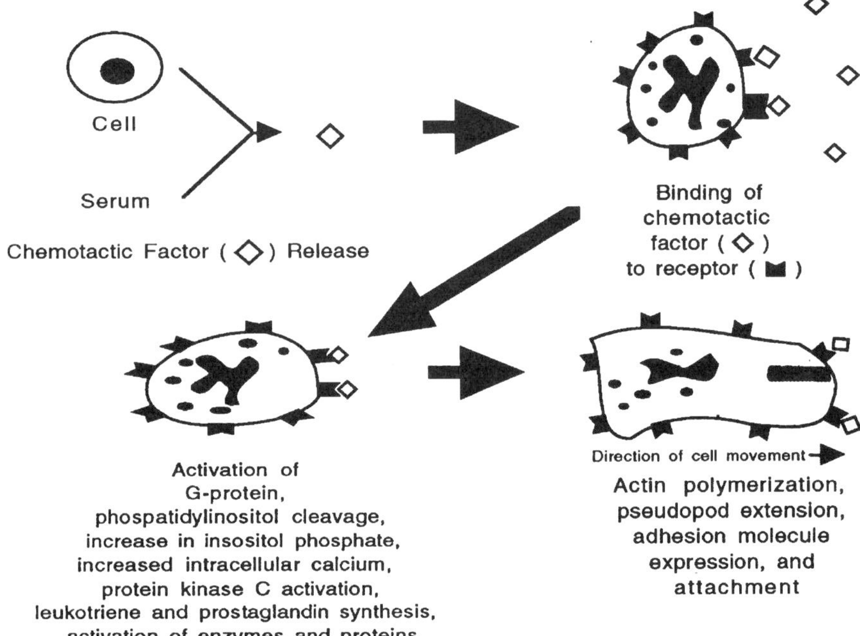

Figure 13.1. Diagrammatic representation of the proposed mechanism of cell movement based on the neutrophil. Release of a chemotactic factor by a stimulated cell or by generation from humoral sources (upper left). The chemotactic factor diffuses to the responding cell and attaches to receptors on the cell surface (upper right). This binding of a chemotactic factor to its receptor (lower left) results in the activation of a pertussis toxin sensitive G-protein. G-protein activation causes cleavage of phophatidylinositol, which releases calcium from intracellular stores, and splitting of diacylglycerol, activation of protein kinase C, an increase in arachidonate, and phosphorylation and activation of many proteins and enzymes, including glycogen phosphorylase, phospholipase A2, and various ion pumps and channels. This, in turn, results in the formation of lamellae, or pseudopods, which extend from the cell in the direction of migration, attach to the surface ahead of the cell, and appear to pull the cell forward (lower right)

ahead of the cell, and pull the cell forward[6,7]. The mechanism by which the cells are pulled forward appears quite complex, but it is known that polymerization of actin is important[7].

In the context of the inhibition of cell migration, several events are believed to be important in the termination of cell movement. When the cell no longer senses a chemotactic gradient, the lamellae are no longer directionally extruded and cell movement stops[6,7]. Chemotactic receptors appear to be eventually downregulated, but the decrease is specific for the chemotactic factor added[6]. This results in "desensitization", or a decrease in the chemotactic response of the cell for the chemoattractant to which it had just been exposed.

Table 13.1. Physiologic inhibitors of cell migration

Complement inhibitors	*Proteinases and antiproteinases*
Clq esterase	α_1 Proteinase inhibitor
C3b inactivator	α_1 Antichymotrypsin
β1H	Antileukoproteinase
Carboxypeptidase N	Neutrophil elastase
GcGlobulin	Cathepsin G
Chemotactic factor inactivator	Elastase generated fragments
C4 derived monocyte	C reactive protein
chemotaxis inhibitor	IgG
Cytokines	*Arachidonic acid metabolites*
Migration inhibitory factor	Prostaglandin E_1
Interferon gamma	Prostacyclin
Tumor necrosis factor α	Lipoxin A4
GM-CSF	
Neutrophil immobilizing factor	*Nitric oxide related*
Leukocyte inhibitory factor	Nitric oxide synthase inhibitors
Human alveolar macrophage leukocyte	Nitric oxide
inhibiting factor	

GM-CSF = Granulocyte macrophage colony stimulating factor.

Table 13.2. Partial listing of the disorders associated with decreased cell movement

Acquired	Congenital
Severe infections	Job's syndrome
Diabetes mellitus	Chediak–Higashi syndrome
Rheumatoid arthritis	Lazy leukocyte syndrome
Burns	Wiskott–Aldridge syndrome
Bone marrow transplantation	Down's syndrome
Cancer	Familial Mediterranean fever
Increased IgA	CD18 deficiency
Liver cirrhosis	Neutrophil actin dysfunction
Alcoholic hepatitis	syndrome
α_1 Antitrypsin deficiency	
Hypersensitivity pneumonitis	
Hemodialysis	
Sarcoidosis	
Systemic lupus erythematosus	

Table 13.3. Partial listing of pharmacologic inhibitors of cell migration

β-Agonists 　Isoproterenol 　Formoterol 　Salmeterol	*Platelet activating factor antagonists* 　WEB-2086 　BN-52021
Anti-inflammatory agents 　Corticosteroids 　Chromolyn sodium 　Nedocromil sodium 　Cyclosporine 　Azathioprine 　FK506 　Non-steroidal anti-inflammatory agents	*Antihistamines* 　Terfenadine 　Ketotifen 　Cetirizine 　Loratidine *Immunotherapy*
Phosphosdiesterase (PDE) inhibitors 　Theophylline 　Rolipram 　WAY-PDA-641 　Zordaverine	*Histamine inhalation*

Although a classification of inhibitors of cell migration based on their mechanisms would be ideal, such a classification is problematic because the mechanisms of many of the inhibitors of cell migration are often speculative or unknown. Therefore, a classification system based on the source of the inhibitor is presented here. This system includes physiologic inhibitors which are normal serum or tissue factors that can attenuate cell migration (Table 13.1), host factors in which an acquired or inherited defect of the responding cell results in a decreased migratory response (Table 13.2), inhibitors derived from micro-organisms which may give the organism an advantage in evading normal host defenses, and pharmacologic inhibitors which may have an inhibition of cell migration as part of the intended therapeutic outcome or as an unintended side effect (Table 13.3).

METHODS FOR MEASURING CELL MOVEMENT

The development of the blindwell chemotaxis chamber by Boyden in 1962 stimulated the modern interest in cell migration[8]. This technique allowed relatively easy *in vitro* testing of chemotaxis, chemotactic factors, and inhibitors of chemotaxis and is reasonably accurate and quantitative. In this blindwell technique, a chemotactic stimulus is placed in the lower of two chambers that are separated by a membrane with pores of a certain diameter. The migrating cells are placed in the upper chamber and either the number of cells which transverse the membrane are counted (Fig. 13.2) or the distance the cells migrate into the membrane is measured (leading front assay[9]). Later, methods examining cell migration under agarose, capillary tube microassays, radiolabeling the migrating cells, or examining individual cells rather than populations were developed[10-13]. Although in general these methods give similar results, there have been excep-

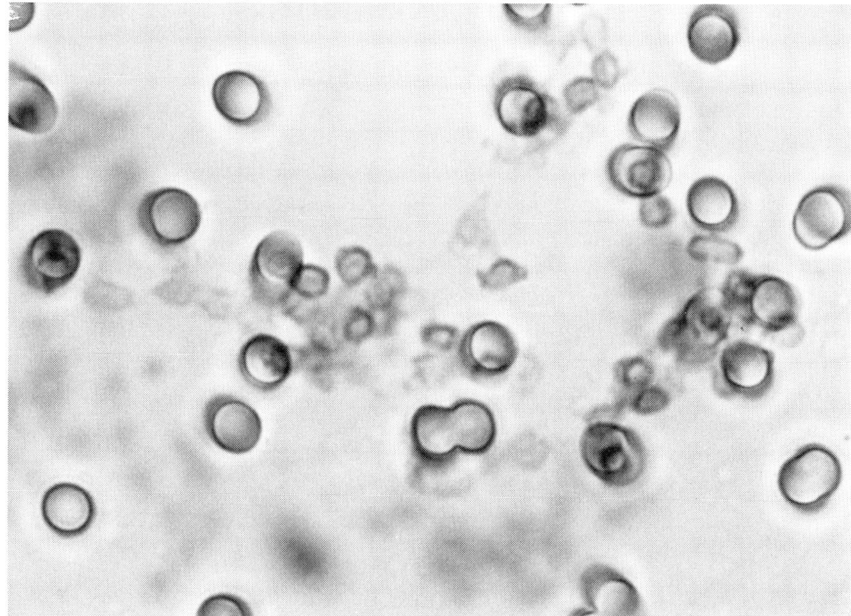

Figure 13.2. Photomicrograph of lymphocytes which have migrated through a nitrocellulose membrane with 8 μm pores, in response to a chemotactic stimulus. The microscope is focused on the lower surface of the membrane. The large structures resembling rings are the pores. The cells sharply in focus represent those which have migrated through the membrane, while the smudge-like shapes represent out of focus cells on the upper portion of the membrane

tions. For example, Otsuka *et al.*[14] examined the effects of recombinant tumor necrosis factor α (TNFα) on neutrophil migration and found opposite effects with the under-agarose and blindwell chamber methods[14]. Observations such as these underscore that these chemotaxis assays are *in vitro* assays, and therefore have limitations.

In recognition of these problems, several inventive assays have been developed to mimic the *in vivo* situation more closely. Casale *et al.*[15] developed a method of culturing cells to confluence on a chemotactic membrane. The radio-labeled cells are added to the top of a blindwell chamber and the number of cells which migrate to the bottom is determined. Using this technique, the investigators have reported that migration of neutrophils through epithelial or endothelial cells grown to confluence on a chemotactic membrane can produce quantitatively variable results, suggesting that the barrier through which the cell is migrating may be important in inhibiting cell movement. In the context of the lung, *in vivo* techniques for repeated quantification of inflammatory cell migration have been developed[16]. Of course, bronchoalveolar lavage and biopsy can sample the lumens of the airways or the submucosal structures and can be useful for determining the *in vivo* activity of a chemotactic factor[17].

PHYSIOLOGIC INHIBITORS

COMPLEMENT

The complement system is a potent source of neutrophil, basophil, monocyte, and eosinophil chemotactic activity[18]. Most of the chemotactic activity can be attributed to generation of C5 fragments[18]. A number of inhibitors can prevent complement pathway activation before the cleavage of C5 and, therefore, might be expected to decrease generation of complement derived chemotactic activity[18]. The initial C5 fragment formed, C5a, is a potent chemotactic factor, but rapidly acted upon by carboxypeptidase-N, cleaving the terminal arginine to form the less potent chemotactic factor $C5a_{desArg}$[18]. $C5a_{desArg}$ can decrease binding to the cochemotaxin, GcGlobulin (vitamin D binding protein), restoring its chemotactic activity to approximate that of $C5a$[19]. Chemotactic factor inactivator, an inhibitor of GcGlobulin binding to $C5a_{desArg}$, can decrease the chemotactic activity of the C5 fragments by binding to GcGlobulin and preventing the GcGlobulin mediated increase in chemotactic activity[20].

PROTEINASES AND ANTIPROTEINASES

The role of proteinases and antiproteinases in cell migration is complex. Studies with the bacterial chemotactic factor, fMLP, have suggested that a neutrophil membrane peptidase activity is necessary for a full chemotactic response[21]. In high doses, α_1 proteinase inhibitor, α_1 antichymotrypsin, and antileukoproteinase can all inhibit neutrophil chemotactic responses, presumably by inhibiting a neutrophil membrane peptidase activity[22,23]. However, recent studies with α_1 proteinase inhibitor have revealed a greater complexity. In low doses, α_1 proteinase inhibitor is chemotactic, suggesting that an inflammatory site α_1 proteinase inhibitor may initially augment neutrophil chemotaxis, but later act to downregulate the inflammatory response as concentrations increase[23]. Adding to the complexity, cleavage of the active site of α_1 proteinase inhibitor or complexing of α_1 proteinase inhibitor with neutrophil elastase can generate neutrophil chemotactic activity[24,25].

CYTOKINES

Historically, the search for physiologic inhibitors of neutrophil migration occurred quite early in cytokine research. A number of cytokines have been studied for their capacity to modulate cell migration. One of the earliest identified was migration inhibitory factor (MIF), which is released from activated T lymphocytes and inhibits the migration of macrophages and monocytes[26]. However, confusion arose as to the identity and relationship of MIF to interferon gamma (IFNγ), which itself can attenuate monocyte migration[27]. More recently, a unique cDNA has been described for human MIF[28], and although IFNγ and MIF both have synergistic effects with the lipid A portion of lipopolysaccharide, they appear to be distinct[29].

As previously mentioned, TNFα has been found to both stimulate and inhibit neutrophil chemotaxis *in vitro*, but when tested *in vivo* appeared to produce predominantly an inhibitory effect[14]. There has been similar controversy regarding granulocyte macrophage colony stimulating factor (GM-CSF), with both chemotactic and chemotactic inhibitory properties being reported for neutrophils when tested *in vitro*[30,31].

A number of cytokines have been described for which the only known function appears to be inhibition of chemotaxis. Lymphocytes have been reported to release a protein that inhibits neutrophil chemotaxis[32]. Sibille *et al.*[33] have identified a low molecular weight inhibitor of neutrophil chemotaxis derived from alveolar macrophages. Cooper *et al.*[34] extended these observations and have identified this inhibitor in normal bronchoalveolar lavage fluid. Recent work has shown this inhibitor to have a high degree of homology with influenza A nucleoprotein which also can inhibit neutrophil migration[35].

ARACHIDONIC ACID METABOLITES

Arachidonic metabolites can modulate cell migration. Prostaglandin E_2 can decrease chemotaxis of neutrophils and fibroblasts, and prostacyclin can decrease migration of neutrophils and monocytes[36,37].

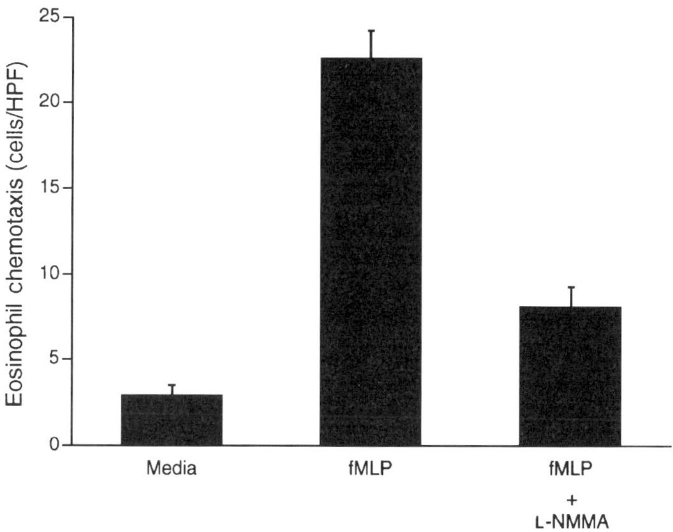

Figure 13.3. Representative experiment demonstrating pharmacologic inhibition of eosinophil chemotaxis. Human eosinophils purified to >95% purity were incubated for 30 min with media or the nitric oxide synthase inhibitor, L-N^G-monomethyl-arginine (L-NMMA, 10^{-4} mol litre^{-1}). Cells incubated in media alone were then evaluated for their background migration without a chemotactic stimulus (media) or their directed migration to a chemotactic stimulus, N-formyl-methionyl-leucyl-phenylalanine, (fMLP, 10^{-6} mol litre^{-1}). Cells incubated with L-NMMA and subsequently allowed to migrate toward fMLP (fMLP + L-NMMA) showed a decrease in migration to fMLP compared with cells incubated in media alone before migration toward fMLP (middle bar). HPF = High power field

IMMUNOGLOBULINS

Van Epps *et al.*[38] noted an association between the presence of negative skin tests to recall antigens and increased levels of IgA. Subsequently, it was determined that neutrophil chemotaxis can be inhibited by IgA myeloma sera, and this was specifically attributable to the IgA M component[39].

Increased IgE has been associated with a neutrophil chemotaxis defect and recurrent staphylococcal infections, which has been termed Job's syndrome[40]. On the basis of the association between decreased neutrophil chemotaxis and increased IgA, it might be logical to assume that increased IgE causes the neutrophil migratory defect. However, studies have failed to support this supposition. There is a poor association between leukocyte responsiveness and serum IgE levels, and IgE does not appear to inhibit neutrophil chemotaxis directly[41].

NITRIC OXIDE

Nitric oxide synthase inhibitors have been associated with a reduction in both neutrophil, monocyte, and eosinophil migration[42,43] (Fig. 13.3, p. 223). Presumably, this results from a reduction in intracellular cyclic guanosine monophosphate, which is often increased when leukocytes are stimulated with chemotactic factors[44]. However, nitric oxide itself may decrease monocyte chemotaxis in relatively high doses[37].

HOST FACTORS

AGE

Neutrophil chemotaxis may be decreased at the extremes of age. Decreases in both neutrophil and monocyte chemotactic activity have been reported in neonates[45]. The defect in neonatal neutrophils can be improved by treatment with cholesteryl hemisuccinate, a plasma membrane rigidifier, suggesting that increased membrane fluidity might potentially account for this defect[45]. In elderly animals or man, decreases in the capacity of neutrophils to migrate have also been reported[46].

DIET

Dietary deficiencies can affect leukocyte migration. Severe protein malnutrition appears to depress neutrophil migration[47]. *In vitro* neutrophil chemotaxis was diminished at early time intervals (<120 min), but normal numbers of cells had migrated by 180 min. Hypophosphatemia has also been associated with defective neutrophil chemotaxis and phagocytosis in a patient receiving hyperalimentation, apparently as a result of ATP depletion, as adenosine and phosphate improved migration[48].

Dietary supplementation has also been shown to affect leukocyte migration. Supplementation with n-3 polyunsaturated fatty acids, such as cod liver oil, has been show to inhibit neutrophil and monocyte chemotaxis in healthy subjects[49]. An extension of these observations has recently been reported in subjects with smoking related chronic obstructive pulmonary disease, a disorder associated with an accumulation of neutrophils in the lung: after control for pack–years of smoking, age, gender, race, height, weight, energy intake, and educational level, the intake of dietary n-3 polyunsaturated fatty acids was inversely related to the risk of cigarette smokers developing chronic obstructive pulmonary disease[50]. Although the association between increased dietary intake of n-3 polyunsaturated fatty acids and a decreased neutrophil influx into the lung was not demonstrated, these observations suggest an *in vivo* extension of the *in vitro* inhibition of neutrophil chemotaxis.

Chicken soup has long been advocated for inflammatory conditions such as asthma[51]. Studies have suggested that there may be a basis for "grandmother's favorite medicine", because chicken soup decreases neutrophil chemotaxis *in vitro*, apparently because of thiosulfinates or cepaenes present from the onions in the soup[52,53].

ACQUIRED DISORDERS

A number of disorders have been reported to be associated with a defect in leukocyte motility (Table 13.2). Severe acute infections have been associated with a decrease in neutrophil chemotaxis[54]. However, others have found an increase in neutrophil migration during bacterial infection[55]. Diabetes mellitus has been associated with mildly depressed neutrophil chemotaxis which can be improved by incubation of the diabetic neutrophils with glucose and insulin[56,57]. In rheumatoid arthritis, a decrease in neutrophil chemotaxis has also been reported[58]. Incubation of normal neutrophils with rheumatoid factor positive serum decreases migration, suggesting that ingestion of rheumatoid complexes may be the cause of the decrease[58]. Depressed neutrophil migration has been found in about 50% of patients after bone marrow transplantation for leukemia or aplastic anemia[59]. These patients were receiving antithymocyte globulin for graft versus host disease and had more severe bacterial infections. Neutrophil migration is also decreased with severe burns[60]. A decrease in chemotactic factor receptors on the neutrophils may explain the decrease in migration[60].

The increased incidence of infection is well recognized as a major cause of morbidity and mortality in patients with cancer[61]. A decrease in neutrophil or monocyte migration has been associated with many malignancies[62]. An increase in chemotactic factor inactivator may explain some of these observations, although other circulating inhibitors may be present[62]. Increased levels of chemotactic factor inactivator have also been suggested to explain decreased neutrophil migration in a variety of disorders including liver cirrhosis, alcoholic hepatitis, α_1 antitrypsin deficiency, hypersensitivity pneumonitis, hemodialysis, and sarcoidosis[63–67].

An inhibitor of C5 derived chemotactic activity in serum obtained from some patients with systemic lupus erythematosus has been described[68]. Presence of this inhibitor has been associated with increased susceptibility to bacterial infections[69]. Subsequent work has shown that the lupus associated inhibitor is complement factor Bb and, in common with chemotactic factor inactivator, exerts its effect by altering cochemotaxin interaction with $C5a_{desArg}$[69].

CONGENITAL DISORDERS

Congenital defects of cellular migration have been described, but appear to be rare. As previously mentioned, decreased neutrophil chemotaxis occurs in the inherited disorder, Job's syndrome[40]. Patients with the rare inherited disorder, Chediak–Higashi syndrome, have recurrent pyogenic infections, partial oculocutaneous albinism, and can have an accelerated lymphoma-like phase[70]. The leukocytes, in addition to other granule bearing cells, contain giant lysosomal granules. Neutrophils and monocytes obtained from patients with Chediak–Higashi syndrome migrate poorly *in vitro*[70]. Another apparently congenital disorder is the "lazy leukocyte" syndrome. Originally described in two children with recurrent fever, oral lesions, severe neutropenia, and a cellular chemotactic defect, it is possible that this syndrome might represent a form of the more recently described actin dysfunction syndrome (see below[71]).

Matzner *et al.* have described an inhibitor specific for C5a in synovial and peritoneal fluid[72]. This factor was found to be deficient in familial Mediterranean fever, an inherited disease characterized by recurrent episodes of unprovoked inflammation involving the joints and pleural and peritoneal cavities[72]. This underscores the principle that a deficiency of an inflammatory inhibitor can result in inappropriate inflammation.

One of the most exciting recent discoveries in biology has been the description of the leukocyte integrins[73]. This family of closely related glycoproteins mediates, at least in part, the adherence of inflammatory cells to endothelial and other cells[73]. The leukocyte integrins consist of one of several α subunits (also called the cluster of differentiation (CD) 11 subunit) non-covalently associated with a common β subunit (also called the CD18 subunit)[73]. Now designated as either the CD11/CD18 complex, or grouped into the larger family of integrin molecules, these adhesion molecules include lymphocyte function associated antigen-1 (LFA-1: LFA-1α, CD11a, alpha$_L$), macrophage-1 (Mac-1: MO-1, CD11b, alpha$_M$), and p150, 95 (CD11c, alpha$_X$) associated with the common β subunit CD18 (β_2). Patients deficient in the common CD18 subunit suffer from recurrent infections because of the inability of their leukocytes to migrate from the bloodstream to phagocytose and kill invading organisms[74].

Actin polymerization is known to be involved in neutrophil migration[7]. A genetic disorder associated with partial impairment of neutrophil actin assembly and a resultant motility and phagocytic defect has been described[75].

INHIBITORS DERIVED FROM INFECTIOUS SOURCES

VIRUSES

Viral infection can result in decreased migration of both neutrophils and monocytes. Neutrophils obtained from patients with measles or hepatitis B have a decreased chemotactic response[76,77]. Human monocytes incubated with a variety of viruses and tested for chemotactic responsiveness had depressed responses after *Herpes simplex* and influenza infection, but vaccinia, polio, and reoviruses did not produce an effect[78]. Consistent with these observations, monocytes obtained from patients with influenza had a decreased chemotactic response compared with normal and febrile controls, and 3 weeks after recovery their monocyte chemotactic activity had returned to normal[79]. More recently, synthetic peptides corresponding to the sequences from gp120 or gp41 of the human immuno-deficiency virus-1 (HIV-1) envelope were found to decrease the migration of neutrophils obtained from HIV-1 infected donors[80]. Although the mechanism(s) of the decrease in leukocyte migration with viral infection remains largely unknown, these observations may explain the increased incidence in bacterial infections after some viral infections.

BACTERIA

Bacteria can release a variety of substances that may modulate cellular migration. Although bacterial products such as fMLP can attract neutrophils, bacteria can also release substances which inhibit cell migration, perhaps giving these bacteria a selective survival advantage. Endotoxins from *Escherichia coli, Salmonella minnesota*, and *Pseudomonas aeruginosa* have all been reported to reduce neutrophil migration, although there is considerable strain to strain variation[81,82]. Consistent with these *in vitro* observations, neutrophils obtained from normal subjects after infusion of *Pseudomonas* endotoxin have decreased migration[83]. The mechanism is unknown, but endotoxin can alter chemotactic receptor numbers on neutrophils[84]. Proteinases released by bacteria may also modulate cell migration. For example, elastase released by *Ps. aeruginosa* can decrease monocyte chemotaxis[85] and both group A and B streptococci can cleave the carboxy-terminal end of C5a, resulting in a decrease in chemotactic activity[86].

PHARMACOLOGIC INHIBITORS

A large body of literature has accumulated pertaining to leukocyte function *in vitro*. Inhibitors of chemotaxis may inhibit the responding cell (Fig. 13.3) or may inactivate the chemotactic stimulus. However, caution must be used in extrapolating these *in vitro* findings to an *in vivo* situation, as many agents used are non-physiologic or used at supraphysiologic concentrations *in vitro*. Furthermore, various cell responses are influenced by multiple factors and by different mechanisms. For example, corticosteroids may have potent effects on neutrophils or eosinophils through indirect mechanisms, by decreasing production of chemotactic factors such as interleukin-3 (IL-3), IL-5, IL-8, or GM-CSF. However, in general, anti-inflammatory agents seem to produce the expected decrease in inflammatory cell migration that is likely to be part of their mechanism of action. Table 13.3 lists some pharmacologic agents which have been reported to affect cell migration.

CORTICOSTEROIDS

Although corticosteroids can reduce inflammation by a number of mechanisms, one mechanism appears to be a reduction in chemotactic activity. Methylpred-nisolone reduces lymphocyte, monocyte, and neutrophil migration to fMLP and

C5a, and dexamethasone inhibits lymphocyte migration to IL-1α and leukotriene B₄[87,88].

Corticosteroids are potent agents in the therapy of allergic rhinitis and asthma, and inhibit the late allergic response and the infiltration of eosinophils into the airways. These agents decrease circulating eosinophils within hours, whereas prolonged administration progressively decreases eosinophils in the bone marrow and airways[89]. This effect is most probably due to inhibition of production of cytokines such as GM-CSF, IL-3 and IL-5, all of which promote the growth of cytokines and inhibit corticosteroid induced programmed cell death or apoptosis[89]. Although eosinophils have high affinity receptors for corticosteroids, most *in vitro* studies show no direct effect on cell function except for survival[89]. In this regard, *in vitro* eosinophil incubation with corticosteroids does not affect adhesion to endothelial cells, whereas *in vivo* administration does inhibit their subsequent *in vitro* chemotaxis and adhesion[89]. Thus most of the effects of corticosteroids on eosinophil function are produced indirectly by their effect on cytokine production. For example, corticosteroids inhibit cytokines and the generation of IL-1β, IL-4 and TNFα, which activate endothelial cells to express intercellular adhesion molecule-1, vascular cell adhesion molecule-1, and endothelial leucocyte adhesion molecule-1 (E-selectin)[89]. In this manner, by inhibiting cytokine production, corticosteroids inhibit the adherence and accumulation of eosinophils at the sites of allergic inflammation.

β-AGONISTS

β-Agonists such as isoproterenol, or newer β-agonists such as formoterol, have been reported to decrease neutrophil or eosinophil chemotaxis[90,91]. This is not surprising, because β-agonists increase cyclic AMP and an increase in cyclic AMP has been associated with a decrease in migration[90]. However, the effect is not universal among β-agonists, because salbutamol fails to inhibit eosinophil chemotaxis[91].

PHOSPHODIESTERASE INHIBITORS

Theophylline, a relatively non-selective phosphodiesterase (PDE) inhibitor, has been reported to inhibit neutrophil migration. This decrease in neutrophil chemotaxis would be consistent with the mechanism proposed for inhibition of chemotaxis by the β-agonists. Like the β-agonists, theophylline increases neutrophil cyclic AMP, although by the mechanism of inhibiting PDE, the enzyme responsible for cyclic AMP degradation[90,92]. Eosinophils and neutrophils contain the PDE isoenzyme, PDE-IV[93]. Tanimoto *et al.*[93] demonstrated the functional importance of PDE-IV by showing that a selective inhibitor of PDE-IV, WAY-PDA-641, decreases human blood eosinophil and neutrophil migration.

ANTI-INFLAMMATORY AGENTS

Azathioprine and other antimetabolites produce reductions in chemotaxis of most inflammatory cells. In contrast, cyclosporine A predominantly reduces lymphocyte migration with modest, if any, effects on neutrophil or monocyte movement[87,88]. Recently, the anti-inflammatory macrolide, FK506, has been shown to inhibit neutrophil migration[94].

The non-steroidal anti-inflammatory drugs have also been shown to decrease neutrophil migration *in vitro*. Diclofenac, indomethacin, piroxicam, and tolfenamic acid decrease neutrophil migration[95]; aspirin, however, appears to stimulate neutrophil movement[96].

CROMOLYN SODIUM AND NEDOCROMIL

Both of these agents have been reported to reduce eosinophil and neutrophil migration[97]. A related compound, lodoxamide tromethamine, also inhibits allergen induced bronchoconstriction in patients with asthma[98]. Both of these agents inhibit the *in vivo* accumulation of eosinophils in man[99] and in guineapigs[100], which may account, at least in part, for their capacity to inhibit the late bronchoconstrictor reaction to allergen challenge.

PLATELET ACTIVATING FACTOR ANTAGONISTS

The effect of platelet activating factor (PAF) and other eosinophil chemotactic factors on eosinophil activation and mediator release has demonstrated PAF to be a very potent chemotactic agent[101]. PAF antagonists such as Ginkogolide B (BN-52021) and the Boehringer compound, WEB-2086, are very potent in inhibiting eosinophil chemotaxis and superoxide production after PAF stimulation[102,103].

ANTIHISTAMINES

Terfenadine has greater inhibitory effects on eosinophil chemotaxis than on neutrophil chemotaxis[104]. At concentrations of 500 and 1000 ng.ml^{-1}, it significantly inhibited PAF induced and fMLP induced eosinophil chemotaxis, whereas 1000 ng.ml^{-1} was necessary to suppress neutrophil chemotaxis. Cetirizine, a new second generation antihistamine, was reported to have non-H$_1$ effects, including inhibition of eosinophil chemotaxis[105]. Loratidine has also been shown to inhibit eosinophil chemotaxis and superoxide production following stimulation with PAF or fMLP[106]. These effects of loratidine were observed at nanomolar concentrations that would be expected to occur with the recommended clinical dose.

IMMUNOTHERAPY

Rak *et al.*[107] reported that immunotherapy abrogates the generation of eosinophil and neutrophil chemotactic activity during the pollen season. These same investigators[108] subsequently observed that immunotherapy inhibited eosinophil number, eosinophil cationic protein levels and chemotactic activity in both serum and bronchoalveolar lavage fluid of patients with asthma during the pollen season. Whereas seasonal pollen exposure normally increases airway reactivity, it did not in these subjects.

 R. A. Robbins and R. G. Townley

HISTAMINE AND HISTAMINE INHALATION

Histamine is known to decrease neutrophil chemotaxis *in vitro*[109]. Bury and Radermecker[110] extended this observation by showing a decline in the movement of neutrophils obtained from healthy or asymptomatic asthmatic patients after histamine inhalation.

SUMMARY

The migration of cells is a complex process. This process can be influenced by a variety of normal physiologic inhibitors, including inhibitors of specific inflammatory pathways such as inhibitors of the complement system, or a variety of non-specific inhibitors, such as proteinases and antiproteinases, cytokines, arachidonic acid metabolites, immunoglobulins, or nitric oxide related inhibitors. These physiologic inhibitors are probably important in the normal termination of an inflammatory reaction which, if left unchecked, could result in severe tissue destruction. In addition, host factors including age, diet, and a variety of acquired disorders may influence cell migration. Infectious agents may release factors that disrupt normal host defenses, including the migration of inflammatory cells, and thus perhaps confer a selective advantage to the organism. Lastly, a number of pharmacologic agents may influence cell migration, which may be an intended part of their therapeutic benefit, or unintentional, resulting in an unwanted decrease in host defense.

REFERENCES

1. Miles A A, Miles E M, Burke J. The value and duration of defense reactions of the skin to the primary lodgement of bacteria. *Br J Pharmacol* 1957; **38**: 79–96.
2. Weiss S J. Tissue destruction by neutrophils. *N Engl J Med* 1989; **320**: 365–376.
3. Goldstein R H, Fine A. Fibrotic reaction in the lung: the activation of the lung fibroblast. *Exp Lung Res* 1986; **11**: 245–261.
4. Zahm J-M, Chevillard M, Puchelle E. Wound repair of human surface respiratory epithelium. *Am J Respir Cell Mol Biol* 1991; **5**: 242–248.
5. Polakis P G, Uhing R J, Snyderman R. The folrmylpeptide chemoattractant receptor copurifies with a GTP-binding protein containing a distinct 40-kDa pertussis toxin substrate. *J Biol Chem* 1988; **263**: 4969–4976.
6. Zigmond S H. Chemotactic response of neutrophils. *Am J Respir Cell Mol Biol* 1989; **1**: 451–453.
7. Stossel T P. On the crawling of animal cells. *Science* 1993; **260**: 1086–1094.
8. Boyden S. The chemotactic effect of mixtures of antibody and antigen on polymorphonuclear leucocytes. *J Exp Med* 1962; **115**: 453–466.
9. Zigmond S H, Hirsch J G. Leukocyte locomotion and chemotaxis: new methods for evaluation and demonstration of cell-derived chemotactic factor. *J Exp Med* 1973; **137**: 387–410.
10. Nelson R D, Quie P G, Simmons R L. Chemotaxis under agarose: a new and simple method for measuring chemotaxis and spontaneous migration of human polymorphonuclear leukocytes and monocytes. *J Immunol* 1975; **115**: 1650–1656.
11. Coyle D E, Brammer P W, Halsall H B. A microcapillary assay (MASS) for macrophage migration inhibition factor. *J Immunol Methods* 1980; **35**: 259–265.
12. Gallin J I, Clark R A, Kimball H R. Granulocyte chemotaxis; an improved *in vitro* assay employing ^{51}Cr-labelled granulocytes. *J Immunol* 1973; **110**: 233–240.

13. Zigmond S H. A new visual assay of leukocyte chemotaxis. In Gallin J I, Quie P G, eds. *Leukocyte Chemotaxis: Methods, Physiology, and Clinical Implications.* New York: Raven Press, 1978; 57–66.

14. Otsuka Y, Nagano K, Nagano K, *et al.* Inhibition of neutrophil migration by tumor necrosis factor: *ex vivo* and *in vivo* studies in comparison with *in vitro* effect. *J Immunol* 1990; **145:** 2639–2643.

15. Casale T B, Abbas M K. Comparison of leukotriene B4-induced neutrophil migration through different cellular barriers. *Am J Physiol* 1990; **258:** C639–C647.

16. Kirsch C M, Sigal E, Pjokic T D, *et al.* An *in vivo* chemotaxis assay in the dog trachea: evidence for chemotactic activity of 8, 15 diHETE. *J Appl Physiol* 1988; **65:** 1792–1795.

17. Martin T R, Pistorese B P, Chi E Y, *et al.* Recruitment of neutrophils into the alveolar space without a change in protein permeability. *J Clin Invest* 1989; **84:** 1609–1610.

18. Müller-Eberhard H J. Molecular organization and function of the complement system. *Annu Rev Biochem* 1988; **57:** 321–347.

19. Kew R R, Webster R O. GcGlobulin (vitamin D-binding protein) enhances the neutrophil chemotactic activity of C5a and C5a des arg. *J Clin Invest* 1988; **82:** 364–369.

20. Robbins R A, Hamel F G. Chemotactic factor inactivator interaction with Gc-globulin (vitamin D-binding protein): a mechanism of modulating the chemotactic activity of C5a. *J Immunol* 1990; **144:** 2371–2376.

21. Painter R G, Dukes R, Sullivan J, *et al.* Function of neutral endopeptidase on the cell membrane of human neutrophils. *J Biol Chem* 1988; **263:** 9456–9461.

22. Stockley R A, Shaw J, Afford S C, *et al.* Effect of alpha-1-proteinase inhibitor on neutrophil chemotaxis. *Am J Respir Cell Mol Biol* 1990; **2:** 163–170.

23. Aoshiba K, Nagai A, Ishihara Y, *et al.* Effects of α_1-proteinase inhibitor on chemotaxis and chemokinesis of polymorphonuclear leukocytes: its possible role in regulating polymorphonuclear leukocyte recruitment in human subjects. *J Lab Clin Med* 1993; **122:** 333–340.

24. Banda M J, Rice A G, Griffin G L, Senior R M. Alpha$_1$ proteinase inhibitor is a neutrophil chemoattractant after proteolytic inactivation by macrophage elastase. *J Biol Chem* 1988; **263:** 4481–4484.

25. Banda M J, Rice A G, Griffin G L, *et al.* The inhibitory complex of human alpha$_1$ proteinase inhibitor and human leukocyte elastase is a neutrophil chemoattractant. *J Exp Med* 1988; **167:** 1608–1617.

26. George M, Vaughn J H. *In vitro* cell migration as a model for delayed hypersensitivity. *Proc Soc Exp Biol Med* 1962; **111:** 514–521.

27. Thurman G B, Braude I A, Gray P W, *et al.* MIF-like activity of natural and recombinant human interferon-γ and their neutralization by monoclonal antibody. *J Immunol* 1985; **134:** 305–309.

28. Weiser W Y, Temple P A, Witek-Giannotti J S, *et al.* Molecular cloning of a cDNA encoding a human macrophage migration inhibitor factor. *Proc Natl Acad Sci USA* 1989; **86:** 7522–7526.

29. Herriottt M J, Jiang H, Steward C A, *et al.* Mechanistic differences between migration inhibitory factor (MIF) and IFN-γ for macrophage activation. *J Immunol* 1993; **150:** 4524–4531.

30. Wang J M, Colella S, Allavena P, *et al.* Chemotactic activity of human recombinant granulocyte-macrophage colony-stimulating factor. *Immunology* 1984; **2:** 257–281.

31. Kownatzki E, Liehl E, Aschauer H, *et al.* Inhibition of chemotactic migration of human neutrophilic granulocytes by recombinant human granulocyte-macrophage colony-stimulating factor. *Immunopharmacology* 1990; **19:** 139–143.

32. Klempner M S, Rocklin R E. Effects of leukocyte inhibitory factor (LIF) on human neutrophil function. *Inflammation* 1983; **7:** 145–153.

33. Sibille Y, Merrill W W, Naegel G P, *et al.* Human alveolar macrophages release a factor which inhibits phagocyte function. *Am J Respir Cell Mol Biol* 1989; **1:** 407–415.

34. Cooper J A D Jr, Sibille Y, Zitnik R, *et al.* Isolation of an inhibitor of neutrophil function from bronchial lavage of normal volunteers. *Am J Physiol* 1991; **260:** L501–L509.

35. Carcelen R I, Cooper J A D Jr. Effects of influenza A nucleoprotein on neutrophil function [Abstract]. *Am J Respir Crit Care Med* 1994; **149:** A123.

36. Takenawa R, Ishitoya I, Nagai Y. Inhibitory effect of prostaglandin E_2, forskolin, and dibutyl cAMP on arachidonic acid release and inositol phospholipid metabolism in guinea pig neutrophils. *J Biol Chem* 1986; **261:** 1092–1098.

37. Bath P M W, Hassall D G, Gladwin A-M, *et al.* Nitric oxide and prostacyclin: divergence of inhibitory effects on monocyte chemotaxis and adhesion to endothelium in vitro. *Arterioscler Thromb* 1991; **11:** 254–260.

38. Van Epps D E, Palmer D L, Williams R C Jr. Characterization of serum inhibitors of neutrophil chemotaxis associated with anergy. *J Immunol* 1974; **113:** 189–200.

39. Van Epps D E, William R C Jr. Suppression of leukocyte chemotaxis by human IgA myeloma components. *J Exp Med* 1976; **144:** 1227–1242.

40. Hill H R, Ochs H D, Quie P G, *et al.* Defect in neutrophil granulocyte chemotaxis in Job's syndrome or recurrent "cold" staphylococcal abscesses. *Lancet* 1974; **2:**617–619.

41. Quie P G, Cates K L. Clinical manifestations of disorders of neutrophil chemotaxis. In: Gallin J I, Quie P G, eds. *Leukocyte Chemotaxis: Methods, Physiology, and Clinical Implications.* New York: Raven Press, 1978; 307–328.

42. Kaplan S S, Billiar T, Curran R D, *et al.* Attenuation of chemotaxis with N^G-monomethyl-L-arginine: a role for cyclic GMP. *Blood* 1989; **74:** 1885–1887.

43. Belenky S N, Robbins R A, Rennard S I, *et al.* Inhibitors of nitric oxide synthase attenuate neutrophil chemotaxis *in vitro*. *J Lab Clin Med* 1993; **122:** 388–394.

44. Hatch G E, Nichols W K, Hill H R. Cyclic nucleotide changes in human neutrophils induced by chemoattractants and chemotactic modulators. *J Immunol* 1977; **119:** 450–456.

45. Wolach B, Ben Dor M, Chomsky O, *et al.* Improved chemotactic ability of neonatal polymorphonuclear cells induced by mild membrane rigidification. *J Leukoc Biol* 1992; **51:** 324–328.

46. McLaughlin B, O'Malley K, Cotter T G. Age-related differences in granulocyte chemotaxis and degranulation. *Clin Sci* 1986; **70:** 59–62.

47. Schopfer K, Douglas S D. Neutrophil function in children with kwasiorkor. *J Lab Clin Med* 1976; **88:** 450–461.

48. Craddock P F R, Yawata Y, Van Santen L, *et al.* Acquired phagocyte dysfunction: a complication of the hypophosphatemia of parenteral hyperalimentation. *N Engl J Med* 1974; **290:** 1403–1407.

49. Lee T H, Hoover R L, Williams J D, *et al.* Effect of dietary enrichment with eicosapentaenoic acid and docosahexaenoic acid on *in vitro* neutrophil migration and monocyte leukotriene generation and neutrophil function. *N Engl J Med* 1985; **312:** 1217–1224.

50. Shahar E, Folsom A R, Melnick S L, *et al.* Dietary n-3 polyunsaturated fatty acids and smoking-related chronic obstructive pulmonary disease. *N Engl J Med* 1994; **331:** 228–233.

51. Muntner S. *The Medical Writings of Moses Maimonides Treatise on Asthma.* Philadelphia: Lippincott, 1963; 13, 18–20, 42, 68.

52. Rennard B O, Ertl R F, Gossman G L, *et al.* Chicken soup inhibits neutrophil chemotaxis [Abstract]. *Am Rev Respir Dis* 1993; **147:** A472.

53. Dorsch W, Schneider E, Bayer T, *et al.* Anti-inflammatory effects of onions: inhibition of chemotaxis of human polymorphonuclear leukocytes by thiosulfinates and cepaenes. *Int Arch Allergy Appl Immunol* 1990; **92:** 39–42.

54. Tellado J M, Christou N V. Critically ill anergic patients demonstrate polymorphonuclear neutrophil activation in the intravascular compartment with decreased cell delivery to inflammatory foci. *J Leukoc Biol* 1991; **50:** 547–553.

55. Hill H R, Gerrard J M, Hogan N A, *et al.* Hyperactivity of neutrophil leukotactic responses during active bacterial infection. *J Clin Invest* 1974; **53:** 996–1002.

56. Mowat A G, Baum J. Chemotaxis of polymorphonuclear leukocytes from patients with diabetes mellitus. *N Engl J Med* 1971; **284:** 621–627.

57. Hill H R, Sauls H S, Dettloff J L, *et al.* Impaired leukotactic responsiveness in patients with juvenile diabetes mellitus. *Clin Immunol Immunopathol* 1974; **2:** 395–403.

58. Mowat A G, Baum J. Chemotaxis of polymorphonuclear leukocytes from patients with rheumatoid arthritis. *J Clin Invest* 1971; **50:** 2541–2549.

59. Clark R A, Johnson F L, Klebanoff S J, *et al.* Defective neutrophil chemotaxis in bone marrow transplant patients. *J Clin Invest* 1976; **58:** 22–31.

60. Bjornson A B, Somers S D. Down-regulation of chemotaxis of polymorphonuclear leukocytes following thermal injury involves two distinct mechanisms. *J Infect Dis* 1993; **168:** 120–127.

61. Levine A S, Schimpff S C, Graw R G Jr, *et al*. Hematologic malignancies and other marrow failure states: progress in the management of complicating infections. *Semin Hematol* 1974; **11:** 141–202.
62. Mandell L A, Afnan M. Chemotactic inhibitors in sera of patients with neoplastic disease. *Clin Invest Med* 1991; **14:** 131–141.
63. Maderazo E G, Ward P A, Quintiliani R. Defective regulation of chemotaxis in cirrhosis. *J Lab Clin Med* 1975; **85:** 621–630.
64. Robbins R A, Zetterman R K, Kendall T J, *et al*. Elevation of chemotactic factor inactivator in alcoholic liver disease. *Hepatology* 1987; **7:** 872–877.
65. Ward P A, Talamo R C. Deficiency of the chemotactic factor inactivator in human sera with α_1-antitrypsin deficiency. *J Clin Invest* 1973; **52:** 516–519.
66. Kreutzer D L, McCormick J R, Thrall R S, *et al*. Elevation of serum chemotactic factor inactivator activity during acute inflammatory reactions in patients with hypersensitivity pneumonitis. *Am Rev Respir Dis* 1982; **125:** 612–614.
67. McCormick J R, Kreutzer D L, Keating H J, *et al*. Alterations in activities of anaphylatoxin inactivator and chemotactic factor inactivator during hemodialysis. *Am J Pathol* 1982; **109:** 283–287.
68. Perez H D, Andron R I, Goldstein I M. Infection in patients with systemic lupus erythematosus: association with a serum inhibitor of complement-derived chemotactic activity. *Arthritis Rheum* 1979; **22:** 1326–1333.
69. Perez H D, Hooper C, Volanakis J, *et al*. Specific inhibitor of complement (C5)-derived chemotactic activity in systemic lupus erythematosus related antigenically to the Bb fragment of human factor B. *J Immunol* 1987; **139:** 484–489.
70. Blume R S, Wolff S M. The Chediak-Higashi syndrome: studies in four patients and a review of the literature. *Medicine* 1972; **51:** 1200–1206.
71. Miller M E, Oski F A, Harris M B. Lazy-leukocyte syndrome: a new disorder of neutrophil function. *Lancet* 1971; **1:** 665–669.
72. Matzner Y, Brzezinski A. C5a-inhibitor deficiency in peritoneal fluids from patients with familial Mediterranean fever. *N Engl J Med* 1984; **311:** 287–290.
73. Kishimoto T K, Larson R S, Corbi A L, *et al*. The leukocyte integrins. *Adv Immunol* 1989; **46:** 149–182.
74. Anderson D C, Springer T A. Leukocyte adhesion deficiency: an inherited deficiency in the MAC-1, LFA-1, and p150,95 glycoproteins. *Annu Rev Med* 1987; **38:** 175–194.
75. Boxer L A, Hedley-Whyte E T, Stossel T P. Neutrophil actin dysfunction and abnormal neutrophil behavior. *N Engl J Med* 1984; **291:** 1093–1099.
76. Anderson R, Sher R, Rabson A R, *et al*. Defective chemotaxis in measles patients. *S Afr Med J* 1974; **7:** 1819–1820.
77. Magliulo E, Benzi-Cipelli R. Impaired leukotaxis in viral hepatitis B. *N Engl J Med* 1975; **293:** 303–304.
78. Kleinerman E K, Snyderman R, Daniels C A. Depression of human monocyte chemotaxis by herpes simplex and influenza viruses. *J Immunol* 1974; **113:** 1562–1567.
79. Kleinerman E K, Snyderman R, Daniels C A. Depression of human monocyte chemotaxis during acute influenza infection. *Lancet* 1975; **2:** 1063–1064.
80. Pinegin B V, Saidov M Z, Scheltsyna T L, *et al*. Peripheral blood neutrophils from HIV-1-infected individuals are armed with factors that cause inhibition of their migration in response to specific antigens. *Immunol Lett* 1993; **36:** 13–17.
81. Dahinden C, Fehr J. Granulocyte activation by endotoxin. I. Correlation between adherence and other granulocyte functions, and role of endotoxin structure on biological activity. *J Immunol* 1983; **130:** 857–862.
82. Kharazmi A, Fomsgaard A, Conrad R S, *et al*. Relationship between chemical composition and biological function of *Pseudomonas aeruginosa* lipopolysaccharide: effect on human neutrophil chemotaxis and oxidative burst. *J Leukoc Biol* 1991; **49:** 15–20.
83. Territo M C, Golde D W. Granulocyte function in experimental human endotoxemia. *Blood* 1976; **47:** 539–544.
84. Goldman D W, Inkel H, Gifford L A, *et al*. Lipopolysaccharide modulates receptors for leukotriene B_4, C5a, and formyl-methionyl-leucyl-phenylalanine on rabbit polymorphonuclear leukocytes. *J Immunol* 1986; **137:** 1971–1976.

85. Kharazmi A, Nielsen H. Inhibition of monocyte chemotaxis and chemiluminescence by *Pseudomonas aeruginosa* elastase. *APMIS* 1991; **99:** 93–95.

86. Bohnsack J F, Mollison K W, Buko A M, *et al.* Group B streptococci inactivate complement component C5a by enzymic cleavage at the C-terminus. *Biochem J* 1991; **273:** 635–640.

87. Wang L F, Adams D H, Elias E, *et al.* Inhibition of leucocyte chemotaxis by immunosuppressive drugs: an important mode of action? *Transplant Proc* 1990; **22:** 2342.

88. Ross J S, Bacon K B, Camp R D R. Potent and selective inhibition of in vitro lymphocyte migration by cyclosporine and dexamethasone. *Immunopharmacol Immunotoxicol* 1990; **12:** 439–455.

89. Schleimer R P. Glucocorticosteroids: their mechanisms of action and use in allergic disease. In: Middleton E J, Reed C E, Ellis E F, *et al.*, eds. *Allergy: Principles and Practice*. St Louis: Mosby, 1988; 739–765.

90. Harvath L, Robbins J D, Russell A A, *et al.* cAMP and human neutrophil chemotaxis: elevation of cAMP differentially affects chemotactic responsiveness. *J Immunol* 1991; **146:** 224–232.

91. Eda R, Sugiyama H, Hopp R J, *et al.* Inhibitory effects of formoterol on platelet-activating factor induced eosinophil chemotaxis and degranulation. *Int Arch Allergy Immunol* 1993; **102:** 391–398.

92. Rivkin I, Rosenblatt J, Becker E L. The role of cyclic AMP in the chemotactic responsiveness and spontaneous motility of rabbit peritoneal neutrophils: the inhibition of neutrophil movement and the elevation of cyclic AMP levels by catecholamines, prostaglandins, theophylline and cholera toxin. *J Immunol* 1975; **115:** 1126–1134.

93. Tanimoto Y, Maruo H, Bewtra A K, *et al.* Effects of phosphodiesterase-IV inhibitor (WAY-PDA-641) on human eosinophil and neutrophil migration *in vitro*. *J Allergy Clin Immunol* 1994; **93:** 570A.

94. Burnett D, Adams D H, Martin T J, *et al.* Inhibition by FK506 of formyl peptide-induced neutrophil activation and associated protein sythesis. *Biochem Pharmacol* 1994; **58:** 1081–1088.

95. Smith M J H, Walker J R. The effects of some antirheumatic drugs on an *in vitro* model of human polymorphonuclear chemokinesis. *Br J Pharmacol* 1984; **69:** 473–478.

96. Kemp A S, Smith J. The effect of salicylate on human leucocyte migration. *Clin Exp Immunol* 1982; **49:** 233–238.

97. Bruijnzeel P L B, Warringa R A J, Kok P T M, *et al.* Inhibition of neutrophil and eosinophil induced chemotaxis by nedocromil sodium and sodium cromoglycate. *Br J Pharmacol* 1990; **99:** 7998–8002.

98. Watt G, Bui T, Townley R. Protective effect of lodoxamide tromethamine on allergen inhalation challenge. *J Allergy Clin Immunol* 1980; **66:** 286–294.

99. Hutson P A, Holgate S T, Church M K, Effect of cromolyn sodium and albuterol on early and late phase bronchoconstriciton and airway leukocyte inflitration after allergen challenge of nonanesthetized guinea pigs. *Am Rev Respir Dis* 1988; **138:** 1157–1163.

100. Schellenberg R R, Ishida K, Thomason R J. Nedocromil sodium inhibits airway hyperresponsiveness on eosinophilic infiltration induced by repeated antigen challenge in guinea pigs. *Br J Pharmacol* 1991; **103:** 1842–1846.

101. Tamura N, Agrawal D K, Suliaman F A, *et al.* Effects of platelet activating factor on the chemotaxis of normodense eosinophils from normal subjects. *Biochem Biophys Res Commun* 1987; **142:** 638–644.

102. Townley R G, Hopp R J, Agrawal D K, *et al.* Platelet-activating factor and airway reactivity. *J Allergy Clin Immunol* 1989; **83:** 997–1010.

103. Tamura N, Agrawal D K, Townley R G, *et al.* Platelet-activating factor, human eosinophils and Ginkogolide B (BN 52051). In: Braquet P, ed. *The Ginkogolides Chemistry, Biology, Pharmacology and Clinical Perspectives*. Barcelona: Prous, 1988; 217–224.

104. Okada C, Hopp R J, Miyagawa H, *et al.* The effect of terfenadine on neutrophil chemotactic activity (NCA) and eosinophil chemotactic activity after inhalation of platelet activating factor (PAF) *in vivo*, and on neutrophil chemotaxis in vitro. *Arch Allergy Immunol* 1992; **97:** 181–186.

105. Townley R G, Okada C. Use of cetirizine to investigate non-H_1 effects of second-generation antihistamines. *Ann Allergy* 1992; **68:** 190–196.

106. Eda R, Sugiyama H, Hopp R J, *et al*. Effect of loratadine on human eosinophil function *in vitro*. *Ann Allergy* 1993; **71**: 373–378.

107. Rak S, Håkanson L, Venge P. Immunotherapy abrogates the generation of eosinophil and neutrophil chemotactic activity during pollen season. *J Allergy Clin Immunol* 1990; **86**: 706–713.

108. Rak S, Bjornson A, Hakanson L, *et al*. The effect of immunotherapy on eosinophil accumulation and production of eosinophil chemotactic activity in the lung of subjects with asthma during natural pollen exposure. *J Allergy Clin Immunol* 1991; **88**: 878–888.

109. Hill H R, Setensen R D, Quie P G, *et al*. Modulation of human neutrophil chemotactic responses by cyclic 3'-5'-GMP and cyclic 3'-5'-AMP. *Metabolism* 1975; **24**: 447–456.

110. Bury T B, Radermecker M F. Depression of polymorphonuclear chemotaxis and T-lymphocyte proliferation following histamine inhalation in man. *Eur Respir J* 1989; **2**: 826–833.

14

Lung Repair

CRAIG A. HENKE AND PETER B. BITTERMAN
University of Minnesota, Minneapolis, USA

INTRODUCTION

The lung is susceptible to injury from a vast array of both exogenous and endogenous noxious agents. The extent of injury sustained depends on a variety of factors, including the toxicity of a particular agent, the quantity of noxious agent, and the duration of exposure. Therefore, the spectrum of injury seen clinically ranges from a small focal area of injury of one lung to a diffuse process involving all lobes of both lungs. Despite this variation in degree and extent of injury, the reparative response of the lung is remarkably similar in most cases, reflecting a uniform pattern of response to injury. This uniform reparative response of the lung to injury, which recapitulates the wound healing response in general, manifests itself in a common pattern of histologic alterations seen pathologically[1].

The focus of this discussion will be on lung repair after acute injury. Acute lung injury can be defined as the rapid onset of a diffuse inflammatory process involving the entire alveolus, including the air–lung interface (epithelium), interstitium, and blood–lung interface (endothelium)[2,3]. It can be elicited by a variety of endogenous and exogenous agents and can produce a spectrum of injury ranging from mild to severe (also termed the acute respiratory distress syndrome, ARDS)[4–6]. Histologically, the hallmark lesion of acute lung injury, independent of the causative agent, is diffuse alveolar damage[1]. The reparative response of the lung to diffuse alveolar damage is also manifested by a stereotypical pattern of repair, and has been classified into two separate phases[7]. The acute phase of repair is termed the exudative phase and is characterized by the accumulation of plasma derived fluid and inflammatory cells in the alveolar wall and airspace. The fibroproliferative phase, or second phase, of repair is characterized by the expansion and accumulation of mesenchymal cells and their connective tissue products within the interstitium and airspace. However, both interesting and perplexing is the observation that, despite similar degrees of injury, patient support, and this uniform reparative response, patient outcomes can

Pulmonary Defences. Edited by Robert A. Stockley.
© 1997 John Wiley & Sons Ltd.

vary from rapid death from a fulminant fibroproliferative response, to complete recovery[8–10].

To understand the mechanisms of lung repair and to provide a basis for beginning to understand the factors critical for restoration of normal lung function, it is necessary to review normal lung structure and the physiological function. This will provide the necessary background for considering how the interaction of cells with the extracellular matrix and polypeptide growth factors may alter cellular phenotype and behavior, and how these interactions in turn determine the morphological pattern of the reparative response and therefore the physiologic outcome of lung repair.

STRUCTURE AND FUNCTION: NORMAL ALVEOLAR ANATOMY AND PHYSIOLOGY

The normal gas exchange apparatus can be conceptualized as consisting of three anatomical compartments: the microvascular endothelium or blood–lung interface, the alveolar epithelium constituting the air–lung interface, and the interstitium, which separates the epithelium from the endothelium. Figure 14.1 shows microscopic views of normal alveolar anatomy.

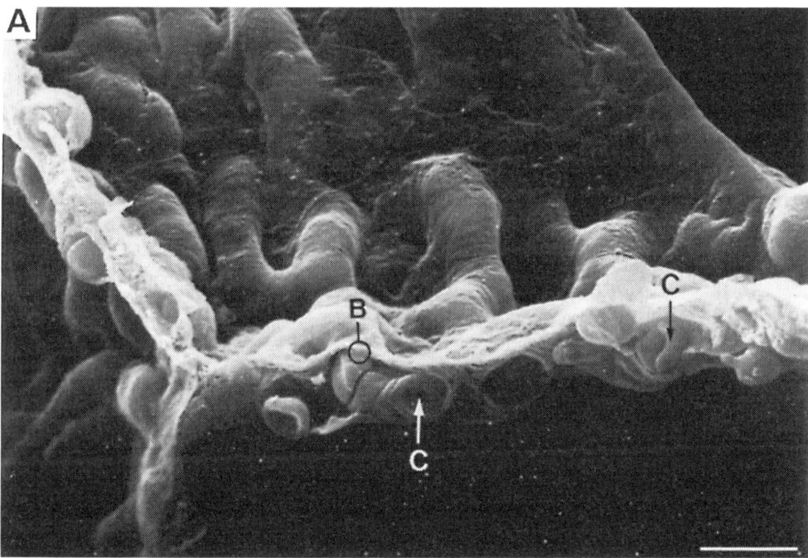

Figure 14.1. Normal alveolar anatomy.   **A:** Scanning electron microscopic view of alveolar wall, showing the very thin tissue barrier (B) separating the airspace from red blood cells within the extensive capillary network in the alveolar wall.   **B** (opposite): Transmission electron microscopic view also illustrating the thin membrane barrier (mB) which separates erythrocytes (EC) in a capillary (C) from the airspace. EN = Endothelial cell nucleus; EP = epithelial cell; F = connective tissue fibrils; fb = fibroblast. Bar = 1 µm. Reproduced from Weibel[11] with permission

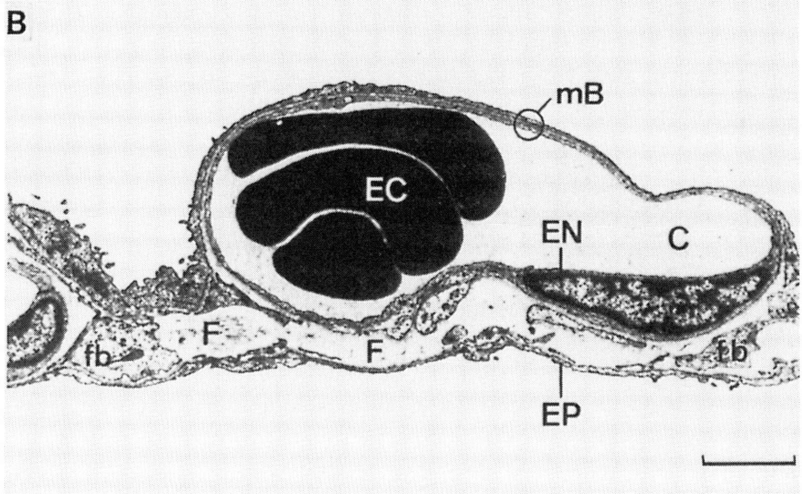

AIR–LUNG INTERFACE

The alveolar epithelium consists predominantly of type I and type II epithelial cells. Type I cells constitute one-third of the alveolar epithelial cell population, yet occupy more than 95% of the epithelial surface area. Morphologically, they are flat and contain attenuated cytoplasm, permitting the distance from air to blood to be as small as 0.3 μm[11]. Tight junctions between type I cells serve as the primary barrier to the flux of solute and water from the interstitium into the alveolar airspace. Type II epithelial cells constitute two-thirds of the alveolar epithelial cell population[12]. They are responsible for the synthesis of surfactant, and are capable of proliferation, thereby replacing senescent or injured type I epithelial cells, which have little or no ability to divide[13–15].

Type II cells contain Na^+, K^+-ATPase, located on their basolateral membrane[16]. This sodium pump utilizes energy derived from the hydrolysis of ATP to drive sodium absorption. Active transport of Na^+ occurs unidirectionally. Sodium moves passively into the cell through apical sodium channels; the Na^+, K^+-ATPase pump then drives it from the cell into the interstium. This facilitates the passive movement of Cl- and water into the interstitium, thereby keeping the alveolar space relatively free of fluid[17].

It has now become appreciated that monolayers of type II cells *in vitro* are also capable of transporting macromolecules across the alveolar epithelium. Although the precise mechanism of macromolecule transport is not known, it is believed to involve vesicular uptake and secretion pathways[18]. The ability of the alveolar epithelium to transport macromolecules such as albumin may be one mechanism by which the net removal of proteins from the alveolar airspace occurs after pulmonary edema.

INTERSTITIUM

The pulmonary interstitium is the space between the alveolar epithelium and the vascular endothelium which serves both to separate and to bind together these two cell layers, and acts as the structural support of the lung. It contains various cell types that serve different functions, a fiber system providing mechanical support, and two basement membranes that form a barrier to the alveolar epithelium and endothelium and support the attachment for these cell layers.

Interstitial Mesenchymal Cells

Three predominant cell types are found in the pulmonary interstitium: fibroblasts, myofibroblasts, and pericytes. Fibroblasts can be found associated with the fiber system of the interstitium; they are capable of synthesizing and secreting collagen, fibronectin, and proteoglycans, which are important components of the interstitial matrix[19]. Myofibroblasts contain abundant bundles of actin microfilaments which serve a contractile function[20]. They can be found in the strong connective tissue rings that surround the "mouths" of alveoli. Although the precise function of contractile myofibroblasts in the pulmonary interstitium is not known, in the granulation tissue of healing cutaneous wounds contractile myofibroblasts are believed to supply the force for wound contraction[21]. Pericytes are myofibroblasts that are closely apposed to the capillary endothelial cell basement membrane[22]. Like myofibroblasts, pericytes contain bundles of actin filaments and may act to impart contractile tone to the microcirculation.

Although the lineage relationship among the interstitial mesenchymal cells is not clear, the development of cytoskeletal differentiation markers provides evidence indicating that phenotypic heterogeneity exists among these cells. This suggests that they may differentiate from one form to another. In this regard, recent work indicates that rat fibroblasts in alveolar septae become α-smooth muscle actin positive myofibroblasts after the administration of bleomycin[23]. Myofibroblasts containing abundant α-smooth muscle actin are the predominant contractile cell present in healing wounds. They are typically found in areas of intra-alveolar fibrosis in fibrosing lung diseases such as hypersensitivity pneumonitis, idiopathic pulmonary fibrosis, and bronchiolitis obliterans with organizing pneumonia[24]. The mechanisms for such phenotypic modulations are not known, but recent work indicates that specific growth factors and the extracellular matrix exert effects on mesenchymal cell functions such as adhesion, migration, and proliferation and therefore may modulate the cytoskeletal state. Such alterations in mesenchymal cell phenotype may have key roles in lung repair and the subsequent development of pulmonary fibrosis.

Interstitial Matrix

The major elements of the interstitial matrix include collagen, elastic fibers, proteoglycans, and fibronectin (Table 14.1). They serve as a structural support for the lung, yet permit mechanical deformation during ventilation. Collagen is the most abundant component of the interstitial matrix[25]. Type I and III collagens represent the major interstitial collagens. Type I collagen has the greatest tensile strength and is believed to serve as a major structural protein in the fiber support system. Elastic fibers, composed of elastin, form a random network in the interstitium that imparts elasticity to the matrix.

Table 14.1. Structure–function relationship of the extracellular matrix (ECM)

Component	Structure	Function	
Collagen	Triple helical chains: 1) Fibrils 2) Helices 3) Short chains	1. 2. 3. 4.	Major structural molecule Supports cell adhesion Binds to other ECM components Promotes cell migration
Elastin	Fibrils with β spirals	1.	Provides elastic properties
Laminin	850 kDa glycoprotein with three subunits (see Fig. 14.2)	1. 2. 3. 4. 5.	Promotes cell adhesion, spreading and migration Modulates cell differentiation and phenotype Binds to other ECM components B1 chain induces capillary tube formation E8 region promotes lung alveolar formation
Fibronectin	440 kDa glycoprotein; disulfide bonded dimer	1. 2. 3.	Promotes cell adhesion, spreading and migration Binds to other ECM components Wound/tissue repair
Proteoglycans	Core protein with attached glycosaminoglycan sidechains; multiple classes	1. 2. 3.	Glycosaminoglycan — specific effects a) Osmotic pressure — modulates fluid balance b) Steric exclusion c) Binds other ECM components d) Binds peptide growth factors Core protein function a) Cell surface receptor b) Supports cell adhesion, spreading and migration Other effects — modulates cell differentiation

Fibronectin is synthesized by fibroblasts and forms fibrils associated with mesenchymal cells and other matrix molecules. In the adult lung it is found primarily in the basement membrane, and around mesenchymal cells[26]. The fibronectin molecule contains specific binding domains that facilitate the adhesion of cells[27]. Through these binding domains, fibronectin is able to influence key cellular functions such as adhesion, migration, proliferation, and differentiation.

Three predominant types of proteoglycans are found in the pulmonary interstitium: heparan, chondroitin, and dermatan sulfate. The proteoglycan molecules are complex and consist of a core protein to which glycosaminoglycan side chains are attached. The proteoglycans serve a variety of functions. They provide a gel-like ground substance that has a tremendous capacity to take up water and therefore can modulate fluid balance and lung compliance[28,29]. In addition, in common with fibronectin, they also can modulate cell adhesion, migration and proliferation[30]. Proteoglycans also are capable of binding growth factor molecules and may serve as growth factor reservoirs, providing growth factor to adhering cells during lung repair[31]. An additional proteoglycan, hyaluronic acid, also is a normal constituent of the lung interstitium and is in dynamic flux. During lung development, hyaluronic acid is present in large quantities and has a major role in cell adhesion and migration. Although the adult lung contains small amounts of hyaluronic acid, marked increases occur after lung injury and may play an important part in cell adhesion and migration during the repair phase[32].

Basement Membranes

The basement membranes are complex structures with many functions. The epithelial and endothelial basement membranes over a large portion of the gas exchange surface are a fused structure excluding other interstitial elements, thereby providing minimal distance for the exchange of gases. They are composed primarily of type IV collagen, laminin, entactin, and heparan and chondroitin sulfate proteoglycan[33]. Each component of the basement membrane has different biologic effects that act in concert to affect cell function. For example, laminin, the major non-collagenous component of the basement membrane contains

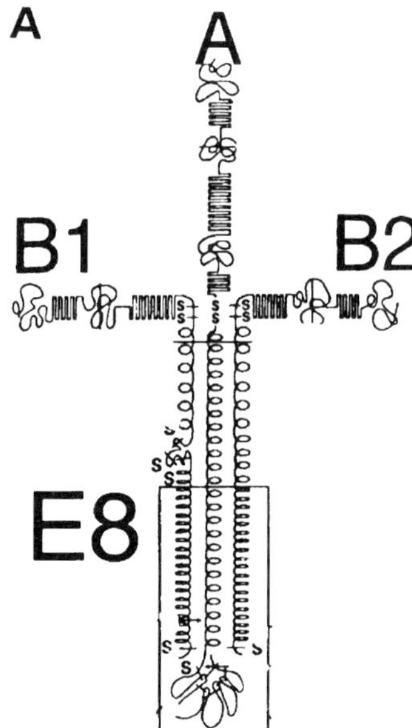

Figure 14.2. Schematic diagram of laminin. Role of laminin in alveolar epithelial and capillary endothelial cell differentiation. **A:** A, B1, and B2 denote each of the laminin chains, and E8 represents the cell adhesion site on laminin that is capable of promoting the assembly of type II cells into alveolar structures **B:** within the A subunit is the RGD domain which supports endothelial cell adhesion, and within the B subunit is a domain which induces the endothelial cell to form a ring or capillary-like structure **C. A** and **B** reproduced from Matter *et al.*[35] by copyright permission of the Rockefeller University Press; **C** reproduced from Sannes[36] with permission

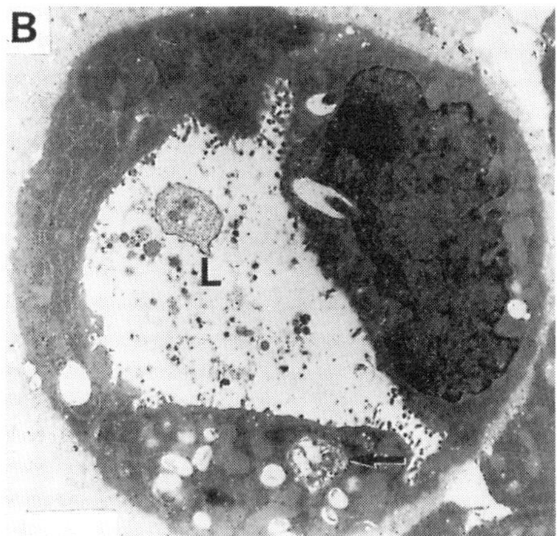

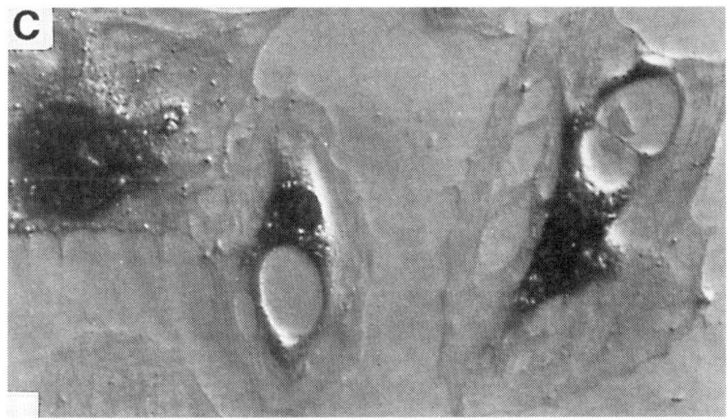

distinct biologic domains with cellular and ligand binding specificity (Fig. 14.2). Through these binding domains, laminin promotes cell adhesion and migration and modulates cell differentiation. The A subunit of laminin contains the RGD peptide sequence which promotes the adhesion of endothelial cells, while a specific site on the B1 subunit induces the endothelial cells to form a ring-like structure with a hollow lumen[34]. Furthermore, another distinct laminin domain, the E8 cell adhesion site, is capable of promoting the assembly of type II epithelial cells into alveolar structures with a central lumen[35].

The composition of the basement membrane varies as a function of both location and developmental state. For example, the basement membrane associated with type I cells differs in composition from that of type II cells. The basement membrane of type I cells contains more sulfated esters (chondroitin sulfate proteoglycan) than the basement membrane of type II cells[36]. When type II cells divide, daughter cells either remain type II or differentiate into type I cells. Such regional differences in the basement membrane may have key roles in these differentiation events.

Clearly, the composition of the basement membrane is vitally important in directing alveolar epithelial and endothelial cell differentiation and function. In addition, the basement membrane forms a support surface for epithelial and endothelial regeneration and a barrier function excluding interstitial cells from the alveolar airspace and capillary lumen. Loss of this support and barrier structure has been identified as one determinant leading to the loss of normal alveolar architecture and function[37,38].

Extracellular Matrix: Structure and Organ Function

The ultimate goal of lung repair is to restore function and promote physiologic recovery. This cannot occur if the architectural structure or the components that comprise the structure are absent or deranged. The components of the extracellular matrix supply critical structural information which modulates cellular phenotype and behavior and the organization of various cell types into a physiologically functioning unit. Within extracellular matrix molecules are specific domains with which matrix receptors on the surface of the cell may interact. The binding of such surface receptors with matrix molecules triggers a variety of post-ligand binding events within the cell that ultimately determine cell behavior. For example, the seven peptide sequence present in the carboxyl terminal of the basement membrane protein, laminin, supports type II cell adhesion and the formation of type II cells into alveolar morphological units[35]. It logically follows that derangements in the message provided by the extracellular matrix as a result of injury may substantially alter the pattern of repair. This alteration in lung morphology may result in maladaptive physiologic functioning of the lung unit, as occurs during the development of pulmonary fibrosis.

BLOOD–LUNG INTERFACE

Compared with the systemic circulation, the pulmonary vasculature has several special characteristics, which reflect its strategic location and function. For example, the pulmonary vessels are low resistance vessels and the arterioles have less developed muscle cells in their wall. Within the pulmonary capillaries, no smooth muscle cells are present[39].

Because of their number and the surface area they occupy, the alveolar capillaries represent the greatest majority of vessels within the lung. Characteristic features of the capillary endothelium include extreme thinness and a small number of organelles. In general, they are relatively long cells oriented in the long axis of the vessel. They represent over 40% of lung cells and occupy $130\,\text{m}^2$ of surface area[40].

Lung endothelial cells are complex cells with many functions relevant to lung injury and repair. Endothelial cells synthesize and release fibrinolytic factors, such as plasminogen activator which is vital in the maintenance of vascular patency[41]. In addition, endothelial cells are a significant source of prostaglandins, which may have a role in the pathophysiology of vascular remodeling seen in pulmonary hypertension[42]. Furthermore, endothelial cells contain a variety of surface receptors. For example, these cells contain surface adhesion receptors for such inflammatory cells as neutrophils and monocytes[43,44]. In addition, low affinity receptors for heparin binding growth factors such as basic fibroblast growth factor (bFGF) have been identified on the endothelium[45]. This growth factor, which has been identified on the alveolar epithelial surface of the lung after lung injury, is a potent growth factor for both endothelial cells and fibroblasts and may play a part in the development of pulmonary fibrosis and in the normal repair of the endothelium. Endothelial cells also contain surface matrix receptors, including integrins and cell surface proteoglycans that have important roles in endothelial cell adhesion and migration on the extracellular matrix during the repair process.

ANATOMY OF ACUTE LUNG INJURY

AIR–LUNG INTERFACE

Alveolar Airspace

Figure 14.3 shows the anatomy of the air–lung interface after acute injury. After alveolar injury, protein-rich fluid, derived from extravasation of plasma from the damaged microvasculature, inhomogenously fills the alveolar airspaces. Within this inflammatory exudate are red blood cells, inflammatory cells such as neutrophils and macrophages, and cell debris. Examples of the protein and lipid components of this exudate include fibrin/fibrinogen, fibronectin, albumin, immunoglobulins, and remnants of surfactant[46,47]. Augmented procoagulant activity, coupled with an absent or markedly decreased fibrinolytic activity, favors the polymerization of fibrinogen to cross linked fibrin[48]. Cross linked fibrin, fibronectin and other proteins form a provisional matrix within the alveolar airspace that clings to and covers the alveolar septum wherever the epithelium is denuded.

After this exudative phase in response to injury, a proliferative phase of repair ensues. This phase of repair is characterized by the migration of activated myofibroblasts into the alveolar airspace and onto the provisional fibrin matrix through gaps in the epithelial basement membrane[37,38]. During this phase of repair, both fibronectin and hyaluronic acid rapidly accumulate in the airspace[32,38,51]. Importantly, both fibronectin and hyaluronic acid support fibroblast migration. Fibroblasts contain cell surface matrix receptors for both fibronectin ($\alpha_4\beta_1$, and $\alpha_5\beta_1$ integrin) and hyaluronic acid (cluster of differentiation (CD) 44, receptor for hyaluronic acid mediated motility (RHAMM)) which bind specific adhesion domains on these molecules[52–55]. It is likely that the interaction between these extracellular matrix proteins and cell surface receptors has a key role in the development of intra-alveolar fibrosis.

Myofibroblast migration into the airspace is followed by the synthesis of connective tissue components on the luminal side of the basement membrane. Biochemical analysis of lung tissue obtained from patients during the proliferative phase of repair reveals a two- to three-fold increase in total collagen content, with a relative increase in type I collagen isotype[56,57]. The synthesis of type I collagen is principally localized to mesenchymal cells within the airspace, rather than the interstitium[51].

Not all alveoli develop intra-alveolar fibrosis during the proliferative phase of repair. Those alveoli without fibrotic lesions are lined by regenerating type II cells

                               C. A. Henke and P. B. Bitterman

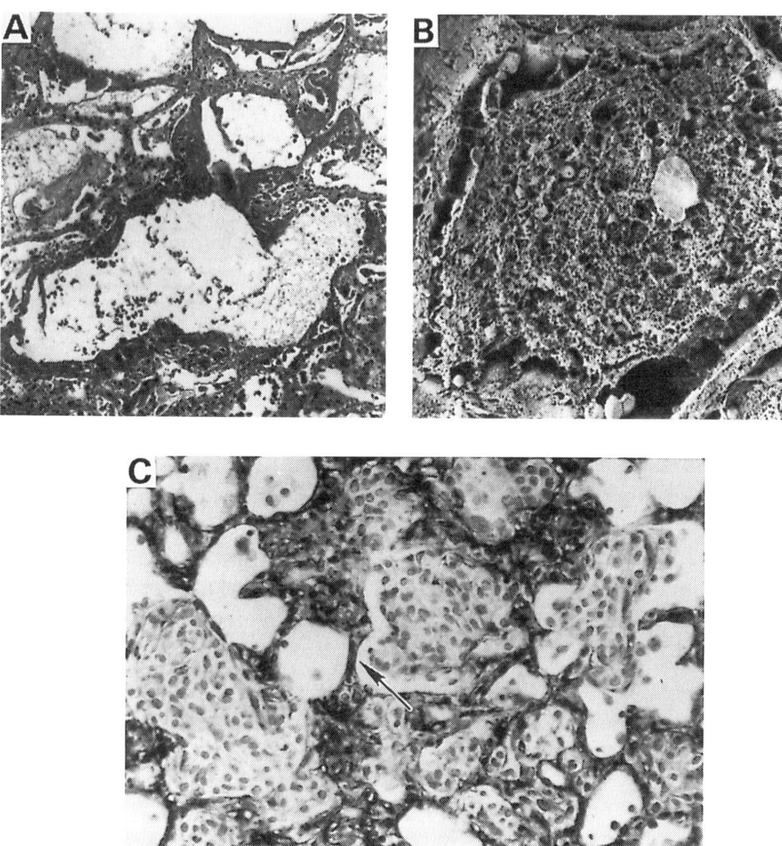

Figure 14.3. Acute lung injury: anatomy of injury to the air–lung interface. **A:** Light microscopic view of fibrin provisional matrix (hyaline membrane) covering denuded alveolar epithelial surface.   **B:** Scanning electron microscopic view illustrating the dense fibrin meshwork covering an injured alveolus.   **C:** Light microscopic view of inflammatory cells within the alveolar airspace. Reproduced from Anderson and Thielen[49] and Lazenby *et al.*[50] with permission

and the architecture of these alveoli become more normal. In contrast, in alveoli with intra-alveolar fibrosis, often the end result is the obliteration of the alveoli by adhesion and coalescence of adjacent alveolar walls, with the subsequent loss of functional alveolar capillary units[1].

Alveolar Epithelium

Ultrastructurally, type I epithelial cell injury is present within hours of disease onset[58]. All stages of epithelial damage may be visible, and range from cytoplasmic swelling to cell death, which is manifested as large areas of the basement membrane denuded of cells.

INTERSTITIUM

During the acute exudative stage, enlargement of the interstitial spaces by the influx of inflammatory cells and local fibrin deposition results in a markedly thickened alveolar septum. In some areas, gaps in the basement membrane develop, leaving the interstitium in direct communication with the alveolar airspace[37,38]. In addition, structural changes in the extracellular matrix components are a prominent feature of interstitial injury. For example, following paraquat toxicity in primate lungs, structural damage to collagen fibrils, elastic fibers, and dissociated and disrupted basement membranes can be found and are associated with marked inflammation[37]. Presumably, such changes result from proteolytic enzymes released by inflammatory cells. Late proliferative changes also are apparent in the interstitium and are characterized by an expanded mesenchymal cell population consisting of groups of activated myofibroblasts[37,38].

BLOOD–LUNG INTERFACE

Typically, overt endothelial cell defects are less conspicuous than epithelial cell defects. Nevertheless, rapid and extensive injury to the capillary endothelium is a characteristic of acute lung injury. Ultrastructural analysis of endothelial cells reveals injury manifested as mitochondrial swelling and dilatation of the endoplasmic reticulum[59]. In areas where endothelial cell death has occurred, these defects are typically covered with fibrin. Complete capillary destruction as a result of occlusion of capillaries by microthrombi is common in lung injury[59]. The number of patent capillaries markedly decreases as endothelial cells are sloughed from the basement membrane, leading to marked impairment of the pulmonary microcirculation[59]. Thromboembolic occlusion of small arterioles is also common. The early intravascular coagulation coupled with subsequent fibroproliferative changes within the vessel walls leads to the characteristic increase in pulmonary vascular resistance which is a predominant physiological abnormality in acute lung injury.

RESPONSE TO TISSUE INJURY

Clinically, the response to acute lung injury is variable. Some patients rapidly repair the transmural injury to the alveolar wall. Effective repair is characterized by resorption of the inflammatory airspace exudate and by re-epithelialization of the alveolar basement membrane by dividing type II cells which later differentiate into type I epithelial cells. Interstitial repair is characterized by a rapid but controlled mesenchymal cell response which results in the repair and restructuring of the damaged extracellular matrix by the synthesis of new connective tissue elements. Effective repair of the microvasculature is characterized by endothelial cell migration and division, which repairs defects in the luminal endothelial cell monolayer of the vessel. The resolution of thrombi restores vascular luminal patency and completes the process of alveolar repair. Unfortunately, the repair response does not always result in a return to normal architecture. In some patients, the normal architecture is distorted by a fibroproliferative response, resulting in the obliteration of alveoli by expanding mesenchymal cells and their connective tissue products. This fibroproliferative response itself may lead to severe gas exchange abnormalities and death from respiratory insufficiency. Detailed morphologic analysis of lungs from patients with acute lung injury has defined the events characterizing effective and unsuccessful lung repair. This information will provide the basis for a discussion of the major determinants which regulate the repair response.

REPAIR OF THE AIR–LUNG INTERFACE

Clearance of the airspace inflammatory exudate and reconstitution of the alveolar epithelium appear to be interrelated. Repopulation of the alveolus with type II cells requires type II cell adhesion and migration onto the airspace provisional matrix or onto the pre-existing basement membrane not covered by the provisional matrix. Ultrastructural studies reveal the presence of type II cells located on the surface of the provisional matrix[49,60] (Fig. 14.4). Furthermore, recent studies indicate that isolated type II cells adhere better to the provisional matrix proteins fibronectin and fibrin than to the basement membrane proteins type IV collagen and laminin, and are capable of migrating on fibronectin coated surfaces[61]. In addition, recent studies indicate that type II cells express a variety of integrin cell surface matrix receptors and preliminary studies indicate that $\alpha_v\beta_3$ integrin and $\alpha_5\beta_1$ integrin are important in mediating type II adhesion to the provisional matrix proteins fibrin and fibronectin, respectively[61,62]. Collectively, these data suggest that type II cell adhesion and migration on the provisional matrix proteins fibrin and fibronectin are important for successful re-epithelialization of the air–lung interface after lung injury. Presumably, once on the surface of the provisional matrix or pre-existing basement membrane, type II cells divide and a subset differentiate into type I epithelial cells. However, the molecular mechanisms regulating epithelial cell population size and composition are currently undefined.

Resolution of the exudative inflammatory fluid is necessary for normal gas exchange to occur. Animal studies indicate that hypoxic injury to rat lungs results in an increase in alveolar Na^+ resorption *in vivo* and increases in Na^+, K^+-ATPase membrane protein[63]. In addition, steady state mRNA levels for the α_1 and β_1 Na^+, K^+-ATPase subunits have been found to be increased, suggesting that hyperoxia increases alveolar epithelial active sodium transport through the increased expression of Na^+, K^+-ATPase[64]. This may also be an important mechanism by which alveolar edema fluid is cleared from the airspace after acute lung injury.

Clearance of the fibrin provisional matrix is important for normal alveolar repair to ensue. Rat pulmonary type II cells in culture express, synthesize, and release urokinase-type plasminogen activator[65]. The expression of urokinase-type plasminogen activator activity has been found to increase as type II cells become flattened, and is upregulated by the presence of the proinflammatory signal, tumor necrosis factor α. As plasminogen activator activity is important in the local generation of plasmin and represents a critical step in fibrinolysis, the pulmonary

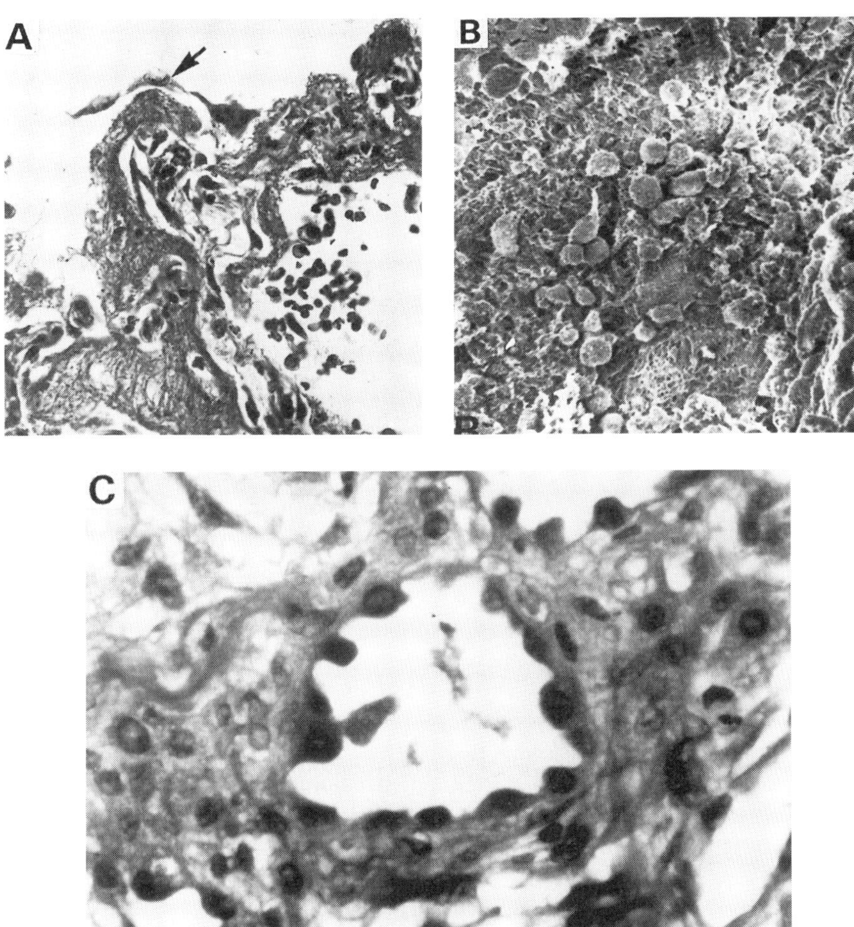

Figure 14.4. Acute lung injury: repair of the alveolar epithelial surface. **A:** Light microscopic view illustrating type II epithelial cells beginning to repopulate the surface of the fibrin provisional matrix. **B:** Scanning electron micrograph also illustrating type II cell re-epithelialization on the fibrin meshwork. **C:** Type II cells re-epithelializing the fibrin surface covering an injured alveolus. Reproduced from Anderson and Theielen[49] and Stanley *et al.*[60] with permission

alveolar epithelium may have a key role in the resolution of the fibrin provisional matrix after lung injury.

REPAIR OF THE INTERSTITIUM

The extracellular matrix is a dynamic microenvironment during tissue repair. Synthesis of new connective tissue elements to repair or replace damaged matrix components is mediated by mesenchymal cells. Expansion of the mesenchymal cell population is a prominent feature of the repair process, and these cells are recruited via chemotactic signals to damaged areas within the airspace, the interstitial matrix of the alveolar wall, and walls of blood vessels. Within these regions, active remodeling of matrix elements occurs through the synthesis of fibronectin and type I and III collagens, and the degradation of other connective tissue elements. During the repair process, the extracellular matrix has two critical roles. First, extracellular matrix molecules or fragments recruit mesenchymal cells to damaged regions by a chemotactic mechanism. Second, specific binding domains on extracellular matrix molecules help mediate such cellular behavior as adhesion, migration, and proliferation. The extracellular matrix supplies information to cells, influencing their conformation, position, and differentiated state and therefore plays a key part in determining the pattern of repair. This dictates the subsequent three dimensional structure of the organ and physiologic function upon the completion of repair.

Remodeling of the Basement Membrane

After lung injury there is an increase in fibronectin in the lung parenchyma and in the alveolar lining fluid[50,51]. In addition to plasma, both fibroblasts and alveolar macrophages are sources of fibronectin, which is deposited into the fibrin provisional matrix lining the denuded basement membrane. Animal models of cutaneous wound healing suggests that deposits of fibronectin on the denuded basement membrane may facilitate re-epithelialization[66]. This is consistent with studies indicating that isolated rat type II cells adhere better to fibronectin than to the basement membrane proteins, type IV collagen and laminin[61].

The synthesis and expression of proteoglycans in lung development and after injury has received considerable attention. In adult lungs, synthesis of proteoglycans is low, with heparan sulfate proteoglycan predominating[67]. However, in developing lung increased synthesis of chondroitin sulfate proteoglycan has been identified[68,69]. Although the precise function of chondroitin sulfate proteoglycan in developing lung is not known, it is thought to be involved in branching morphogenesis and cell migration. Recent immunohistochemical studies reveal that intense staining for chondroitin sulfate proteoglycan is found in basement membranes in later stages of lung development, where it is thought to influence epithelial cell differentiation[33]. These data suggest that local and regional differences in basement membrane composition might also occur during lung repair and may have a key role in alveolar epithelial cell differentiation. This is consistent with data indicating that the basement membrane is a complex structure, varying in molecular content and function depending on the location and developmental state.

Remodeling of the Interstitial Matrix

After lung injury, structural changes indicating damage or destruction of connective tissue within the interstitium are prominent. Various proteolytic enzymes derived from inflammtory cells are able to damage type I, III, and IV collagens and elastin[70]. In response to interstitial injury there is a marked expansion of mesenchymal cells. These cells are capable of synthesizing and repairing the damage to the interstitial connective tissue elements.

Defining the signals that regulate the synthesis and degradation of the newly repaired extracellular matrix is critical for a thorough understanding of the reparative process. One of the best characterized signals that modulates fibrosis is transforming growth factor β (TGFβ). TGFβ can both enhance connective tissue deposition and inhibit its degradation. It is released from degranulating platelets and is synthesized by wound macrophages[71,72]. Although its role in interstitial repair after lung injury has not been defined, TGFβ appears to be important in modulating connective tissue deposition after acute lung injury. In addition, it has been implicated as a profibrotic signal in the development of pulmonary fibrosis in patients with idiopathic pulmonary fibrosis (IPF)[73].

The mechanism by which TGFβ modulates interstitial connective tissue repair has been partially elucidated, revealing a complex process. Both fibronectin and type I collagen gene transcription are increased by TGFβ, resulting in an increase in their steady state mRNA levels and protein synthesis[74]. In addition, TGFβ may promote collagen accumulation, not only by increasing its synthesis, but also by decreasing its degradation. TGFβ inhibits the proteolytic degradation of collagen by decreasing the expression of the fibroblast metalloproteinase collagenase, and by increasing the expression of the collagenase inhibitor, tissue inhibitor of metalloproteinase-1 (TIMP-1)[75].

During wound repair, there is active remodeling of the connective tissue stroma. Both metalloproteinases, a family of enzymes capable of degrading most matrix elements, and TIMP can be found in different sites within a healing wound[76]. Furthermore, both the enzymes and the inhibitors can be produced by a variety of cell types, including fibroblasts, epithelial cells, endothelial cells and macrophages[76]. Although both metalloproteinases and TIMP can be found within the lung after murine lung injury resulting from hyperoxia, their precise role in modulating connective tissue remodeling has not been defined[77]. In healing skin wounds, epithelial cells near the site of the resorbing wound edge have been found to express interstitial collagenase, suggesting that they are capable of degrading and remodeling the adjacent stroma[76]. It is likely that precise topographical and temporal controls of the enzymes and inhibitors exist, acting to regulate the remodeling process.

REPAIR OF THE BLOOD–LUNG INTERFACE

The precise sequence of events constituting effective repair of the microvasculature after lung injury is largely unknown. That effective repair can occur is suggested by the near normal recovery of physiologic function in many survivors of acute lung injury. In this disorder, injury to the vascular bed is widespread and extensive, and is characterized by endothelial cell injury and death, with marked loss of capillaries. By inference, effective repair must include regeneration of an intact endothelial cell layer in damaged vessels and, probably, angiogenesis or new capillary formation to regenerate lost capillaries[59]. In addition, the extensive damage to the microvasculature is accompanied by remodeling of extra-alveolar vessels[59]. In most patients there is a muscularization and intimal fibrosis of intra-acinar microvessels that frequently extends also to larger arteries[59].

In vitro studies of wounded large vessel endothelial cells indicate that repair of small denuded areas of basement membrane occur by endothelial cell migration[78]. Larger denuded regions are re-endothelialized by a combination of migration and proliferation of surrounding non-damaged endothelial cells[79]. When endothelial cells migrate into the wounded area, their orientation is parallel to the axis of blood flow[80]. Endothelial cell cues to orientation appear to be derived from both the underlying extracellular matrix and the axis of blood flow[80]. These studies suggest that information supplied both by the extracellular matrix and by biophysical signals such as flow or sheer stress are important in large vessel repair.

The role of angiogenesis in the repair of the microvasculature after lung injury is uncertain but inferential, in that effective lung repair must have a means of regenerating the marked loss of capillaries that is so predominant a feature of severe lung injury. Previous work has shown that capillary proliferation can occur after acute lung injury[81–83]. However, it is uncertain whether these capillaries are only a part of the granulation tissue response to extensive injury, or whether they become an essential component in the regeneration of the markedly rarefied microvasculature. Lending further support to the role of angiogenesis in capillary repair, polypeptide growth factors capable of regulating endothelial cell migration and proliferation have been recovered from the air–lung interface after lung injury and include bFGF and platelet derived growth factor (PDGF)[84–86]. In addition, angiogenic proteins capable of stimulating new vessel formation *in vivo* have been identified in patients after lung injury[84]. However, the role of these endothelial cell modulating factors in directing the regeneration of new capillary networks remains to be determined.

MALADAPTIVE REPAIR: FACTORS LEADING TO THE LOSS OF NORMAL ARCHITECTURE AND THE DEVELOPMENT OF INTRA-ALVEOLAR FIBROSIS

Pulmonary fibrosis after acute lung injury results from the organization of the fibrin provisional matrix in the airspace by myofibroblasts, with subsequent deposition of collagen. The development of intra-alveolar fibrosis is the predominant mechanism leading to the loss of normal alveolar architecture and functional alveolar capillary units. Clearly, the loss of normal alveolar structure results in physiologic dysfunction. Intra-alveolar fibrosis can thus be considered a form of maladaptive repair that, clinically, leads to respiratory insufficiency and death in 15–40% of patients with severe acute lung injury[87–89]. Alveolar fibrosis can be considered maladaptive in that fibroproliferation occurs in a critical anatomic location, thereby causing organ dysfunction. However, it should not be considered maladaptive because it is an abnormal biologic process. The fibroproliferative response after acute lung injury is a stereotypical response recapitulating the normal biologic response of wound healing.

The intensity and duration of the injurious agent and the resulting intensity and duration of the inflammatory response are the major determinants of the degree of lung injury. Furthermore, damage to the basement membrane has been identified as one determinant leading to intra-alveolar fibrosis[37,38]. Breaks within the basement membrane allow activated myofibroblasts to move into the airspace and disruption of the basement membrane may influence subsequent epithelial cell regeneration (Fig. 14.5). Flooding of the alveolar airspace with fibrin, resulting in collapse of the airspace and permanent apposition of the alveolar walls, also leads to pulmonary fibrosis[1] (Fig. 14.5). In addition, extensive destruction of lung structures and the subsequent formation of granulation tissue can lead to permanent fibrosis. Table 14.2 summarizes the factors likely to influence loss of normal alveolar architecture.

Although many patients who develop intra-alveolar fibrosis have severe respiratory insufficiency and die, some patients with intra-alveolar fibrosis are capable of resolving their fibrotic lesions and recover without significant physiologic impairment[90]. An examination of the factors that initiate and drive the fibroproliferative response will provide insight into how this stereotypical morphologic pattern of the reparative response results in maladaptive repair and physiologic organ dysfunction in some patients, yet may be reversible without significant physiologic dysfunction in others[90].

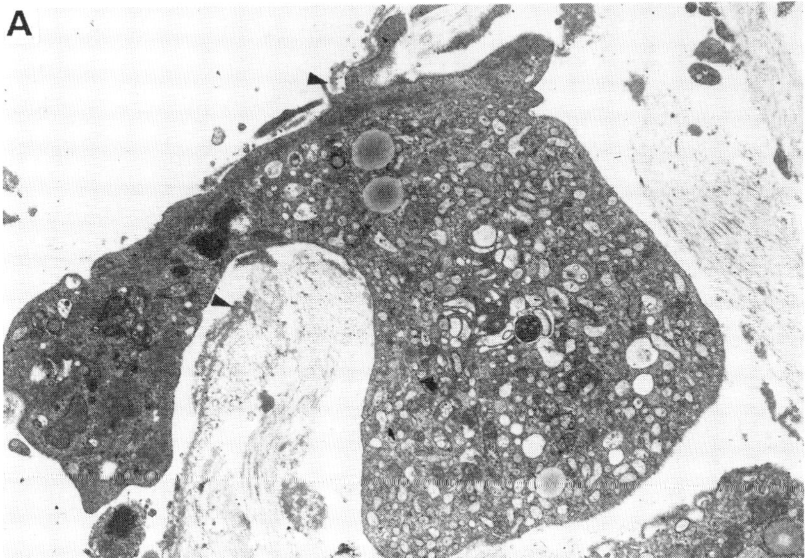

Figure 14.5. Maladaptive repair following acute lung injury: intra-alveolar fibrosis. **A:** Migration of a myofibroblast from the interstitium through a gap in the basement membrane into the alveolar airspace. **B** (opposite): Light microscopic view showing complete obliteration of the alveolus by intra-alveolar fibrous tissue. **A** reproduced from Fukuda *et al.*[38] and **B** from Burthardt[1] with permission

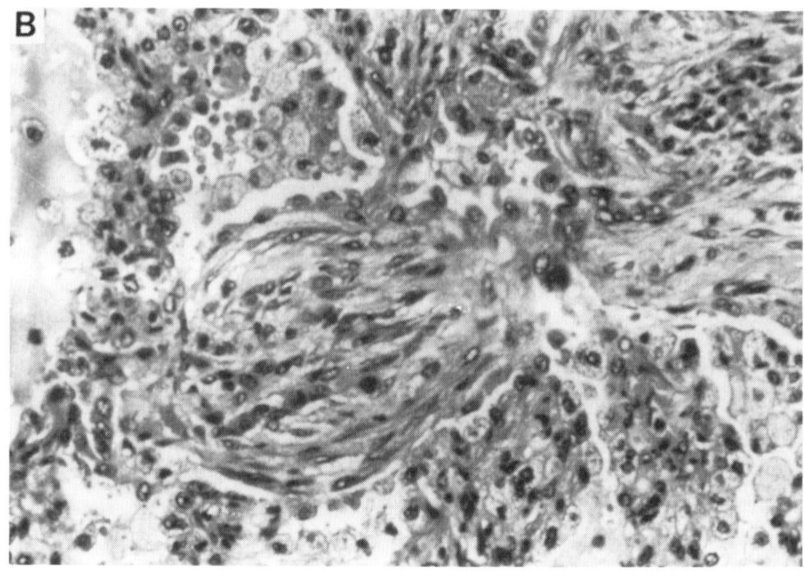

Figure 14.5. (*Continued*)

Table 14.2. Probable factors predisposing to loss of normal
alveolar architecture

Greater intensity of injurious agent
Longer duration of exposure to injurious agent
Greater intensity of inflammatory response
Longer duration of inflammatory response
Damage to basement membrane with gap formation
Deficiency of surfactant
Collapse of alveolar walls and permanent apposition
Flooding of airspace with fibrin and provisional matrix formation
Extensive injury with intra-alveolar granulation tissue formation
Impaired re-epithelialization of alveolar basement membrane
Extensive damage to capillary bed

ROLE OF POLYPEPTIDE GROWTH FACTORS IN THE DEVELOPMENT OF INTRA-ALVEOLAR FIBROSIS

Inflammatory signals initiate the mesenchymal cell repair response to injury. During the early phase of lung injury, large numbers of alveolar macrophages accumulate in the airspaces. Alveolar macrophages are capable of synthesizing a number of polypeptide growth factors for mesenchymal cells including bFGF, PDGF, and fibronectin[85,91,92]. Within the airspace, high local concentrations of growth factors influence mesenchymal cell function. These peptide growth factors, as a result of their ability to modulate migration and proliferation, have key roles in the development of airspace fibrosis (Table 14.3). It is important to note, however, that our current understanding of the signals that regulate the

A   Inflammation/Injury

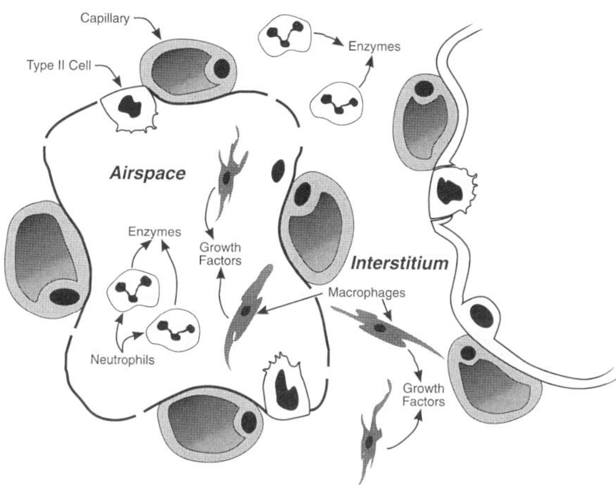

Figure 14.6. Schematic diagram illustrating the sequential processes of alveolar injury, response to injury, and outcome of the repair processes. **A:** Inflammatory response with neutrophils and macrophages accumulating in the airspace and interstitium. Release of enzymes by neutrophils results in injury to the air–lung interface and flooding of the alveolar compartment. Macrophages are recruited to the injured alveolus and release multiple growth factors which modulate the repair response. **B:** In response to growth factors, mesenchymal cells proliferate within the interstitium and repair the disrupted interstitial matrix. They can also migrate through gaps in the basement membrane onto the fibrin provisional matrix within the injured airspace. **C:** Effective repair occurs when the inflammatory response abates and epithelial cells repopulate the alveolar surface. Apoptosis of mesenchymal cells within the airspace and interstitium may be one means by which excess cells are eliminated during resolution of the repair process. Unsuccessful repair occurs in the face of continued inflammation, with progressive formation of fibrous tissue in the airspace. In addition, in the absence of continued inflammation and exogenous growth factors, an altered proliferative phenotype of mesenchymal cells may also contribute to an exuberant fibroproliferative response

fibroproliferative response to lung injury is limited. The specific signals that mediate specific parenchymal cell behaviors, their sources within the alveolar microenvironment, and the temporal and spatial patterns of their release remain to be determined. To illustrate their mode of action, we will focus on PDGF related peptides, bFGF, and fibronectin, which have all been recovered from the alveolar epithelial surface during the repair phase after acute lung injury.

PDGF exists as a dimer composed of two chains. It is a potent chemoattractant for mesenchymal cells and recruits non-proliferating mesenchymal cells into the cell cycle by stimulating the G_0–G_1 transition[93]. PDGF has been implicated in the pathogenesis of acute and chronic fibrotic lung disease[86]. The source of PDGF within the airspace depends on the phase of repair considered. In early stages during the exudative phase of lung repair, degranulating platelets are probably the major source of PDGF. Later during the fibroproliferative phase, alveolar

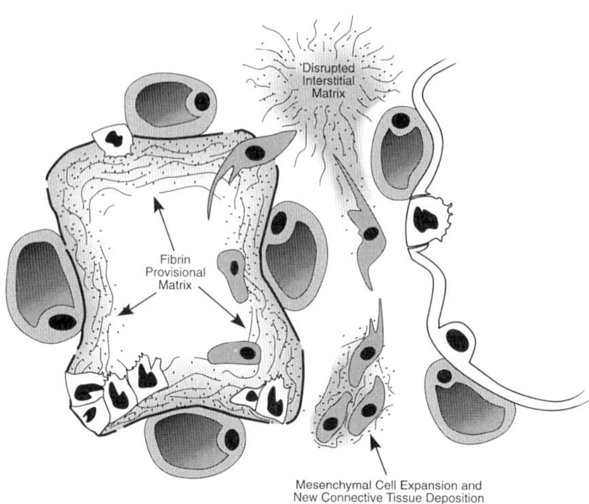

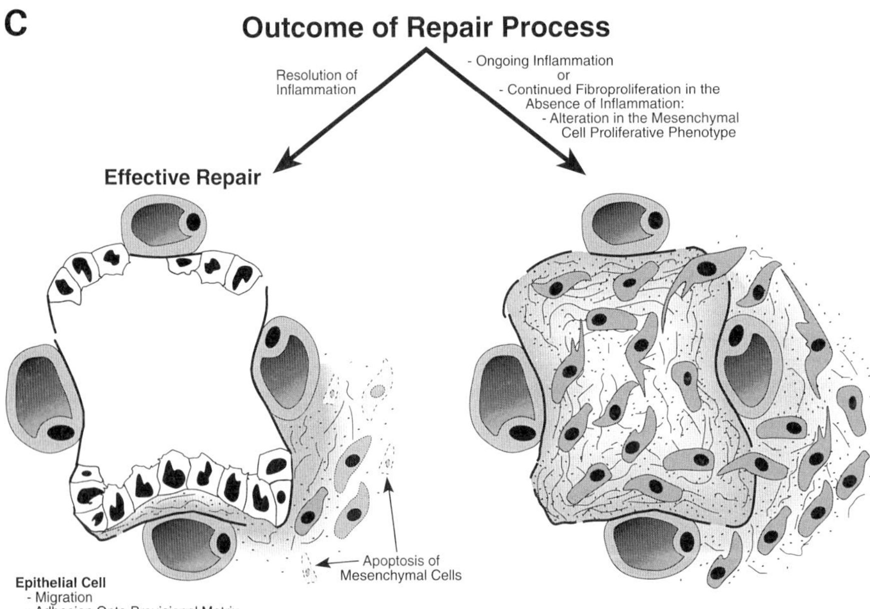

Figure 14.6. (*Continued*)

macrophages increase in number within the airspace and preliminary data indicate that they are a source of PDGF related peptides.

bFGF, like PDGF, is a potent stimulator of mesenchymal cell growth. It is an 18 kDa peptide and has been found in markedly increased amounts in the alveolar airspace during the fibroproliferative phase of repair after acute lung injury[84,85].

Table 14.3. Pathogenesis of intra-alveolar fibrosis: role of peptide growth factors

Growth factor	Action
PDGF	Chemoattractant for mesenchymal cells Induces mesenchymal cell proliferation (stimulates G_0–G_1 transition) Binds to ECM components
bFGF	Stimulates mesenchymal cell proliferation Alters cellular phenotype Promotes cell migration Binds to proteoglycans in ECM

PDGF = Platelet derived growth factor; ECM = extracellular matrix; bFGF = basic fibroblast growth factor.

Alveolar macrophages recovered from the air–lung interface after lung injury have been found to synthesize and release 18 kDa bFGF[85]. In common with PDGF, bFGF has been implicated as an important biologic factor regulating the granulation tissue reponse during normal wound healing[94].

Immunohistochemical analysis of lung tissue from patients after acute lung injury has revealed fibronectin to be abundant within regions of evolving airspace fibrosis[38]. Fibronectin, a 440 kDa glycoprotein, is generally considered to be a component of the extracellular matrix. However, in common with PDGF, it can act as a stimulus for mesenchymal cells to enter into the G_1 phase of the cell cycle. The source and isoforms of fibronectin within the airspace remain unknown. The relative contribution of plasma derived versus local cellular sources of fibronectin probably depends on the temporal phase of repair, with plasma derived fibronectin predominating early, and locally produced fibronectin being important during the later fibroproliferative phase. Cellular sources that may contribute to locally produced fibronectin include alveolar macrophages and intra-alveolar mesenchymal cells. In IPF, alveolar macrophage expression of fibronectin mRNA is increased, as is the release of fibronectin, and increased amounts of fibronectin can be found at the alveolar epithelial surface in patients with IPF[95].

ROLE OF FIBRIN PROVISIONAL MATRIX IN THE DEVELOPMENT OF INTRA-ALVEOLAR FIBROSIS

After severe lung injury, alterations of both the coagulation and fibrinolytic pathways have been demonstrated in the alveolar compartment, and predispose to the formation and persistence of fibrin deposition on the denuded alveolar epithelial lining[48] (Table 14.4). Importantly, the pattern of deposition of fibrin and fibronectin correlates with the location of subsequent intra-alveolar fibrosis[37,38]. Although traditionally viewed as structural molecules which form the framework of the extracellular matrix, extracellular molecules such as fibrinogen and fibrin have also been shown to promote cell adhesion and migration. Mesenchymal cells such as fibroblasts and endothelial cells migrate on extracellular matrix proteins such as fibrinogen and fibrin via cell surface matrix receptors that interact with distinct domains on extracellular matrix proteins. Recent work has

Table 14.4. Pathogenesis of intra-alveolar fibrosis: Role of extracellular matrix molecules

Extracellular matrix molecule	Action
Fibrin/fibrin degradation products	Forms provisional matrix in airspace after injury Chemoattractant for mesenchymal cells Supports cell adhesion, spreading and migration Promotes angiogenesis Binds other ECM components
Hyaluronic acid	Supports cell adhesion and migration Accumulates in alveolar airspace during repair
Chondroitin sulfate proteoglycan	Accumulates in ECM during wound repair Promotes cell migration
Fibronectin	Extracellular matrix molecule that functions as growth factor Accumulates in fibrin provisional matrix during repair Induces mesenchymal cell proliferation (stimulates G_0-G_1 transition) Promotes cell adhesion, spreading and migration

ECM = Extracellular matrix.

identified a specific receptor on acute lung injury fibroblasts and from wound endothelial cells, termed CD44 related chondroitin sulfate proteoglycan, that mediates the ability of these cells to migrate and invade into fibrin matrices[96,97]. It is a transmembrane proteoglycan matrix receptor that is capable of binding a variety of extracellular matrix proteins, including fibronectin, fibrinogen, and hyaluronic acid. Furthermore, work by Dvorak *et al.* has demonstrated that fibrin is capable of eliciting an angiogenic response and the formation of granulation tissue[98]. Collectively, these data suggest that CD44 related chondroitin sulfate proteoglycan interaction with fibrin may have an important role in directing mesenchymal cell migration and invasion into the fibrin provisional matrix during lung repair.

In further support of the role of the provisional matrix in the fibroproliferative response to injury, proteolytically derived cleavage fragments of fibrin, fibronectin, elastin, and collagen are potent chemoattractants for mesenchymal cells[99–102]. In addition, proteases can be found in exaggerated amounts within the airspaces after lung injury, lending further support to the role of the extracellular matrix in regulating the fibrotic response[103].

Hyaluronic acid is a matrix proteoglycan associated with cell migration that accumulates within the alveolar airspace after lung injury[32,104]. Fibroblasts have been found to contain multiple cell surface matrix receptors capable of interacting with hyaluronic acid including CD44, CD44 related chondroitin sulfate proteoglycan, and RHAMM[54,55,96,105]. CD44 has been shown to be the primary adhesion receptor for hyaluronic acid[106]. Both CD44 related chondroitin sulfate proteoglycan and RHAMM have been associated with fibroblast migration. These data provide evidence that the fibrin provisional matrix is more than just a scaffold for cellular organization during fibroproliferation; provisional matrix molecules themselves have critical roles in regulating the fibroproliferative response after lung injury.

FACTORS LEADING TO THE PERPETUATION OF THE FIBROPROLIFERATIVE RESPONSE

In that subset of patients with severe acute lung injury who develop progressive intra-alveolar fibrosis and organ dysfunction, two factors which may lead to the perpetuation of the fibroproliferative response have been identified. First, an ongoing protracted inflammatory response has been identified as one factor leading to a relentless fibroproliferative response. Second, an altered stable proliferative phenotype of mesenchymal cells isolated from patients dying from fibroproliferation after severe acute lung injury has been identified. The processes of injury, response, and successful or unsuccessful repair are summarized in Fig. 14.6, pp. 255–6.

Inflammation

Inflammation is the primary process which initiates the fibroproliferative response. Much of our knowledge in this area is derived from observations and studies on patients with chronic inflammatory lung disorders such as IPF. In IPF, continuing inflammation is the primary driving force stimulating the fibroproliferative response[107]. In such disorders, paracrine signals derived from inflammatory cells direct mesenchymal cell function. In patients with acute lung injury, observational studies suggest that persistent inflammation during repair may be one driving force behind the progressive fibrotic response[108,109]. In a pilot study, Meduri *et al.* treated patients with severe ARDS, approximately 2 weeks into the course of the disease process, with systemic corticosteroids[109]. A subset of patients rapidly responded to this treatment with improvement in physiologic function. It was found that the histologic pattern of preserved alveolar architecture and the presence of myxoid (cellular) type fibrosis predicted a good outcome, allowing the investigators to speculate that treatment intervention before the intra-alveolar fibrotic response progressed to the late acellular phase (dense collagenous scar) may facilitate resolution of the fibrotic response.

Alteration in Mesenchymal Cell Proliferative Phenotype

A second factor may play a part in the progressive fibrotic response of patients with severe acute lung injury. Mesenchymal cells, isolated from patients dying after lung injury, were found to have an altered proliferative phenotype[110]. These cells were capable of sustained division in defined medium lacking exogenous growth factors. Autocrine factor release did not account for these findings. The growth factor independent proliferation of myofibroblasts may be explained by an initial alteration of resident mesenchymal cells by trophic signals (e.g. peptide growth factors) in the injured lung, conferring upon them a stable differentiated state manifested by an intrinsically enhanced proliferative phenotype, or by the occurrence of selective expansion of a normally resident minority mesenchymal cell population.

Although the fundamental mechanisms that permit acute lung injury myofibroblasts to proliferate independently of exogenous growth factors is not known, one possible explanation may be derived from the striking alterations that occur in the extracellular matrix during the repair process. Mesenchymal cells contain cell surface matrix receptors that interact with the extracellular matrix and which influence cell behaviors, including proliferation. The mesenchymal cell proliferative phenotype may be altered by the presence of growth factors during the initial inflammatory response. Alterations in cell surface matrix receptors may accompany this change in phenotype. After abatement of the inflammatory response, the striking alterations in the extracellular matrix that occur within the interstitium and the alveolar airspace may convey information to mesenchymal cells via surface matrix receptors that results in a continued proliferative response. Obviously, additional work examining the key phenotypic properties of "fibrotic" fibroblasts and the ability of selected extracellular matrix molecules to modulate mesenchymal cell phenotype will be required to examine this hypothesis.

Immunohistochemical analysis of subpopulations of myofibroblasts has proven useful in classifying mesenchymal cells phenotypically. Such analysis of these cells supports the hypothesis that a subset of phenotypically altered mesenchymal cells may be involved in the pathogenesis of intra-alveolar fibrosis. For example, the expression of α-smooth muscle actin has been used as a marker of wound repair fibroblasts. Investigations of lung tissue obtained both from animals after exposure to bleomycin and from humans with IPF indicate that airspace myofibroblasts stain positive for α-smooth muscle actin[23,24]. Therefore, α-smooth muscle actin expressing myofibroblasts appear to be a phenotypically altered fibroblast involved in wound repair and the development of airspace fibrosis.

RESOLUTION OF INTRA-ALVEOLAR FIBROSIS

POSSIBLE ROLE OF PROGRAMMED CELL DEATH

Available clinical studies, in addition to animal models of lung injury, indicate that alveolar remodeling can be virtually complete, with restoration of normal or near normal anatomy and function[90,108,109,111]. This raises a key question in the natural history of lung repair: what happens to the intra-alveolar myofibroblasts and endothelial cells that form fibrous or granulation tissue in the airspaces? One important physiologic mechanism for the elimination of cells during wound and tissue remodeling is programmed cell death. It is important to note that the cellular degradation which characterizes programmed cell death is not accompanied by an inflammatory response, permitting orderly cell removal without derangement of adjacent tissue. Experimental wound healing studies in rats have revealed that activated myofibroblasts and endothelial cells, which form granulation tissue during wound healing, undergo a form of programmed cell death termed apoptosis[112]. In this regard, Polunovsky *et al.*, examining bronchoalveolar lavage fluid obtained from patients during the repair phase of acute lung injury, have found bioactive proteins capable of inducing fibroblast and endothelial cell programmed cell death[113]. Furthermore, on histologic examination of lung tissue obtained from patients with severe acute lung injury during the repair phase, apoptotic cells were present within airspace granulation tissue[113]. While the bioactive factor(s) and their source have yet to be identified, these results suggest that programmed cell death may be one important mechanism in the remodeling process which facilitates the resolution of intra-alveolar fibrotic tissue[114].

ROLE OF MESENCHYMAL–EPITHELIAL CELL INTERACTIONS IN LUNG REPAIR

Mesenchymal–epithelial cell interactions are an integral component of organ development. The exchange of information, regulated by autocrine, paracrine, and juxtacrine peptide growth factors and by the extracellular matrix, are critical factors which regulate cell proliferation and differentiation. For example, in the developing mouse lung, the mesenchyme provides paracrine support to the epithelium that stimulates cell proliferation and branching morphogenesis[115]. In this regard, Fukuda *et al.* found that the re-establishment of epithelial–mesenchymal interactions in paraquat induced fibrotic lesions seemed to correlate with recovery from injury[37]. Consistent with this hypothesis, Adamson *et al.* found that epithelial cell proliferation in mouse explants which had been exposed to hyperoxic conditions were preferentially retarded, while fibroblast growth became predominant[116]. They hypothesized that severe injury and the hyperoxic environment retarded repair of the alveolar epithelium, which in turn perturbed normal epithelial–fibroblast interaction, resulting in promotion of the fibrotic process. In support of this hypothesis, detailed analysis of lung cell kinetics in mice exposed to hyperoxic conditions has shown that hyperoxia substantially delays epithelial cell proliferation[117]. One possible explanation for the regulatory role of the alveolar epithelium in limiting the fibrotic response could be the production of negative regulatory signals that counteract such profibrotic signals as TGFβ. The role of mesenchymal–epithelial cell interaction during lung repair is not clearly defined, but these results suggest that this interaction may be crucial in the re-establishment of normal alveolar anatomy.

SUMMARY AND FUTURE DIRECTIONS

This review of lung repair has highlighted and focused on the concept of repair as a complex process involving the co-ordinate interaction of cells with other cell types, the extracellular matrix, and peptide growth factors. These interactions in turn result in changes in cellular phenotype and therefore influence such cellular behavior as adhesion, migration, and proliferation. The pattern of these responses in turn determines the structural outcome of repair and whether these changes result in physiologic recovery or progressive fibrosis.

Further delineation of the precise roles of peptide growth factors and extracellular matrix molecules in regulating the repair process will supply critical information needed to design effective therapeutic approaches capable of modulating the repair response and improving patient outcome. A major unresolved issue revolves around whether there is redundancy in the repair process, with various

                    C. A. Henke and P. B. Bitterman

growth factors and extracellular matrix molecules acting individually to bring about similar modulations in cellular function. A competing hypothesis contends that the repair response consists of a network of molecules, each with a distinct effect, that act co-ordinately to bring about the repair response. If each specific growth factor and extracellular matrix molecule has distinct effects on cellular function and no overlap exists, then targeting a specific molecule may prove successful in modulating cellular behavior and the repair process. However, if redundancy exists, then effective therapy is likely to need to target specific cellular behavior such as adhesion, migration, or proliferation, rather than targeting a specific molecule.

REFERENCES

1. Burkhardt A. Alveolitis and collapse in the pathogenesis of pulmonary fibrosis. *Am Rev Respir Dis* 1989; **140:** 513–524.
2. Murray J F, Matthay M A, Luce J M, *et al*. An expanded definition of the adult respiratory distress syndrome. *Am Rev Respir Dis* 1988; **138:** 720–723.
3. Petty T L, Ashbaugh D G. The adult respiratory distress syndrome. *Chest* 1971; **60:** 233–239.
4. Fowler A A, Hamman R F, Zerbe G O, *et al*. Adult respiratory distress syndrome: prognosis after onset. *Am Rev Respir Dis* 1985; **132:** 472–478.
5. Kaplan R L, Sahn S A, Petty T L. Incidence and outcome of the repiratory distress syndrome in gram-negative sepsis. *Arch Intern Med* 1979; **139:** 867–869.
6. Fowler A A, Hamman R F, Good J T, *et al*. Adult respiratory distress syndrome: risk with common predispositions. *Ann Intern Med* 1983; **98:** 593–597.
7. Balk R, Bone R C. The adult respiratory distress syndrome. *Med Clin North Am* 1983; **67:** 685–699.
8. Montgomery A B, Stager M A, Carrico C J, *et al*. Causes of mortality in patients with the adult respiratory distress syndrome. *Am Rev Respir Dis* 1985; **132:** 485–489.
9. Alberts W M, Priest G R, Moser K M. The outlook for survivors of ARDS. *Chest* 1983; **84:** 272–274.
10. Lakshminarayan S, Stanford R E, Petty T L. Prognosis after recovery from adult respiratory distress syndrome. *Am Rev Respir Dis* 1976; **113:** 7–15.
11. Weibel E R, ed. The pathway for oxygen. In: *Structure and Function in the Mammalian Respiratory System*. Cambridge, MA and London, UK: Harvard University Press, 1984; 314–315.
12. Crapo J D, Barry B E, Gehr P, *et al*. Cell number and cell characteristics of the normal lung. *Am Rev Respir Dis* 1982; **125:** 332–337.
13. Bowden D H. Cell turnover in the lung. *Am Rev Respir Dis* 1983; **128:** S46–48.
14. Evans M J, Cabral L J, Stephens R J, *et al*. Transformation of alveolar type 2 cells to type 1 cells following exposure to NO_2. *Exp Mol Pathol* 1975; **22:** 142–150.
15. Voelker D R, Mason R J. Alveolar type II epithelial cells. In: Massaro D, ed. *Lung Cell Biology: Lung Biology in Health and Disease*, Vol 41. New York: Marcel Dekker, 1989; 487–538.
16. Schneeberger E E, McCarthy K M. Cytochemical localization of Na^+, K^+-ATPase in rat type II pneumocytes. *J Appl Physiol* 1986; **60:** 1584–1589.
17. Cheek J M, Kim K J, Crandall E D. Tight monolayers of rat alveolar epithelial cells: bioelectric properties and active sodium transport. *Am J Physiol* 1989; **256:** C688–C693.
18. Kim K J, Cheek J M, Crandall E D. ^{14}C-albumin transport across rat alveolar epithelial monolayers [Abstract]. *Am Rev Respir Dis* 1989; **139:** A477.
19. Bradley K H, Kawanami H O, Crystal R G. The fibroblast of human lung alveolar structures: a differentiated cell with a major role in lung structure and function. *Methods Cell Biol* 1980; **21A:** 37–64.
20. Kapanci Y, Assimacopoulos A, Irle C, *et al*. "Contractile interstitial cells" in pulmonary alveolar septa: a possible regulator of ventilation–perfusion ratio? Ultrastructural, immunofluorescence, and *in vitro* studies. *J Cell Biol* 1974; **60:** 375–392.

21. Sappino A P, Schurch W, Gabbiani G. Biology of disease. Differentiation repertoire of fibroblastic cells: expression of cytoskeletal proteins as marker of phenotypic modulations. *Lab Invest* 1990; **63:** 144–161.

22. Weibel ER. On pericytes, particularly their existance on lung capillaries. *Microvasc Res* 1974; **8:** 218–235.

23. Vyalov S L, Gabbiani G, Kapanci Y. Rat alveolar myofibroblasts acquire α-smooth muscle actin expression during bleomycin-induced pulmonary fibrosis. *Am J Pathol* 1993; **143:** 1754–1765.

24. Leslie K, King T E Jr, Low R. Smooth muscle actin is expressed by airspace fibroblast-like cells in idiopathic pulmonary fibrosis and hypersensitivity pneumonitis. *Chest* 1991; **99:** 47S–48S.

25. Sobin S S, Fung Y C, Tremer H M. Collagen and elastin fibers in human pulmonary alveolar walls. *J Appl Physiol* 1988; **64:** 1659–1675.

26. Torikata C, Villiger B, Kuhn C, *et al.* Ultrastructural distribution of fibronectin in normal and fibrotic human lung. *Lab Invest* 1985; **52:** 399–408.

27. Pierschbacher M, Ruoslahti E. Synthetic peptide with cell attachment activity of fibronectin. *Proc Natl Acad Sci USA* 1983; **80:** 1224–1227.

28. Wiederhielm C A, Fox J R, Lee D R. Ground substance mucopolysaccharides and plasma proteins: their role in capillary water balance. *Am J Physiol* 1976; **230:** 1121–1125.

29. Bhattacharya J, Cruz T, Bhattacharya S, *et al.* Hyaluronan affects extravascular water in lungs of unanesthetized rabbits. *J Appl Physiol* 1989; **66:** 2595–2599.

30. Tool B P. Glycosaminoglycans in morphogenesis. In: Hay E, ed. *Cell Biology of the Extracellular Matrix*. New York: Plenum Press, 1981; 259–294.

31. Ruoslahti E, Yamasguchi Y. Proteoglycans as modulators of growth factor activities. *Cell* 1991; **64:** 867–869.

32. Bray B A, Sampson P M, Osman M, *et al.* Early changes in lung tissue hyaluronan (hyaluronic acid) and hyaluronidase in bleomycin-induced alveolitis in hamsters. *Am Rev Respir Dis* 1991; **143:** 284–288.

33. Sannes P L, Burch K K, Khosla J, *et al.* Immunohistochemical localization of chondroitin sulfate, chondroitin sulfate proteoglycan, heparan sulfate proteoglycan, entactin, and laminin in basement membranes of postnatal developing and adult rat lungs. *Am J Respir Cell Mol Biol* 1993; **8:** 245–251.

34. Grant D S, Tashiro K I, Segui-Real B, *et al.* Two different laminin domains mediate the differentiation of human endothelial cells into capillary-like structures *in vitro*. *Cell* 1989; **58:** 933–943.

35. Matter M L, Laurie G W. A novel laminin E8 cell adhesion site required for lung alveolar formation *in vitro*. *J Cell Biol* 1994; **124:** 1083–1090.

36. Sannes P L. Differences in basement membrane-associated microdomains of type I and type II pneumocytes in the rat and rabbit lung. *J Histochem Cytochem* 1984; **32:** 827–833.

37. Fukuda Y, Ferrans V J, Schoenberger C I, *et al.* Patterns of pulmonary structural remodeling after experimental paraquat toxicity. The morphogenesis of intraaveolar fibrosis. *Am J Pathol* 1985; **118:** 452–475.

38. Fukuda Y, Ishizaki M, Masuda Y, *et al.* The role of intraalveolar fibrosis in the process of pulmonary structural remodeling in patients with diffuse alveolar damage. *Am J Pathol* 1987; **126:** 171 182.

39. Meyrick B. The structure and ultrastructure of the pulmonary microvasculature. In: Will J A, Dawson C A, Weir E K, *et al.*, eds. *The Pulmonary Circulation in Health and Disease*. Orlando: Academic Press, 1987; 27–39.

40. Weibel E R. Lung cell biology. In: *Handbook of Physiology. The Respiratory System*, Vol 1. Baltimore: Williams and Wilkins Company, 1985; 47–91.

41. Gerard R D, Meidell R S. Regulation of tissue plasminogen activator expression. *Annu Rev Physiol* 1989; **51:** 245–262.

42. Meyrick B, Niedermeyer M E, Ogletree M L, *et al.* Pulmonary hypertension and increased vasoreactivity caused by repeated indomethacin. *J Appl Physiol* 1985; **59:** 443–452.

43. Bevilacqua M P, Pober J S, Mendrick D L, *et al.* Identification of an inducible endothelial leukocyte adhesion molecule, ELAM 1. *Proc Natl Acad Sci USA* 1987; **84:** 9238–9242.

44. Lasky L A. Selectins: interpreters of cell-specific carbohydrate information during inflammation. *Science* 1992; **258**: 964–969.

45. Saksela O, Rifkin D B. Release of basic fibroblast growth factor-heparan sulfate complexes from endothelial cells by plasminogen activator-mediated proteolytic activity. *J Cell Biol* 1990; **110**: 767–775.

46. Bachofen M, Weibel E R. Structural alterations of lung parenchyma in the adult respiratory distress syndrome. *Clin Chest Med* 1982; **3**: 35–56.

47. Schnells G, Voigt W H, Redl H, *et al.* Electron-microscopic investigation of lung biopsies in patients with post-traumatic respiratory insufficiency. *Acta Chir Scand* 1980; **499** (suppl): 9–20.

48. Idell S, James K K, Levin E G, *et al.* Local abnormalities in coagulation and fibrinolytic pathways predispose to alveolar fibrin deposition in the adult respiratory distress syndrome. *J Clin Invest* 1989; **84**: 695–705.

49. Anderson W R, Thielen K. Correlative study of adult respiratory distress syndrome by light, scanning, and transmission electron microscopy. *Ultrastruct Pathol* 1992; **16**: 615–628.

50. Lazenby A J, Crouch E C, McDonald J A, *et al.* Remodeling of the lung in bleomycin-induced pulmonary fibrosis in the rat. *Am Rev Respir Dis* 1990; **142**: 206–214.

51. Kuhn C III, Boldt J, King T E, *et al.* An immunohistochemical study of architectural remodeling and connective tissue synthesis in pulmonary fibrosis. *Am Rev Respir Dis* 1989; **140**: 1693–1703.

52. Hynes R O. Integrins: versatility, modulation, and signaling in cell adhesion. *Cell* 1992; **69**: 11–25.

53. Schmidt C E, Horwitz A F, Lauffenburger D A, *et al.* Integrin–cytoskeletal interactions in migrating fibroblasts are dynamic, asymmetric, and regulated. *J Cell Biol* 1993; **123**: 977–991.

54. Messadi D V, Bertolami C N. CD44 and hyaluronan expression in human cutaneous scar fibroblasts. *Am J Pathol* 1993; **142**: 1041–1049.

55. Turley E A, Torrance J. Localization of hyaluronate and hyaluronate-binding protein on motile and non-motile fibroblasts. *Exp Cell Res* 1984; **161**: 17–18.

56. Zapol W M, Trelstad R L, Coffey J W, *et al.* Pulmonary fibrosis in severe acute respiratory failure. *Am Rev Respir Dis* 1979; **119**: 547–554.

57. Last J A, Siefkin A D, Reisel K M. Type I collagen content is increased in lungs of patients with adult respiratory distress syndrome. *Thorax* 1983; **38**: 364–368.

58. Pietra G G, Ruttner J R, Wust W, *et al.* The lung after trauma and shock: fine structure of the alveolar capillary barrier in 23 autopsies. *J Trauma* 1981; **21**: 454–462.

59. Tomashefski J F, Davies P, Boggis C, *et al.* The pulmonary vascular lesions of the adult respiratory distress syndrome. *Am J Pathol* 1983; **112**: 112–126.

60. Stanley M W, Henry-Stanley M J, Gajl-Peczalska K J, *et al.* Hyperplasia of type II pneumocytes in acute lung injury. Cytologic findings of sequential bronchoalveolar lavage. *Am J Clin Pathol* 1992; **97**: 669–677.

61. Kim H J, Ingbar D H, Henke C A. Integrin mediation of type II cell adherence to provisional matrix proteins. *Am J Phys* 1996; **271**: L277–L286.

62. Lwebuga-Mukasa J S, Nielsen L. Integrin profiles of freshly isolated rat alveolar type II cells [Abstract]. *Am J Respir Crit Care Med* 1994; **149**: A1002.

63. Nici L, Dowin R, Gilmore-Hebert M, *et al.* Upregulation of rat lung Na-K-ATPase during hyperoxic injury. *Am J Physiol* 1991; **261**: L307–314.

64. Carter E P, Duvick S E, Wendt C H, *et al.* Hyperoxia increases active Na^+ resorption *in vivo* and type II cell Na, K-ATPase *in vitro*. *Chest* 1994; **105** (suppl): 75S–78S.

65. Gross T J, Simon R H, Sitrin R G. Expression of urokinase-type plasminogen activator by rat pulmonary alveolar epithelial cells. *Am J Respir Cell Mol Biol* 1990; **3**: 449–456.

66. Clark R A, Mason R J, Folkvord J M, *et al.* Fibronectin mediates adherence of rat alveolar type II epithelial cells via the fibroblastic cell-attachment domain. *J Clin Invest* 1986; **77**: 1831–1840.

67. Horwitz A L, Crystal R G. Content and synthesis of glycosaminoglycans in the developing lung. *J Clin Invest* 1975; **56**: 1312–1318.

68. Rutten T L, van Kuppevelt T H, Janssen H M, *et al.* Ultrastructural localization of a chondroitinase-sensitive, cuprolinic blue-positive filament in developing mouse lung. *Eur J Cell Biol* 1987; **45**: 256–261.

69. Juul S E, Hodson W A, Wight T N. Proteoglycan changes with development in the non-human primate (Macaca nemestrina) lung. *J Cell Biol* 1989; **109:** 233a.

70. Spragg R G, Smith R M. Biology of acute lung injury. In: Crystal RG, West JB, eds. *The Lung: Scientific Foundations.* New York: Raven Press, 1991; 243–257.

71. Sporn M B, Roberts A B, Wakefield L M, *et al.* Some recent advances in the chemistry and biology of transforming growth factor-beta. *J Cell Biol* 1987; **105:** 1039–1045.

72. Rappolee D A, Werb Z. mRNA phenotyping for gene expression in small numbers of cells: platelet-derived growth factor and other factors in wound derived macrophages. *Am J Respir Cell Mol Biol* 1990; **2:** 3–10.

73. Broekelmann T J, Limper A H, Colby T V, *et al.* Transforming growth factor β_1 is present at sites of extracellular matrix gene expression in human pulmonary fibrosis. *Proc Natl Acad Sci USA* 1991; **88:** 6642–6646.

74. Ignotz R A, Endo T, Massague J. Regulation of fibronectin and type I collagen mRNA levels by transforming growth factor β. *J Biol Chem* 1987; **262:** 6443–6446.

75. Edwards D R, Murphy G, Reynolds J J, *et al.* Transforming growth factor beta modulates the expression of collagenase and metalloproteinase inhibitor. *EMBO J* 1987; **6:** 1899–1904.

76. Saarialho-Kere U K, Chang E S, Welgus H G, *et al.* Distinct localization of collagenase and tissue inhibitor of metalloproteinases expression in wound healing associated with ulcerated pyogenic granuloma. *J Clin Invest* 1992; **90:** 1952–1957.

77. Piedboeuf B, Johnston C J, Watkins R H, *et al.* Increased expression of tissue inhibitor of metalloproteinases (TIMP-I) and metallothionein in murine lungs after hyperoxic exposure. *Am J Respir Cell Mol Biol* 1994; **10:** 123–132.

78. Wong M K K, Gotlieb A I. *In vitro* reendothelialization of a single-cell wound. Role of micro-filament bundles in rapid lamellipodia-mediated wound closure. *Lab Invest* 1984; **51:** 75–81.

79. Coomber B L, Gotlieb A I. *In vitro* endothelial cell wound repair. Interaction of cell migration and proliferation. *Arteriosclerosis* 1990; **10:** 215–222.

80. Jackman R W. Persistence of axial orientation cues in regenerating intima of cultured aortic explants. *Nature* 1982; **296:** 80–83.

81. Haselton P S. Adult respiratory distress syndrome: a review. *Histopathology* 1983; **7:** 307–332.

82. Haselton P S, McWilliam L, Haboubi N Y. The lung parenchyma in burns. *Histopathology* 1983; **7:** 333–347.

83. Pratt P C. Pulmonary capillary proliferation induced by oxygen inhalation. *Am J Pathol* 1958; **34:** 1033–1050.

84. Henke C, Fiegel V, Peterson M, *et al.* Identification and partial characterization of angiogenesis bioactivity in the lower respiratory tract after acute lung injury. *J Clin Invest* 1991; **88:** 1386–1395.

85. Henke C, Marinelli W, Jessurun J, *et al.* Macrophage production of basic fibroblast growth factor in the fibroproliferative disorder of alveolar fibrosis after lung injury. *Am J Pathol* 1993; **143:** 1189–1199.

86. Snyder L S, Hertz M I, Peterson M S, *et al.* Acute lung injury: pathogenesis of intraalveolar fibrosis. *J Clin Invest* 1991; **88:** 663–673.

87. Zapol W M, Trelstad R L, Coffey J W, *et al.* Pulmonary fibrosis in severe acute respiratory failure. *Am Rev Respir Dis* 1979; **119:** 574–584.

88. Montgomery A B, Stager M A, Carrico C J, *et al.* Causes of mortality in patients with the adult respiratory distress syndrome. *Am Rev Respir Dis* 1985; **132:** 485–489.

89. Suchyta M R, Clemmer T P, Elliot C G, *et al.* The adult respiratory distress syndrome: a report of survival and modifying factors. *Chest* 1992; **101:** 1074–1079.

90. Suchyta M R, Eliott C G, Colby T, *et al.* Open lung biopsy does not correlate with pulmonary function after the adult respiratory distress syndrome. *Chest* 1991; **99:** 1232–1237.

91. Marinelli W M, Henke C A, Harmon K R, *et al.* Acute lung injury: macrophage production of a 14 kD peptide related to platelet-derived growth factor [Abstract]. *Am Rev Respir Dis* 1993; **147:** A356.

92. Rennard S I, Hunninghake G W, Bitterman P B, *et al.* Production of fibronectin by the human alveolar macrophage: mechanism for the recruitment of fibroblasts to sites of tissue injury in interstitial lung disease. *Proc Natl Acad Sci USA* 1981; **78:** 7147–7151.

93. Deuel T F. Polypeptide growth factors: roles in normal and abnormal cell growth. *Annu Rev Cell Biol* 1987; **3**: 443–492.

94. Pierce G F, Tarpley J E, Yanagihara D, *et al.* Platelet-derived growth factor (BB homodimer), transforming growth factor-β_1, and basic fibroblast growth factor in dermal wound healing. *Am J Pathol* 1992; **140**: 1375–1388.

95. Rennard S I, Crystal R G. Fibronectin in human bronchopulmonary lavage fluid. Elevation in patients with interstitial lung disease. *J Clin Invest* 1981; **69**: 113–122.

96. Henke C A, Rourgta U, Mickelson D J, Knutson J R, McCarthy J B. CD44-related chondroitin sulfate proteoglycan, a cell surface receptor implicated with tumour cell invasion, mediates endothelial cell migration on fibrinogen and invasion into a fibrin matrix. *J Clin Invest* 1996; **97**: 2541–2552.

97. Svec K, White J, Vaillant P, *et al.* Acute lung injury fibroblast migration and invasion into a fibrin matrix is mediated by CD44. *J Clin Invest* 1996; **98**: 1713–1727.

98. Dvorak H F, Harvey V S, Estrella P, *et al.* Fibrin containing gels induce angiogenesis. Implications of tumor stroma generation and wound healing. *Lab Invest* 1987; **57**: 673–686.

99. Mundy G R, DeMartino S, Rowe D W. Collagen and collagen-derived fragments are chemotactic for tumor cells. *J Clin Invest* 1981; **68**: 1102–1105.

100. Postlethwaite A E, Keski-Oja J, Balian G, *et al.* Induction of fibroblast chemotaxis by fibronectin. *J Exp Med* 1981; **153**: 494–499.

101. Senior R M, Griffin G L, Mecham R P. Chemotactic activity of elastin-derived peptides. *J Clin Invest* 1980; **66**: 859–862.

102. Thompson W D, Evans A T, Campbell R. The control of fibrogenesis: stimulation and suppression of collagen synthesis in the chick chorioallantoic membrane with fibrin degradation products, wound extracts, and proteases. *J Pathol* 1986; **148**: 207–215.

103. Lee C T, Fein A M, Lippman M, *et al.* Elastolytic activity in pulmonary lavage fluid from patients with adult respiratory distress syndrome. *N Engl J Med* 1981; **304**: 192–196.

104. Hallgren R, Samuelsson T, Laurent T C, *et al.* Accumulation of hyaluronan (hyaluronic acid) in the lung in adult respiratory distress syndrome. *Am Rev Respir Dis* 1989; **139**: 682–687.

105. Turley E A. Hyaluronan and cell locomotion. *Cancer Metastasis Rev* 1992; **11**: 21–30.

106. Aruffo A, Stamenkovic I, Melnick M, *et al.* CD44 is the principal cell surface receptor for hyaluronate. *Cell* 1990; **61**: 1303–1313.

107. Crystal R G, Ferrans V J, Basset F. Biologic basis of pulmonary fibrosis. In: Crystal R G, West J B, eds. *The Lung. Scientific Foundations.* New York: Raven Press, 1991; 271–286.

108. Meduri G U, Belenchia J M, Estes R J, *et al.* Fibroproliferative phase of ARDS: clinical findings and effects of corticosteroids. *Chest* 1991; **100**: 943–952.

109. Meduri G U, Chinn A J, Leeper K V, *et al.* Corticosteroid rescue treatment of progressive fibroproliferation in late ARDS. Patterns of response and predictors of outcome. *Chest* 1994; **105**: 1516–1527.

110. Chen B, Polunovsky V, White J, *et al.* Mesenchymal cells isolated after acute lung injury manifest an enhanced proliferative phenotype. *J Clin Invest* 1992; **90**: 1778–1785.

111. Kapani Y, Weibel E R, Kaplan H P, *et al.* Pathogenesis and reversibility of the pulmonary lesions of oxygen toxicity in monkeys. *Lab Invest* 1969; **20**: 101–118.

112. Darby I, Skalli O, Gabbiani G, *et al.* α-Smooth muscle actin is transiently expressed by myofibroblasts during experimental wound healing. *Lab Invest* 1990; **63**: 21–29.

113. Polunovsky V A, Chen B, Henke C, *et al.* Role of mesenchymal cell death in lung remodeling after injury. *J Clin Invest* 1993; **92**: 388–397.

114. Bitterman P B, Polunovsky V A, Ingbar D H. Repair after lung injury. *Chest* 1994; **105** (suppl): 118S–121S.

115. Schuger L, Varani J, Mitra R, *et al.* Retinoic acid stimulates mouse lung development by a mechanism involving epithelial–mesenchymal interaction and regulation of epidermal growth factor receptors. *Devel Biol* 1993; **159**: 462–473.

116. Adamson I Y R, Young L, Bowden D H. Relationship of alveolar epithelial injury and repair to the induction of pulmonary fibrosis. *Am J Pathol* 1988; **130**: 377–383.

117. Haschek W M, Reiser K M, Klein-Szanto A J P, *et al.* Potentiation of butylated hydroxytoluene-induced acute lung damage by oxygen: cell kinetics and collagen metabolism. *Am Rev Respir Dis* 1993; **127**: 28–34.

15

Pathogenic Mechanisms of Bacteria Causing Bronchial Infections

ROBERT WILSON AND CHARLOTTE F. J. RAYNER

Imperial College of Science, Technology and Medicine, National Heart and Lung Institute, London, UK

INTRODUCTION

Respiratory tract infections are common, despite the protection provided by a sophisticated system of interrelated lung defences. The lungs have developed from the foregut during evolution and therefore the local defences have been adapted from those formerly protecting foregut in more primitive forms of life, and have not been custom built for this purpose in humans. For example, the site of the entry into the lung lies in a vulnerable position between the oropharynx and gullet. Furthermore, because of its function of gas exchange, the lung is constantly exposed to noxious substances and potentially infective agents from the environment. Infection may occur because of the malfunction of a defence mechanism, which may be inherited (for example cystic fibrosis, hypogammaglobulinaemia or primary ciliary dyskinesia) or acquired (for example viral infection or cigarette smoking), or because of the virulence of a micro-organism. Infections of the airways are more commonly caused by the former, and acute pneumonia by the latter, although this is not always the case[1].

Some of the respiratory tract defence mechanisms are local and "first line", whereas others are only called upon if the first line defences are breached. Their normal function ensures that the healthy lung is sterile from the first bronchial division to the alveoli. In this chapter we will consider the pathogenic mechanisms operating during infections of the airways. We will principally address bronchial infections, although many of the mechanisms may also operate in the upper respiratory tract.

Only relatively few bacterial species are commonly associated with bronchial infections. These are usually relatively non-virulent bacteria that commonly

---

Pulmonary Defences. Edited by Robert A. Stockley.
© 1997 John Wiley & Sons Ltd.

form part of the commensal flora of the upper respiratory tract. Non-typable *Haemophilus influenzae* is a common inhabitant of the nasopharynx of healthy individuals, but is also the most common isolate from patients with infective exacerbations of chronic bronchial disease. The next most frequently isolated bacteria are *Streptococcus pneumoniae*, followed by *Moraxella catarrhalis* and other haemophilus species. *Pseudomonas aeruginosa* infects patients with more severe impairment of host defences, such as cystic fibrosis and other forms of bronchiectasis, or patients receiving assisted ventilation[2].

HOST–BACTERIAL INTERRELATIONSHIPS

Because the bacteria which cause bronchial infections are commonly carried in the upper respiratory tract of healthy people, their pathogenicity must be examined in the wider context of the conditions which are permissive for their colonisation of the respiratory tract and which reflect coevolution of the microbe and host[3]. The dynamic nature of this relationship is demonstrated by the genetic diversity of natural populations of bacteria[4] and the polymorphic nature of the human immune responses against infection. The encounters between bacteria and man are resolved in outcomes that range from the establishment of a commensal relationship (carrier state) to potentially lethal disease, during which the role of specific microbial determinants may differ and phenotypic expression may vary. The pathogenicity of bacteria that cause airway infections should be considered in the wider context of conditions which allow their perpetuation on mucosal surfaces.

The commensal microbe is highly adapted to its host, and deploys strategies to ensure its survival, proliferation and dissemination. In the carrier state, this may result in no discernible damage to the host, but on occasions the organism may multiply and spread into the lower respiratory tract, resulting in disease of varying severity. The carrier state can be thought of as a balance which is altered during disease, usually by a change in the host state rather than by a change in bacterial properties. A variety of circumstances, singularly or in concert, may create these permissive circumstances allowing bacteria to multiply and spread contiguously within the airways. The success of the bacteria in colonising the airways and evading the remaining host defences depends on a variety of pathogenic mechanisms. The bacterial infection stimulates the host to mount an inflammatory response. If this fails to clear the bacteria and bacterial colonisation continues, the inflammatory response may persist. Large numbers of polymorphonuclear leucocytes migrate into the bronchial tree[5], and spillage of proteolytic enzymes[6] and toxic oxidants[7] may damage the airway epithelium. This will in turn encourage bacterial persistence and multiplication, and result in further stimulation of the inflammatory response. A self perpetuating "vicious circle"[1] of host mediated, bacteria stimulated lung damage can occur (Fig. 15.1).

Studies of bacterial pathogenicity should assess the role of potential virulence factors in biologically relevant systems, so that the results of such studies can be interpreted in the context of their role in human infections. This council of perfection is difficult to satisfy, particularly for bacterial pathogens such as

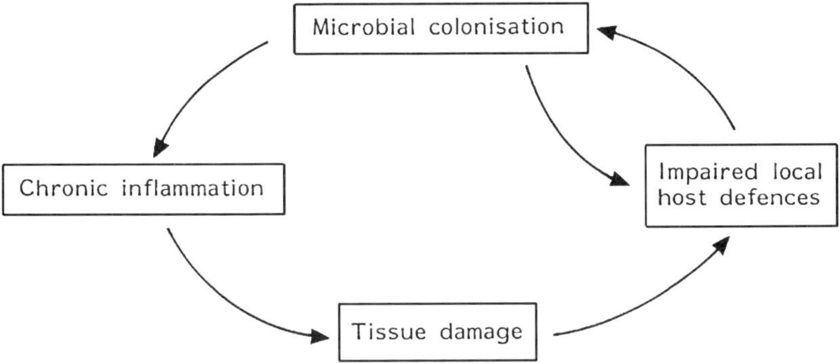

Figure 15.1. The "vicious circle" of host mediated, bacteria stimulated inflammatory damage to the respiratory tract during chronic infection

H. influenzae which are uniquely adapted to humans. The biological relevance of *in vitro* systems and animal models to human disease must be interpreted cautiously, and consideration given to the influence of the conditions of the experiment and the origin of the tissue being used, for example in the consideration of the molecular basis of bacterial attachment to cell surface receptors.

MUCOCILIARY CLEARANCE

Mucociliary clearance (Fig. 15.2) is an important first line defence mechanism of the respiratory tract, protecting the respiratory mucosa against inhaled particles, including bacteria, by transporting them towards the pharynx, trapped in mucus. Each cilium performs an arc-like effective stroke propelling mucus forward, and is withdrawn back to its starting point in a curved fashion within the periciliary fluid beneath the mucus. Efficient mucociliary transport requires coordinated ciliary beating, and the production of the correct quantity and quality of mucus and periciliary fluid[8]. Mucociliary clearance is slow in a number of conditions (Table 15.1), which gives inhaled bacteria the time to multiply and interact with the respiratory mucosa[9–12]:

Primary ciliary dyskinesia and cystic fibrosis are two congenital abnormalities of mucociliary clearance. In patients with either of these conditions, chronic bacterial colonisation of the airways occurs from a young age, leading to chronic sinusitis, cough and sputum production. In primary ciliary dyskinesia the ciliary beat is slow or absent and the beat pattern may be dyskinetic. This is usually associated with an abnormality of ciliary ultrastructure[13]. In cystic fibrosis, abnormal ion transport across the epithelium leads to abnormalities in the periciliary fluid, mucus, or both. Cigarette smoking, viral infection and asthma are common acquired abnormalities of mucociliary clearance. Irritation by the components of cigarette smoke may result in metaplasia of the bronchial epithelium, pronounced hypertrophy and hyperplasia of mucus glands, and an increase in the number and proportion of goblet cells at the expense of ciliated cells. The excessive

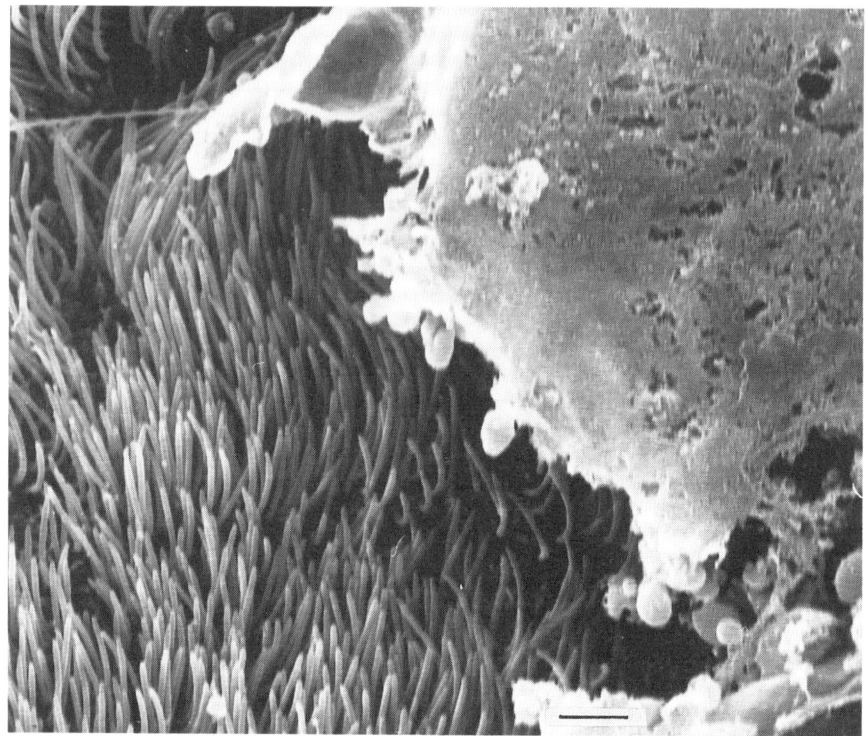

Figure 15.2. Scanning electron micrograph of the ciliated respiratory mucosa. Horizontal bar represents 2.5 μm

Table 15.1. Conditions in which mucociliary clearance is delayed

Condition	Mechanism
Cystic fibrosis	Primary. Abnormal ion transport
Primary ciliary dyskinesia	Primary. Impaired ciliary beating
Young's syndrome	Probably secondary
Bronchiectasis	Secondary. Bacterial products and inflammation, slow ciliary beating and damaged epithelium. Increased production of viscous mucus
Chronic bronchitis/cigarette smoking, pollution	Secondary. Mucus gland hypertrophy, increased proportion of goblet cells, loss of ciliated cells, impaired ciliary function
Virus infection	Secondary. Loss of cilia and ciliated cells, increased production of watery mucus
Asthma	Secondary. Inflammatory mediators impair ciliary function and eosinophil basic proteins damage epithelium

production of mucus combined with the loss of ciliated cells results in slow mucociliary clearance, and in addition there may be a direct effect of cigarette smoke on ciliary function. Viral infection reduces the elasticity of mucus making it less transportable, increases mucus production, destroys ciliated cells and reduces the number of cilia on ciliated cells[9,14].

Bacteria are inhaled from the nasopharynx or from the environment. Normally, they are rapidly cleared via the mucociliary escalator. When this defence mechanism is impaired, it gives bacteria the opportunity to use a variety of pathogenic mechanisms to establish infection of the mucosa. When the impairment is severe, as in cystic fibrosis, this single abnormality may be sufficient to permit infection. More commonly, a number of coincidental events may need to occur before bacterial infection is established. For example, a cigarette smoker may have delayed mucociliary clearance as a result of chronic bronchitis which is then exacerbated by a viral infection, making the airways of the lower respiratory tract more prone to infection by bacteria colonising the nasopharynx. The chance of infection will be increased if the inhaled bacterium is a strain which has not previously been encountered by the smoker's immune system.

Chronic inflammation as a result of infection can impair the mucociliary system by altering the orientation of cilia. Cilia on a single cell usually beat in the same direction, which is called the ciliary axis. This can be assessed by electron microscopy, either from a line drawn through the central microtubules of the cilium (the ciliary axis is perpendicular to this line) or from a line bisecting the basal body and foot process (Fig. 15.3A). However, cilia on biopsy specimens of epithelium from sites of chronic inflammation have axes that point in different directions (Fig. 15.3B). The cilia lack efficacy because their beat direction is disorientated. The metachronal wave of ciliary beating therefore fails to propagate, and hence mucociliary transport is inefficient[15]. Delayed mucociliary clearance correlates very well with the severity of the disorientation. In one patient with chronic mucopurulent sinusitis, 3 months of treatment with antibiotics and topical corticosteroids led to ciliary reorientation and mucociliary clearance returning to normal. Ciliary disorientation has also been described in patients with asthma, chronic bronchitis, and after viral infection; and it has also been suggested that ciliary disorientation may be inherited without any other abnormality of ciliary function or ultrastructure and cause a primary ciliary dyskinesia syndrome.

Bacterial products, or the inflammatory response to infection, may impair mucociliary clearance by affecting one of its component parts. These effects will be described in the following sections.

CILIARY FUNCTION

Ciliated epithelium lines the upper (nasal passages, sinuses, middle ear, and Eustachian tube) and lower (trachea to respiratory bronchioles) respiratory tracts. Ciliary beating provides the major mechanism by which mucus is cleared, and also protects the epithelial surface from the approach of bacteria that might otherwise adhere to it. Certain bacteria produce factors, some of which have been

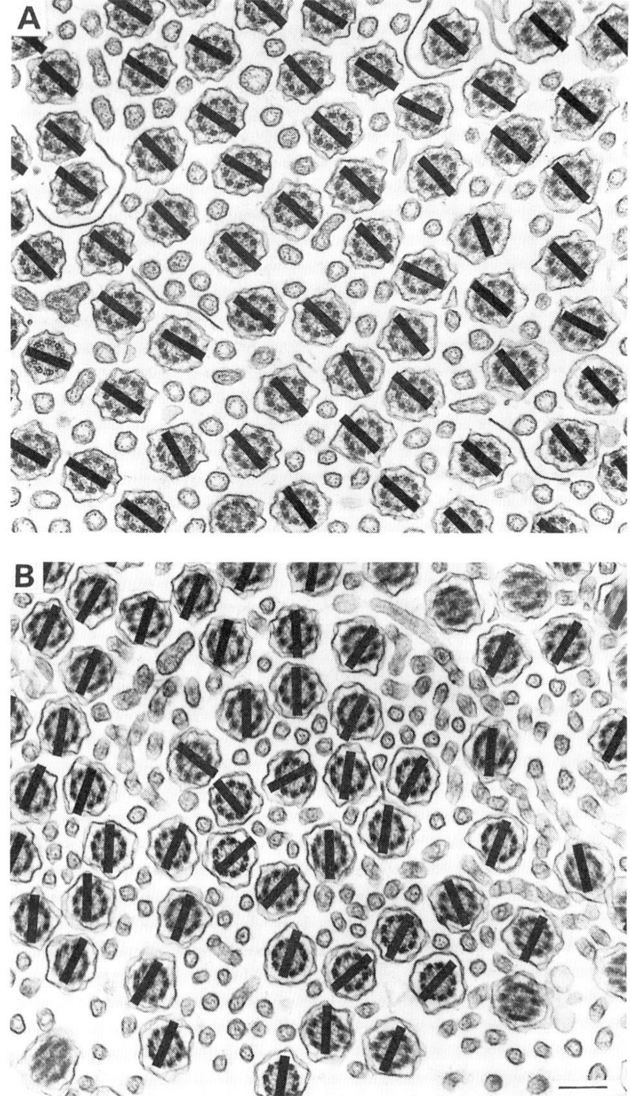

Figure 15.3. Measurement of ciliary orientation by electron microscopy. Cilia are seen in cross section and the direction of ciliary beat (the ciliary axis) is perpendicular to a line drawn through the central microtubules.   **A:** Normal orientation of cilia from a single cell.   **B:** The cilia are disorientated. Horizontal bar represents 0.25 µm

characterised, that slow and disorganise ciliary beating. Some of these factors at higher concentrations, or over longer periods of time, cause damage to epithelial cells; production of these factors *in vivo* would facilitate bacterial colonisation and might permit adherence to and invasion of the epithelium. At present, most of the observations have been made *in vitro*, but identification of the factors that have been characterised in sputum, and demonstration that they are active *in vivo* in animal models, provide indirect evidence of their importance.

The ciliotoxins of *Ps. aeruginosa* have been the best characterised, although factors with similar properties have also been described for other bacterial species which colonise ciliated mucosal surfaces, such as *H. influenzae, Str. pneumoniae, Mycoplasma pneumoniae, Bordetella pertussis, Neisseria meningitidis* and *N. gonorrhoea*[9]. *Ps. aeruginosa* culture filtrates slow ciliary beating and disorganise the beat pattern so that the beat becomes dyskinetic, with adjacent cilia beating in different directions. Prolonged incubation of cells with culture filtrate produced ciliary stasis and epithelial disruption[16]. Only the phenazine pigment content of the filtrates correlated with ciliary slowing activity; the concentrations of other known virulence factors did not. Gel filtration yielded only one peak of ciliary slowing activity which coeluted with phenazine pigments, and the accumulation of phenazines during bacterial culture correlated with the increase in ciliary slowing activity. Two phenazine pigments, pyocyanin and 1-hydroxyphenazine, were extracted from cultures and purified. 1-Hydroxyphenazine caused immediate onset of ciliary slowing and dyskinesia, which was not associated with epithelial disruption. Pyocyanin, however, caused a gradual slowing of ciliary beating associated with epithelial disruption. Both these compounds have been extracted from the sputum of patients infected by *Ps. aeruginosa* at concentrations similar to those required to produce an effect *in vitro*[17], and both slowed mucociliary clearance in the trachea of guineapigs *in vivo*[18].

The mechanism of action of ciliotoxins has been investigated[19]. Pyocyanin-induced slowing of ciliary beat frequency occurred after 2 h, without any damage to the cells, and was completely reversible after the pyocyanin was washed away. Ciliary slowing was associated with a significant decrease in intracellular cyclic AMP and ATP, and was prevented by agents such as isobutyl methyl xanthine and forskolin which increase intracellular cyclic AMP, and by the cyclic AMP analogue, dibutyryl cyclic AMP. ATP is an essential energy source for beating cilia, and it is possible that the effects of pyocyanin are directly mediated through a decrease in ATP concentrations. Pyocyanin has a zwitterionic structure that allows it to donate and accept electrons. It undergoes intracellular substrate cycling with the formation of superoxide and loss of NADH, and this loss of reducing power could cause a decrease in ATP levels. The concentration of intracellular cyclic AMP appeared to be a controlling factor in the effect of pyocyanin on ciliary beating, and it has been suggested that cyclic AMP may affect the availability or use of ATP by the ciliary axoneme[20]. 1-Hydroxyphenazine, in contrast, acts as a mitochondrial poison[21], which also leads to a decrease in intracellular ATP, and suggests a common final mechanism for both ciliotoxins.

There is an increasing awareness that, in the pathogenesis of a wide range of acute and chronic lung disorders, not only is the tissue injury by foreign material or invading micro-organisms important, but the host response to such agents may well contribute to the disease process. For example, toxic oxidants and proteolytic enzymes generated by activated phagocytes are unable to discriminate between microbial pathogens and host cells and proteins. Consequently, bystander cells in close proximity to activated phagocytes are vulnerable to oxidative damage.

Nevertheless, injury to bystander cells is usually minimised by the transient, self-limiting nature of the acute inflammatory response and the protection provided by biological defence systems that neutralise it. If, however, the inflammatory response is ineffectively downregulated, or misdirected, leading to hyperacute or chronic activation of neutrophils, host defences may be overwhelmed, predisposing to host tissue damage. This is believed to occur during chronic infection of the airways (Fig. 15.1).

Exposure of human nasal ciliated epithelium to reactive oxidants generated by enzyme systems, or to reagent hydrogen peroxide or hypochlorous acid, results in ciliary beat slowing and ciliary dyskinesia[7]. 3-Amino benzamide, an inhibitor of the DNA repair enzyme, poly-ADP-ribose polymerase, prevents hydrogen peroxide mediated inhibition of ciliary beat, indicating that oxidant mediated damage to DNA may well be the basis of the effects of hydrogen peroxide on ciliary function. The consequence of oxidative damage to DNA is activation of the DNA repair enzyme which utilises NAD as a cofactor. This could lead to interference with energy metabolism as a result of the depletion of intracellular NAD, an essential cofactor in the Krebs cycle and mitochondrial generation of ATP. In greater concentrations, hydrogen peroxide, in addition to damaging DNA, also directly inactivates glyceraldehyde-3-phosphate dehydrogenase, an important enzyme in this cycle. Thus energy depletion may, as with bacterial ciliotoxins, underlie the mechanism of hydrogen peroxide induced ciliary dysfunction[7].

There may be complex interactions between bacterial products and the inflammatory response. Pyocyanin and 1-hydroxyphenazine both enhance neutrophil oxidative metabolism and degranulation[22]. Pyocyanin primes human neutrophils for increased oxygen consumption, and for generation of superoxide on subsequent exposure of the cells to stimuli of membrane associated oxidative metabolism. 1-Hydroxyphenazine primes neutrophils for enhanced release of myeloperoxidase, and may promote an elastase–antielastase imbalance by increasing the release of neutrophil elastase and by enhancing oxidative inactivation of α_1 proteinase inhibitor[23]. Increased generation of hypochlorous acid as a direct result of enhanced release of myeloperoxidase by 1-hydroxyphenazine sensitised neutorphils appears to be the mediator of this process. Therefore, not only do pyocyanin and 1-hydroxyphenazine compromise ciliary function, they also enhance host mediated damage by the inflammatory response.

BACTERIAL INTERACTIONS WITH MUCUS

The first contact of inhaled bacteria with the mucosal surface is to become trapped in mucus which is subsequently moved cephalad by ciliary beating. An immunohistopathological study of lungs removed from patients with cystic fibrosis showed that, even in severe bronchial infections, the majority of *Ps. aeruginosa* were intraluminal and associated with secretions, rather than attached to the epithelial surface[24]. The observation that *Ps. aeruginosa* has an increased affinity for the mucins from patients with cystic fibrosis may afford one reason that bacteria remain within mucus[25]. Many different micro-organisms demonstrate an affinity for airway mucus[26,27], including *Str. pneumoniae* and

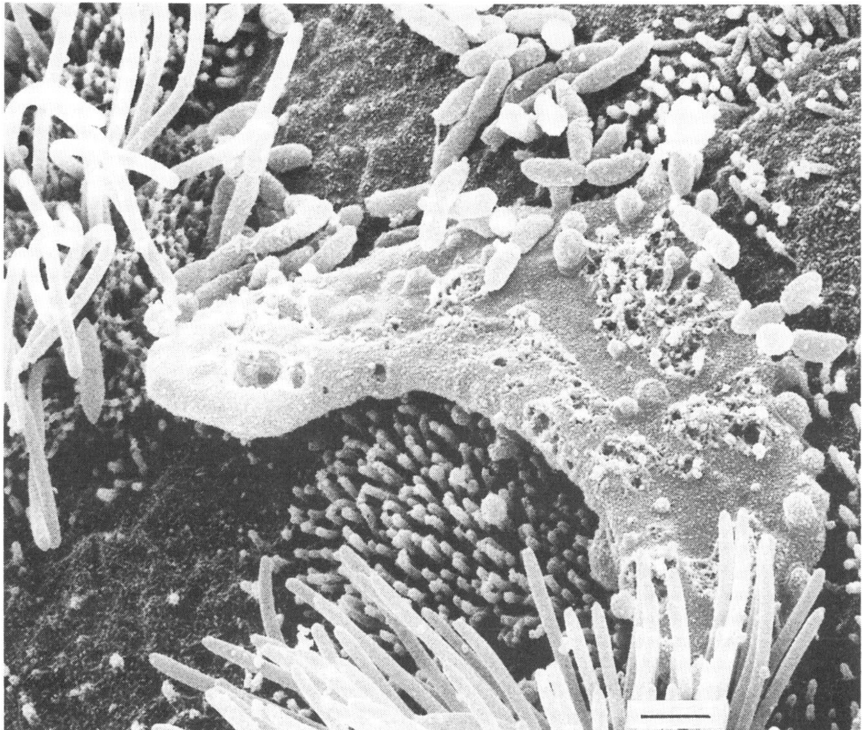

Figure 15.4. Non-typable *Haemophilus influenzae* exhibiting tropism for mucus in an organ culture of human respiratory mucosa. Horizontal bar represents 1 μm

non-typable *H. influenzae* (Fig. 15.4). Airway mucus is rich in potential carbohydrate receptors for bacteria, and in the case of *Ps. aeruginosa* both bacterial adhesins and carbohydrate receptors have been characterised[27,28].

Bacterial adherence to mucus may disadvantage the bacterium in the healthy bronchial tree when mucus is cleared normally. In situations in which mucus is slow moving or static, however, bacterial adherence to mucus could confer a colonisation advantage. There may be areas in the upper respiratory tract, such as those overlying the adenoid and tonsil, where pools of mucus form; in the lower respiratory tract mucus clearance is impaired in chronic bronchitis, bronchiectasis and cystic fibrosis (Table 15.1). A number of bacterial species, including *Ps. aeruginosa*, non-typable *H. influenzae*, and *Str. pneumoniae*, produce factors that stimulate mucus production[29,30]. By stimulating mucus production, impairing ciliary function, and causing damage to epithelium, bacteria may therefore create an environment conducive to their own persistence and spread. Adherence to mucus may also protect bacteria, as mucin has been shown to protect *Ps. aeruginosa* from opsonin mediated phagocytosis[31].

The volume of mucus produced increases during infection of the airways. The causes of this are mucus gland hypertrophy, increase in goblet cell numbers, and stimulation of increased mucus secretion by both bacterial products and the host inflammatory response[32]. If the mucus layer is too thick it may uncouple, so that the inner layer is moved normally by the ciliary beating, but the outer layer is stationary[33]. The rheology of mucus also changes during chronic infection, so that it becomes more viscous and less elastic, and is therefore less well transported by cilia[34]. This change is largely due to the complexing of DNA released by dead inflammatory cells in the mucus.

ION TRANSPORT

Efficient mucociliary clearance depends not only on the characteristics of mucus and its interrelations with cilia, but also on the characteristics of the periciliary fluid. Changes in the depth of periciliary fluid may prevent effective propulsion of mucus by cilia. Simplistically, if there is not enough periciliary fluid the cilia may become entangled, and if there is too much the mucus may be lifted above the tips of the cilia. Furthermore, normal epithelial ion transport across cell membranes is essential for normal epithelial cell secretions. A major role for normal ion transport in effective mucociliary clearance is strongly indicated by studies in cystic fibrosis; airway chloride secretion is reduced and sodium absorption increased, which may be responsible for the characteristic accumulation of airway secretions[35].

Periciliary fluid is difficult to analyse and measure, and it is only recently that techniques for measuring ion transport have been developed[36]. The effect of infection on ion transport has received little attention to date, although it may be important. For instance a haemolysin termed "rhamnolipid", released by *Ps. aeruginosa*, has been shown to interfere with epithelial ion transport *in vitro*[37,38], at concentrations similar to those measured in sputum[30,39].

ADHERENCE TO EPITHELIUM

The airway epithelium forms a continuous but heterogeneous lining of the airways. The ability of bacteria to adhere to mucosal surfaces is an important determinant of colonisation and the pathogenesis of most infections[40,41]. Adherence offers protection from mucociliary clearance and results in the close proximity of bacteria to epithelial cells, allowing toxins to reach concentrations sufficient to influence cell functions[42]. Adherence also increases the ability of bacteria to take up nutrients liberated by damaged host cells, and may be the first step in penetration of the mucosal surface before invasion.

As bacteria approach the epithelial surface, specific molecular interactions may occur. Human cells express many potential receptors for adhesion which include saccharide residues, glycoproteins, glycolipids and proteoglycans[43]. However, whether bacterial adherence to normal ciliated respiratory epithelium occurs *in vivo* is uncertain. There is evidence that *Myco. pneumoniae* and *Bord. pertussis*[44–46] adhere along the ciliary membranes of functional ciliated cells. *Bord. pertussis* filamentous haemagglutinin and pertussis toxin act as adhesins and establish a bridge between the bacteria and one or more carbohydrate containing receptors on cilia[47].

Bacteria use a wide range of adherence mechanisms; examples include lectin-like substances which are found embedded in the outer membrane, the secretion of exopolysaccharide, or the expression of hair-like outgrowths called fimbriae. Fimbriae enhance *H. influenzae* adherence to buccal cells. However, in an organ culture of human nasal turbinate tissue[26], *H. influenzae* did not adhere to normal epithelium, and were seen to adhere only when the epithelium was damaged. Under these experimental conditions, fimbriae did not permit adherence to normal epithelium, nor enhance adherence to damaged epithelium. The result suggests that fimbriae do not play a part, and that epithelial damage is critical. *Ps. aeruginosa* and *Str. pneumoniae* also require epithelial damage before adherence to cells occurs[24,27,48,49]. Some bacterial pathogens have a number of different potential adhesins[50,51], and the epithelial cell receptors available for adherence change in different parts of the respiratory tract[52], suggesting that the interactions are likely to be complicated. This may be of therapeutic importance, as it is unlikely that the binding process can be interrupted by a single intervention aimed at a universal adhesin or receptor. A therapeutic intervention that changes the microenvironment of the mucosa and in doing so influences bacterial interactions (airways pH, mucus biochemistry or protease activity in secretions) seems more likely to be successful.

The condition of the host, and the effect of bacterial products, may also influence bacterial adherence. Adherence of *Ps. aeruginosa* to tracheal cells of patients with tracheostomies who were studied in intensive care units showed a negative correlation with nutritional status[53] and correlated with the acquisition of pneumonitis. The binding of *Ps. aeruginosa* to epithelial surfaces is enhanced by bacterial elastase, alkaline protease and phospholipase C[54,55]. *Ps. aeruginosa* proteases degrade fibronectin, and thus could remove a blocking function of fibronectin, allowing enhanced binding of bacteria to newly exposed receptors[56].

Epithelial cells from patients with recurrent respiratory infections have more adherent bacteria on their surface and bind more bacteria *in vitro*[57]. This suggests that there may be a host predisposition to infection. Recruitment of inflammatory cells to sites of mucosal inflammation involves leucocyte adhesion molecules. Expression of E-selectin on vessels and intercellular adhesion molecule-1 on basal epithelial cells is increased in patients with chronic bronchitis with airflow obstruction[58]. This indicates a continuing inflammatory response to a persistent stimulus which is independent of infection. The effect of this process on bacterial adhesion has yet to be explored.

The interaction of *Str. pneumoniae* with the respiratory mucosa of mice was affected by infection with influenza virus. Pneumococci did not adhere to intact epithelium; however, adherence was significantly increased 6 days after viral infection at sites where there had been desquamation of viral infected cells[59]. Receptors for bacterial adhesins may be unmasked by factors produced by respiratory pathogens which interfere with the structure and integrity of the epithelium. For example, *Ps. aeruginosa* proteases[6], rhamnolipid[60] and pyocyanin[16], *Bord. pertussis* tracheal cytotoxin[46], and *Str. pneumoniae* pneumolysin[61] damage human respiratory epithelium *in vitro*, and this damage may lead to increased adhesion.

However, a number of factors need to be taken into account in studies of bacterial adherence. Most importantly, it is critical to use human tissue whenever possible. Furthermore, bacterial interactions with the bronchial mucosa may differ from those in the nasopharynx, as the epithelial cell receptors may change[52]. Finally, better protection is afforded by the mucociliary system in the lower airways compared with the nasopharynx, where large areas of unciliated epithelium may occur[3,26], and the immune system at the two sites may be different[3]. Future studies of the adherence of respiratory pathogens to epithelium should use well characterised strains, so that results can be interpreted in terms of the molecular structure of the bacterial surface, and adherence can be compared under different experimental conditions. They should also pay particular attention to the source of the tissue and the experimental conditions. *Ex vivo* studies may offer the best opportunity to study the location of bacteria in the airways[24]. The presence of cell culture medium may alter bacterial interactions with the mucosa, therefore systems with an air interface[48] are more physiological and have some advantages when studying adherence. Clinical isolates may stop expressing adhesins during passage in the laboratory, and the tissue may influence the expression of virulence factors by bacteria.

IgA PROTEASES

Secretory immunoglobulins are important humoral factors which protect against bacterial invasion of mucosal surfaces[62]. They neutralise the action of bacterial toxins and prevent bacterial adherence. Secretory IgA is believed to bind to bacterial surface antigens which mediate adherence, thus blocking bacterial attachment, and may also facilitate complement activation and bacterial killing through direct lysis or opsonophagocytosis.

Several bacterial species that colonise mucosal surfaces, including *Str. pneumoniae*, *H. influenzae* and *N. meningitidis*, produce a protease enzyme that cleaves IgA1 at a specific site in the hinge region of the α chain, releasing Fab and Fc fragments[63]. These enzymes are not produced by less virulent but closely related species such as *H. sanguis* and *H. parainfluenzae*. However, the mechanism by which cleavage of IgA1 promotes bacterial colonisation remains to be elucidated, because IgA1 forms only part of the total secretory immunoglobulins present in mucus. Nevertheless, it is possible that, by cleaving IgA1, bacteria become coated with a non-functioning antibody which blocks effective opsonisation[64]. An identical mechanism has been proposed for *Ps. aeruginosa* proteases that similarly cleave immunoglobulin, creating non-functional Fab fragments which may act as blocking antibodies[65]. Another possible mechanism is that IgA1 protease enzyme, which is expressed on the surface of the bacterium, could act as a novel adhesin for bacteria to IgA in mucus[66].

COMPLEMENT

The role of the complement cascade in the host defence against bacterial infection includes opsonisation, bacterial killing, and generation of acute inflammation. Bacteria may interfere with normal complement activity either by inactivation of complement components, or conversely by inducing a misdirected excessive inflammatory response which reduces overall complement activity.

Ps. aeruginosa proteases can inactivate complement components and cleave the C3b receptor from neutrophils[67]. Treatment of human serum with pneumolysin of *Str. pneumoniae* results in activation of the classical complement pathway, in the absence of specific antibody, with concomitant depletion of serum opsonic activity[68].

INTERACTIONS WITH PHAGOCYTES

Bacterial infections of the lower respiratory tract are characterised by rapid infiltration of the airways by activated neutrophils[5], which have been shown in animal models to be crucial for bacterial clearance[69]. The stimulus for this inflammatory response is the generation of host (e.g. C5A, leukotriene B_4 and interleukin-8) and bacterial derived chemotactic factors[70]. Although some bacterial products are proinflammatory, a fundamental requirement for bacterial persistence is to escape detection and elimination by phagocytes. Several bacterial species isolated from lung infections, including *Ps. aeruginosa*, *H. influenzae*, *Staphylococcus aureus* and *Bord. pertussis*, generate factors that affect neutrophil and macrophage function[71]. Some of these substances are cytotoxic, but others, such as pertussis toxin and adenylate cyclase from *Bord. pertussis*, interfere with cellular transduction mechanisms without affecting viability[72,73].

Peptidoglycans constitute an integral part of the cell wall of both Gram negative and Gram positive bacteria. They are structurally complex molecules that consist of long chains of *N*-acetyl muramic acid and *N*-acetyl glucosamine residues cross linked by amino acids. Peptidoglycan fragments of various sizes are released by cell wall turnover during bacterial growth, and although the majority are reincorporated, a percentage are lost into the surrounding milieu. Peptidoglycan fragments have been shown to have numerous biological functions, including activation of complement via the alternate pathway, neutrophil recruitment and generation of pulmonary inflammation in animal models, and stimulation of the release of the inflammatory cytokine interleukin-1α from blood monocytes.

The function of peptidoglycan fragments appears diverse, however, and depends, among other things, on their molecular weight. Tracheal cytotoxin is a fully characterised low molecular weight peptidoglycan fragment released by *Bord. pertussis* that, in addition to being cytotoxic to epithelial cells when present in greater concentrations also inhibits neutrophil chemotaxis *in vitro* at lower concentrations[71]. Low molecular weight peptidoglycan fragments of non-typable *H. influenzae* have also been shown to inhibit neutrophil chemotaxis *in vitro*[74]. The production of these factors *in vivo* would impair neutrophil function and might be one mechanism by which bacteria evade clearance from the airways. Thus, although infection would recruit neutrophils into the airway, their movement towards bacteria may be impaired in the microenvironment of the respiratory mucosa, and phagocytosis avoided. Furthermore, the activated neutrophils may still secrete their contents, damaging bystander lung tissue[6,7] and facilitating bacterial adherence. These interactions are outlined in Fig. 15.5.

An alternative mechanism by which bacteria may avoid clearance is by altering their external surface so they are no longer recognised by immunological surveillance[75]. The surface of non-typable *H. influenzae* has been investigated in

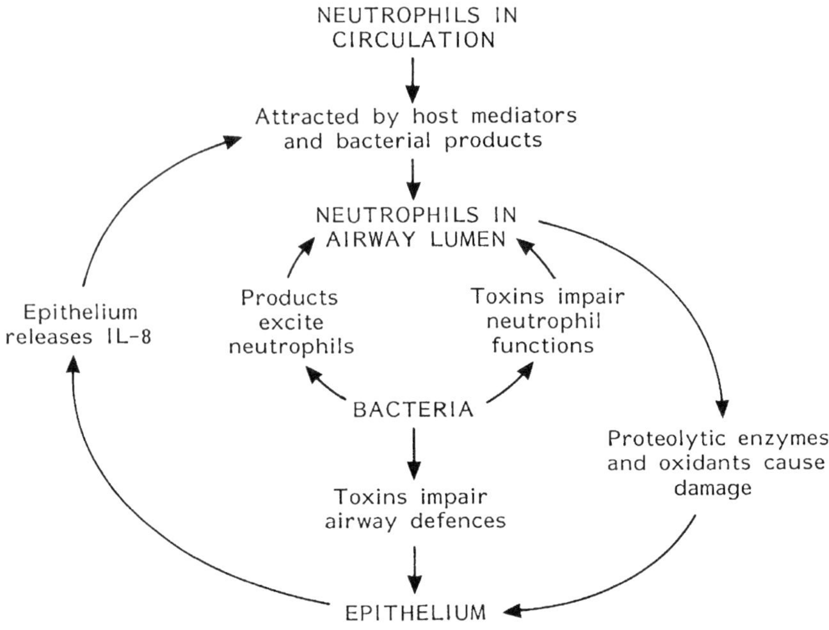

Figure 15.5. Schematic diagram of interactions between neutrophils and bacteria in the airway lumen. IL-8 = Interleukin-8

recent years and consists of outer membrane proteins, lipo-oligosaccharide and fimbriae. The outer membrane proteins have a variety of functions, including selective permeability, preventing attack by enzymes, and providing receptors for binding specific nutrients. P2 is the major protein in the outer membrane and comprises approximately 50% of the protein content of that membrane. Analysis of strains using monoclonal antibodies has indicated that the P2 of individual strains contains an immunodominant and highly strain specific epitope on the bacterial surface[76]. The lipo-oligosaccharide of *H. influenzae* contains short oligosaccharide side chains compared with those of the lipopolysaccharide of the enterobacteriaceae. This structure, also known as endotoxin, is an important virulence factor for many Gram negative bacteria, because it is a biologically active molecule and a potent mediator of inflammation. The lipo-oligosaccharide of non-typable *H. influenzae* is a major surface antigen and demonstrates extensive antigenic heterogeneity amongst strains[77].

The surface of non-typable *H. influenzae* is extremely heterogeneous and phenotypic changes in immunodominant epitopes may encourage the persistence of different strains in the lower respiratory tract of patients with chronic lung disease by allowing particular strains to evade antibody dependent host defence mechanisms[75]. In a longitudinal study involving repeated sampling of sputum from patients, major outer membrane proteins differed from those of the initial isolates, suggesting that changes in outer membrane proteins occur during persistent infection[78,79]. These changes occurred primarily in the strain specific epitope of P2 protein expressed on the bacterial surface[75]. The abundant expression of an immunodominant determinant on the bacterial surface could induce a strain specific immune response, and this might hide conserved determinants that would otherwise induce antibodies that would protect against infection[75]. The heterogeneity of P2 of non-typable *H. influenzae* may be a very important mechanism by which this bacterium evades host defences, and is due to non-synonymous single point mutations in the gene sequence of the surface exposed parts of the protein which results in antigenic drift[80].

Another mechanism by which organisms such as *H. influenzae* could evade host defences would be to evade intracellular killing. This has recently been shown to occur in adenoid tissue, where up to 200 bacteria were seen in macrophage-like cells in the subepithelial layers[81].

THE PATHOGENESIS OF BRONCHIAL INFECTIONS

Current knowledge suggests that the pathogenesis of airway infections is dependent upon the following sequence of events. Relatively non-virulent bacteria are carried in the nasopharynx as part of the commensal flora. Although the exact site of carriage is not known, it is probably in locations rich in non-ciliated epithelium. Bacteria are constantly inhaled from the nasopharynx into the lower respiratory tract yet, in health, effective host defence mechanisms, of which mucociliary clearance may be the most important first line defence, keep the bronchial tree sterile. A variety of circumstances may create permissive conditions, allowing the numbers of bacteria in the nasopharynx to increase and bacteria to spread within the respiratory tract. For example, viral infection and cigarette smoking can perturb the respiratory mucosa, delaying mucociliary clearance and enabling inhaled bacteria to multiply. Although some conditions predisposing to bronchial infections are recognised (Table 15.1), there are probably others, some inherited and some acquired, yet to be determined.

The first interaction of inhaled bacteria is with mucus, to which bacteria bind both specifically and non-specifically. Adherence to the epithelial surface may subsequently occur, which would permit a more stable colonisation that may require damage to occur first. New surface receptors for bacterial adhesion may appear, leading to susceptibility to infection. Bacterial products may influence the pathogenic process by disabling host defence mechanisms and by causing epithelial damage which may expose receptors to which the bacteria adhere. The heterogeneous outer surface of the bacterium may allow it to avoid local immune mechanisms. Bacterial species which possess these pathogenic properties will have an advantage during colonisation and multiply at the expense of other species.

The multiplication and spread of bacteria stimulates the host to mount an inflammatory response. If this fails to clear the bacteria and bacterial colonisation continues, the inflammatory response becomes persistent, and the lymphocyte population of the bronchial wall increases; this, together with the epithelium, may produce cytokines which maintain and amplify the inflammatory response[82,83]. Large numbers of polymorphonuclear leucocytes migrate into the bronchial tree, and secretion of proteolytic enzymes and toxic oxygen radicals may cause further mucus production and damage to the epithelium. An environment is generated that is conductive to the persistence and contiguous spread of the bacteria.

The bacteria causing bronchial infections have an armamentarium of pathogenic mechanisms, outlined in this chapter, which enables them to persist within the airways. In general, these bacteria are relatively non-virulent, as they do not invade the bloodstream and do not cause acute life-threatening illness. They can be thought of as efficient parasites that are able to exploit permissive conditions in the lower respiratory tract. The insidious damage that occurs to the airways is mainly mediated by the host chronic inflammatory response. It seems unlikely that a single pathogenic mechanism can explain why a small number of species are isolated from bronchial infections, and it is more likely that it is the combination of these different mechanisms that provides the identikit of the successful bacterium. Two examples are worth considering in more detail.

H. influenzae type b is carried much less frequently in the nasopharynx of healthy people than are unencapsulated non-typable strains, and causes a very different spectrum of disease, predominantly in children who have not yet developed protective antibodies to the type b capsule (Fig. 15.6). Capsulate *H. influenzae* rarely cause infections of the bronchial tree. When pairs of type b capsulate and non-capsulate strains of *H. influenzae*, which were otherwise identical, were studied in an organ culture of human respiratory mucosa, the results were very different[84]: non-capsulate organisms caused significant epithelial damage, whereas capsulate strains did not. Non-capsulate bacteria adhered to areas of damaged epithelium but, in contrast, capsulate organisms were

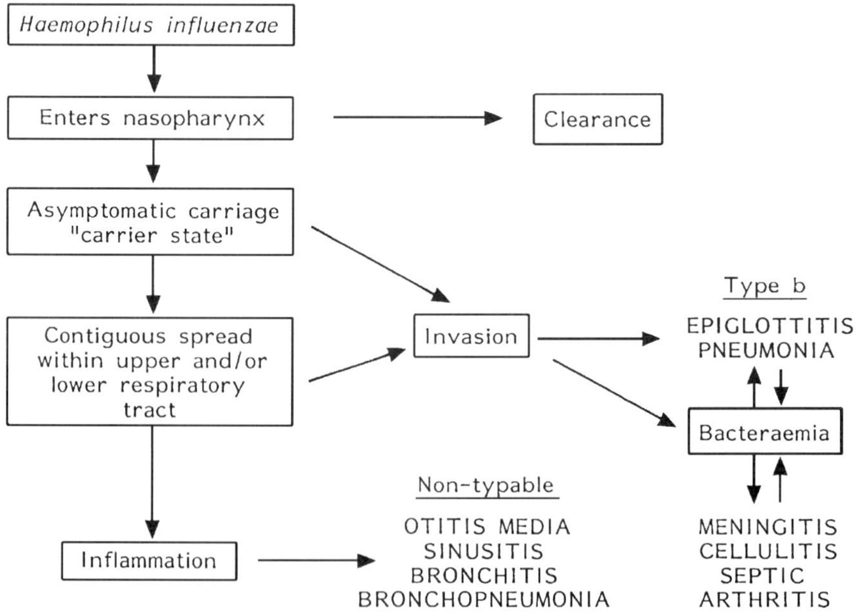

Figure 15.6. Schematic diagram of the pathogenesis of unencapsulated non-typable *Haemophilus influenzae* and *H. influenzae* type b

associated with a thick gel-like matrix above the normal epithelial surface. These observations strongly suggest that the polyribosyl-ribitol phosphate capsule of *H. influenzae* type b makes the organism less efficient at colonising the nasopharynx and prevents dissemination in the bronchial tree. We have observed that culture filtrates from isogenic capsulate and non-capsulate strains have similar effects on respiratory epithelium, so it is likely that the hydrophilic capsule prevents adherence to the mucosa, which in turn alters the pathogenesis of the two types of *H. influenzae*. The capsule, however, protects the bacterium from phagocytosis once it enters the blood stream, leading to more severe disease in young children who lack protective antibody.

Ps. aeruginosa frequently infects the bronchial tree of patients with cystic fibrosis and other forms of bronchiectasis, or patients with the trachea intubated who are receiving assisted ventilation. Once colonisation is established, the bacterium is rarely eliminated, despite antibiotic treatment, and chronic infection leads to a more rapid decline in the patient's condition. Antibiotic resistance of *Ps. aeruginosa* contributes to the difficulty in eradicating the bacterium but, in addition, the bacterium has a large number of pathogenic mechanisms that contribute to its persistence[1,2,16]. However, despite possessing these mechanisms, *Ps. aeruginosa* is almost never isolated from the healthy bronchial tree and only rarely in chronic bronchitis. While there may be a particular association of *Ps. aeruginosa* infection with cystic fibrosis, these observations suggest that the impairment of the bronchial defences has to be severe before *Ps. aeruginosa* is able to colonise. The reason for this is unclear, but two observations may be relevant. First, the presence of *Ps. aeruginosa* in cystic fibrosis sputum is unusual in the presence of *Staph. aureus*[85]. This suggests that *Ps. aeruginosa* is unable to compete with *Staph. aureus* for the ecological niche, and it has been observed that regular use of antistaphylococcal antibiotics in cystic fibrosis leads to earlier colonisation by *Ps. aeruginosa*[86]. Therefore, use of potent broad spectrum antibiotics may eradicate other species and predispose to *Ps. aeruginosa* infection. Second, numerous studies in different systems have noted the complete inability of *Ps. aeruginosa* to adhere to normal epithelium[24,48], but highlighted its affinity for mucus and damaged epithelium. This may predispose to infection in bronchiectasis and cystic fibrosis, when mucociliary clearance is severely impaired and the epithelium may already be damaged.

ACKNOWLEDGEMENTS

The authors would like to thank Mr Andrew Rutman, who provided the electron micrographs, and Miss Jane Burditt for preparation of the manuscript.

REFERENCES

1. Wilson R, Cole P. Respiratory tract infections. In: Barnes P J, ed. *Royal Brompton Review Series Volume 2: Respiratory Medicine —Recent Advances*, chapter 6. London: Butterworths, 1993; 95–122.

2. Fick R B. Pathogenesis of the pseudomonas lung lesion in cystic fibrosis. *Chest* 1989; **96:** 158–164.

3. Wilson R, Moxon E R. Molecular basis of *Haemophilus influenzae* pathogenicity in the respiratory tract. In: Griffiths E, Donachie W, Stephen J, eds. *Bacterial Infections of Respiratory and Gastrointestinal Mucosa.* Reading: Society for General Microbiology, 1988; 29–40.

4. Musser J M, Granoff D M, Pattison P E, *et al.* A population genetic framework for the study of invasive diseases caused by serotype b strains of *Haemophilus influenzae. Proc Natl Acad Sci USA* 1985; **82:** 5078–5082.

5. Currie D C, Peters A M, Garbett N D, *et al.* Indium-III labelled granulocyte scanning to detect inflammation in the lungs of patients with chronic sputum expectoration. *Thorax* 1990; **45:** 541–544.

6. Amitani R, Wilson R, Read R, *et al.* Effects of human neutrophil elastase and bacterial proteinase enzymes on human respiratory epithelium. *Am J Respir Cell Mol Biol* 1991; **4:** 26–32.

7. Feldman C, Anderson R, Kanthakumar K, *et al.* Oxidant-mediated ciliary dysfunction in human respiratory epithelium. *Free Radic Biol Med* 1994; **17:**1–10.

8. Sleigh M A, Blake J R, Liron N. The propulsion of mucus by cilia. *Am Rev Respir Dis* 1988; **137:** 726–741.

9. Wilson R. Secondary ciliary dysfunction. *Clin Sci* 1988; **75:** 113–120.

10. Cole P J. Host–microbe relationships in chronic respiratory disease. In: Reeves D, Geddes A M, eds. *Recent Advances in Infection.* Edinburgh: Churchill Livingstone, 1989; 141–151.

11. Seybold Z V, Mariassy A T, Stroh D, *et al.* Mucociliary interaction *in vitro:* effects of physiological and inflammatory stimuli. *J Appl Physiol* 1990; **68:** 1421–1426.

12. Pavia D, Bateman J R M, Sheaham N F, *et al.* Tracheobronchial mucociliary clearance in asthma: impairment during remission. *Thorax* 1985; **40:** 171–175.

13. Greenstone M, Rutman A, Dewar A, *et al.* Primary ciliary dyskinesia: cytological and clinical features. *Q J Med* 1988; **67:** 405–430.

14. Wilson R, Alton E, Rutman A, *et al.* Upper respiratory tract viral infection and mucociliary clearance. *Eur J Respir Dis* 1987; **70:** 272–279.

15. Rayner C F J, Rutman A, Dewar A, *et al.* Ciliary disorientation in patients with chronic upper respiratory tract infection. *Am J Respir Crit Care Med* 1995; **151:** 800–804.

16. Wilson R, Pitt T, Taylor G, *et al.* Pyocyanin and 1-hydroxyphenazine produced by *Pseudomonas aeruginosa* inhibit human ciliary beating *in vitro. J Clin Invest* 1987; **79:** 221–229.

17. Wilson R, Sykes D A, Watson D, *et al.* Measurement of *Pseudomonas aeruginosa* phenazine pigments in sputum and assessment of their contribution to sputum sol toxicity for respiratory epithelium. *Infect Immun* 1988; **56:** 2515–2517.

18. Munro N, Barker A, Rutman A, *et al.* The effect of pyocyanin and 1-hydroxyphenazine on *in vivo* tracheal mucus velocity. *J Appl Physiol* 1989; **76:** 316–323.

19. Kanthakumar K, Taylor G, Tsang K W T, *et al.* Mechanism of action of *Pseudomonas aeruginosa* pyocyanin on human ciliary beat *in vitro. Infect Immun* 1993; **61:** 2848–2853.

20. Lansley A B, Sanderson M J, Dirksen E R. Control of the beat cycle of respiratory tract cilia by Ca++ and cAMP. *Am J Physiol* 1992; **263:** L232–L242.

21. Armstrong A V, Stewart-Tull D E S, Roberts J S. Characterisation of the *Pseudomonas aeruginosa* factor that inhibits mouse liver mitochondrial respiration. *J Med Microbiol* 1971; **4:** 249–262.

22. Ras G J, Anderson R, Taylor G W, *et al.* Proinflammatory interactions of pyocyanin and 1-hydroxyphenazine with human neutrophil *in vitro. J Infect Dis* 1990; **162:** 178–185.

23. Ras G J, Theron A J, Anderson R, *et al.* Enhanced release of elastase oxidative inactivation of alpha-1-protease inhibitor by stimulated human neutrophils to the *Pseudomonas aeruginosa* pigment 1-hydroxyphenazine. *J Infect Dis* 1992; **166:** 568–573.

24. Baltimore R S, Christie C D C, Walker-Smith G J. Immunohistopathologic localisation of *Pseudomonas aeruginosa* in lungs from patients with cystic fibrosis. *Am Rev Respir Dis* 1989; **140:** 1650–1661.

25. Carnoy C, Ramphal R, Scharjman A, *et al.* Altered carbohydrate composition of salivary mucins from patients with cystic fibrosis and the adhesion of *Pseudomonas aeruginosa. Am J Respir Cell Mol Biol* 1993; **9:** 323–334.

26. Read R C, Wilson R, Rutman A, *et al.* Interaction of non typable *Haemophilus influenzae* with human respiratory mucosa *in vitro. J Infect Dis* 1991; **163:** 549–558.

27. Plotkowski M C, Bajolek-Laudinat O, Puchelle E. Cellular and molecular mechanisms of bacterial adhesion to respiratory mucosa. *Eur Respir J* 1993; **6:** 903–916.

28. Sampson D A, Ramphal R, Lory S. Genetic analysis of *Pseudomonas aeruginosa* adherence: distinct genetic loci control attachment to epithelial cells and mucins. *Infect Immun* 1992; **60:** 3771–3779.

29. Adler K B, Hendley D D, Davis G S. Bacteria associated with obstructive pulmonary disease elaborate extracellular products that stimulate mucus secretion by explants of guinea pig airways. *Am J Pathol* 1986; **125:** 501–514.

30. Somerville M, Taylor G W, Watson D, *et al.* Release of mucus glycoconjugates by *Pseudomonas aeruginosa* rhamnolipids into feline trachea *in vivo* and human bronchus *in vitro. Am J Respir Cell Mol Biol* 1992; **6:** 116–122.

31. Vishwanath S, Ramphal R. Adherence of *Pseudomonas aeruginosa* to human tracheobronchial mucin. *Infect Immun* 1984; **45:** 197–202.

32. Nadel J A. Role of mast cell and neutrophil proteases in airway secretion. *Am Rev Respir Dis* 1991; **144:** S48–S51.

33. Wanner A. Clinical aspects of mucociliary transport. *Am Rev Respir Dis* 1977; **116:** 73–125.

34. Lethem M I, James S L, Marriott C, *et al.* The origin of DNA associated with mucus glycoproteins in cystic fibrosis sputum. *Eur Respir J* 1990; **3:** 19–23.

35. Welsh M J, Fick R B. Cystic fibrosis. *J Clin Invest* 1987; **80:** 1523–1526.

36. Boucher R C. Human airway ion transport. *Am J Respir Crit Care Med* 1994; **150:** 581–593.

37. Stutts M J, Schwab J H, Chen M G, *et al.* Effects of *Pseudomonas aeruginosa* on bronchial epithelial ion transport. *Am Rev Respir Dis* 1986; **134:** 17–21.

38. Graham A, Steel D, Wilson R, *et al.* Effects of purified pseudomonas rhamnolipids on ion transport across sheep tracheal epithelium. *Exp Lung Res* 1993; **19:** 77–89.

39. Kownatzki R, Tummler B, Doring G. Rhamnolipid of *Pseudomonas aeruginosa* in sputum of cystic fibrosis patients. *Lancet* 1987; **2:** 1026–1027.

40. Beachey E H. Bacterial adherence: adhesin–receptor interactions mediating the attachment of bacteria to mucosa surfaces. *J Infect Dis* 1981; **143:** 325–345.

41. Niederman M S. Bacterial adherence as a mechanism of airway colonisation. *Eur J Clin Microbiol Infect Dis* 1989; **8:** 15–20.

42. Middlethrope J M, Witholt B. K-88 mediated binding of *Escherichia coli* outer membrane fragments to porcine intestinal epithelial cell brush borders. *Infect Immun* 1981; **31:** 42–51.

43. Sharon N, Eshdat Y, Silverblatt F J, *et al.* Bacterial adherence to cell surface sugars. In: Elliot K, O'Connor M, Wheelan L, eds. *Microbial Adhesion and Pathogenicity. Ciba Foundations Symposium.* London: Pitman Press, 1986; 119–141.

44. Tuomanen E, Hendley J O. Adherence of *Bordetella pertussis* to human respiratory epithelial cells. *J Infect Dis* 1983; **148:** 125–130.

45. Almagor M, Kahane I, Wiesel J M, *et al.* Human ciliated epithelial cells from nasal polyps as an experimental model of *Mycoplasma pneumoniae* infection. *Infect Immun* 1985; **48:** 552–555.

46. Wilson R, Read R, Thomas M, *et al.* Effects of *Bordetella pertussis* infection on human respiratory epithelium *in vivo* and *in vitro. Infect Immun* 1991; **59:** 337–345.

47. Tuomanen E. Piracy of adhesins: attachments of superinfecting pathogens to respiratory cilia by secreted adhesins of *Bordetella pertussis. Infect Immun* 1986; **54:** 905–908.

48. Tsang K W T, Rutman A, Kanthakumar K, *et al.* Interaction of *Pseudomonas aeruginosa* with human respiratory mucosa *in vitro. Eur Respir J* 1994; **7:** 1746–1753.

49. Rayner C F J, Jackson A D, Rutman A, *et al.* The interaction of pneumolysin sufficient and deficient isogenic variants of *Streptococcus pneumoniae* with human respiratory mucosa. *Infect Immun* 1995; **63:** 442–447.

50. Sable N S, Connor E M, Hall C B, *et al.* Variable adherence of fimbriated *Haemophilus influenzae* type b to human cells. *Infect Immun* 1985; **48:** 119–123.

51. Bakeletz L O, Tallan B M, Hoepf T, *et al*. Frequency of fimbriation of non-typable *Haemophilus influenzae* and its ability to adhere to chinchilla and human respiratory epithelium. *Infect Immun* 1988; **56:** 331–335.

52. Christensen T G, Breuer R, Lucey E C, *et al*. Lectin cytochemistry reveals differences between hamster trachea and bronchus in the composition of epithelial surface glycoconjugates and in the response of secretory cells to neutrophil elastase. *Am J Respir Cell Mol Biol* 1990; **3:** 61–69.

53. Niederman M S, Rafferty T, Saskaki C, *et al*. Comparison of bacterial adherence to ciliated and squamous cells obtained from the human respiratory tract. *Am Rev Respir Dis* 1983; **127:** 85–90.

54. Saiman L, Ishimoto K, Lory S, *et al*. The effect of pilation and exoproduct expression on the adherence of *Pseudomonas aeruginosa* to respiratory epithelial monolayers. *J Infect Dis* 1990; **161:** 541–548.

55. Nicas T I, Iglewski B H. The contribution of exproducts to virulence of *Pseudomonas aeruginosa*. *Can J Microbiol* 1986; **24:** 260–264.

56. Woods D E. Role of fibronectin in the pathogenesis of Gram-negative bacillary pneumonia. *Rev Infect Dis* 1987; **9** (suppl 4): S317–S321.

57. Taylor D C, Clancy R L, Cripps A W, *et al*. An alteration in the host-parasite relationship in subjects with chronic bronchitis prone to recurrent episodes of acute bronchitis. *Immunol Cell Biol* 1994; **72:** 143–151.

58. Stefano A D, Maestrelli P, Roggeri A, *et al*. Upregulation of adhesion molecules in the bronchial mucosa of subjects with chronic obstructive bronchitis. *Am J Crit Care Med* 1994; **149:** 803–810.

59. Plotkowski M C, Puchelle E, Beck G, *et al*. Adherence of type I *Streptococcus pneumoniae* to tracheal epithelium of mice infected with influenza A/PR8 virus. *Am Rev Respir Dis* 1986; **134:** 1040–1044.

60. Read R C, Roberts P, Munro N, *et al*. Effect of *Pseudomonas aeruginosa* rhamnolipids on mucociliary transport and ciliary beating. *J Appl Physiol* 1992; **72:** 2271–2277.

61. Steinfort C, Wilson R, Mitchell T, *et al*. The effect of *Streptococcus pneumoniae* on human respiratory epithelium *in vitro*. *Infect Immun* 1989; **57:** 2006–2013.

62. Brantzaeg P. Humoral immune response patterns of human mucosae. Induction and relation to bacterial respiratory tract infections. *J Infect Dis* 1992; **165** (suppl 1): S167–S176.

63. Plaut A G. The IgA proteases of pathogenic bacteria. *Am Rev Microbiol* 1983; **37:** 603–622.

64. Paton J C, Andrew P W, Boulnois G J, *et al*. Molecular analysis of the pathogenicity of *Streptococcus pneumoniae*: the role of pneumococcal proteins. *Annu Rev Microbiol* 1993; **47:** 89–115.

65. Fick R B, Baltimore R S, Squier S U, *et al*. IgG proteolytic activity of *Pseudomonas aeruginosa* in cystic fibrosis. *J Infect Dis* 1985; **151:** 589–598.

66. Moxon E R, Wilson R. The role of *Haemophilus influenzae* in the pathogenesis of pneumonia. *Rev Infect Dis* 1991; **13:**(suppl 6): S518–S527.

67. Berger M, Sorensen R U, Tosi M F, *et al*. Complement receptor expression on neutrophils at an inflammatory site, the pseudomonas-infected lung in cystic fibrosis. *J Clin Invest* 1989; **84:** 1302–1313.

68. Paton J C, Rowan-Kelly B, Ferrante A Activation of human complement by the pneumococcal toxin pneumolysin. *Infect Immun* 1984; **43:** 1085–1087.

69. Toews G B, Vial W C, Hansen E J. Role of C5 and recruited neutrophils in early clearance of non-typable *Haemophilus influenzae* from murine lungs. *Infect Immun* 1985; **50:**207–212.

70. Ras G, Wilson R, Todd H, *et al*. The effect of bacterial products on neutrophil migration *in vitro*. *Thorax* 1990; **45:** 276–280.

71. Cundell D R, Kanthakumar K, Taylor G W, *et al*. The effect of tracheal cytotoxin from *Bordetella pertussis* on human neutrophil function *in vitro*. *Infect Immun* 1994; **62:** 639–643.

72. Becker E L, Kermode J C, Naccache P H, *et al*. The inhibition of neutrophil granule enzyme secretion and chemotaxis by pertussis toxin. *J Cell Biol* 1985; **100:** 1641–1646.

73. Confer D L, Eaton J W. Phagocyte–host jujitsu; phagocyte impotence caused by internalised bacterial adenylate cyclase. *Trans Assoc Am Physicians* 1983; **45:** 1–7.

74. Cundell D R, Taylor G W, Tabaqchali S, *et al*. Inhibition of *in vitro* human neutrophil migration by low molecular weight products of non-typable *Haemophilus influenzae*. *Infect Immun* 1993; **61:** 2419–2424.

75. Murphy T F, Sethi S. Bacterial infection in chronic obstructive pulmonary disease. *Am Rev Respir Dis* 1992; **146:** 1067–1083.

76. Haase E M, Campagnari A A, Sarwar J, *et al*. Strain specific and immunodominant surface epitopes of the P2 porin protein of non-typable *Haemophilus influenzae*. *Infect Immun* 1991; **59:** 1278–1284.

77. Campagnari A A, Gupta M R, Dudas K C, *et al*. Antigenic diversity of lipooligosaccharides of non-typable *Haemophilus influenzae*. *Infect Immun* 1987; **55:** 882–887.

78. Groeneveld K, van Alphen L, Eijk P P, *et al*. Changes in outer membrane proteins of non-typable *Haemophilus influenzae* in patients with chronic obstructive pulmonary disease. *J Infect Dis* 1988; **158:** 360–365.

79. van Alphen L, Eijk P, Geelen-van den Broek L, *et al*. Immunochemical characterisation of variable epitopes of outer membrane protein P2 of non-typable *Haemophilus influenzae*. *Infect Immun* 1991; **59:** 247–252.

80. Dulm B, van Alphen L, Eijk P, *et al*. Antigenic drift of non-encapsulated *Haemophilus influenzae* major outer membrane protein P2 in patients with chronic bronchitis is caused by point mutations. *Mol Microbiol* 1994; **11:** 1181–1189.

81. Forsgren J, Samuelson A, Ahlin A, *et al*. *Haemophilus influenzae* resides and multiplies intracellularly in human adenoid tissue as demonstrated by *in situ* hybridisation and bacteria viability assay. *Infect Immun* 1994; **62:** 673–679.

82. Lapa e Silva J R, Jones J A H, Cole P J, *et al*. The immunological component of the cellular inflammatory infiltrate in bronchiectasis. *Thorax* 1989; **44:** 668–673.

83. Bedard M, McClure C D, Schiller N I, *et al*. Release of interleukin-8, interleukin-6, and colony-stimulating factors by upper airway epithelial cells: implications for cystic fibrosis. *Am J Respir Cell Mol Biol* 1993; **9:** 455–462.

84. Read R C, Rutman A, Jeffery P K, *et al*. Interaction of capsulate *Haemophilus influenzae* with human airway mucosa *in vitro*. *Infect Immun* 1992; **60:** 3244–3252.

85. Machan Z A, Taylor G W, Pitt T L, *et al*. 2-Heptyl-4-hydroxyquinoline *N*-oxide, an antistaphylococcal agent produced by *Pseudomonas aeruginosa*. *J Antimicrob Chemother* 1992; **30:** 615–623.

86. Loening-Baucke V A, Mischler E, Myers M G. A placebo controlled trial of cephalexin therapy in the ambulatory management of patients with cystic fibrosis. *J Pediatr* 1979; **95:** 630–637.

16

Viral Infections

R. L. SMYTH

Royal Liverpool Children's Hospital, Liverpool, UK

L. K. BORYSIEWICZ

University of Wales College of Medicine, Cardiff, UK

INTRODUCTION

The large surface area presented by the pulmonary epithelium makes it an important site of entry for respiratory pathogens, including viruses. Through this portal of entry a variety of viral infections can be established; infection can be asymptomatic, result in clinical injury which could be local or systemic, or the virus infection may become locally or systemically persistent. Viral respiratory infections are common (Table 16.1), but in each instance the virus has evolved specific measures to counteract and adapt to this route of entry.

LOCAL BARRIERS TO VIRUS INFECTION OF THE RESPIRATORY TRACT

Respiratory viruses are spread by aerosolised droplets. Therefore, even before viruses encounter the respiratory epithelium, the requirement for droplet spread between infected individuals places a considerable constraint on virion particles to resist desiccation. Coughing and sneezing produce droplets of different sizes which can penetrate all levels of the respiratory tract: those less than 5 mm can gain access to the lower airways and alveoli, and slightly larger particles can deposit elsewhere in the respiratory tract,[1,2]. Small droplets remain suspended for long periods and can be spread over considerable distances by air currents. The stability of these particles is affected by the ambient temperature and humidity[3]. Within the droplet, the structure of the virus particle itself will influence the ability of a virus to gain access to the respiratory tract: enveloped viruses can resist desiccation better than non-enveloped viruses[4]. This has been suggested

Pulmonary Defences. Edited by Robert A. Stockley.
© 1997 John Wiley & Sons Ltd.

Table 16.1. Respiratory virus infection

Virus	Nucleic acid	Envelope	Proposed cell receptor	Disease association
Upper respiratory tract				
Rhinovirus	RNA	Non-enveloped	ICAM-1	35% of URTI
Coronavirus	RNA		? Aminopeptidase N or sialic acid	>10%of URTI
Parainfluenza virus	RNA	Enveloped	Sialic acid on glycoproteins or gangliosides	Laryngotracheal bronchitis (croup) and URTI
RSV	RNA	Enveloped	?	<10% URTI
Large airways				
Influenza	RNA	Enveloped	Sialic acid	Influenza and acute bronchitis
Adenovirus	DNA	Non-enveloped	Integrin $\alpha_v\beta_3$ and $\alpha_v\beta_5$ (type 2)	Acute bronchitis and URTI
RSV	RNA	Enveloped	?	Acute bron- chiolitis/ bronchitis
Viral pneumonia				
Children				
RSV	RNA	Enveloped	?	Common
Parainfluenza 1, 2, 3	RNA	Enveloped	Sialic acid glycoproteins or gangliosides	Common
Adenovirus 1, 2, 3, 5	DNA	Non-enveloped	Integrin $\alpha_v\beta_3$ and $\alpha_v\beta_5$ (type 2)	Uncommon
Influenza B	RNA	Enveloped	Sialic acid	Uncommon
Rhinovirus	RNA	Non-enveloped	ICAM-1	Uncommon
Adults				
Influenza A	RNA	Enveloped	Sialic acid	Common
Influenza B	RNA	Enveloped	Sialic acid	Common
Adenovirus 4, 7	DNA	Non-enveloped	?	Common
Adenovirus 1, 2, 3, 5	DNA	Non-enveloped	Integrin $\alpha_v\beta_3$ and $\alpha_v\beta_5$ (type 2)	Uncommon
RSV	RNA	Enveloped	?	Uncommon
Herpesviruses: VZV, CMV, HSV etc	DNA	Enveloped	? Heparan sulphate, CD21 (EBV)	

RNA, DNA = ribo-and deoxyribonucleic acids; ICAM-1 = intercellular adhesion molecule-1; URTI = upper respiratory tract infection; RSV = respiratory syncytial virus; VZV = Varicella zoster virus; CMV = cyto-megalovirus; HSV = Herpes simplex virus, EBV = Epstein–Barr virus.

as an explanation for the predominance of enveloped viruses causing disease in the lower respiratory tract, compared with upper respiratory tract infections[5] (Table 16.1).

The respiratory tract then presents important physical barriers. The first is the mucociliary carpet that, constantly propelled to the oro-pharynx by ciliary action, removes foreign particulate material. If this barrier is impaired, for example by drugs[6], then the individual is more susceptible to virus infection. Intrinsic defects enhance the susceptibility of mice to pulmonary infection with Sendai virus, which is linked to a genetic polymorphism associated with impaired mucociliary function[7].

In this barrier there are a number of secreted products, the most specific in relation to virus infection being virus specific secreted immunoglobulin A (IgA). IgA is the dominant antibody in the nasopharynx and major bronchi, but is replaced by a transudate of IgG and IgM lower in the respiratory tract. The importance of secreted IgA is largely inferred by extrapolation from the protection afforded by IgA against poliovirus in the gastrointestinal tract. In fact, most patients with selective IgA deficiency have no increased susceptibility to respiratory virus infection[8]. One explanation for this may be a substitution of secreted IgM for IgA that is found in patients with selective IgA deficiency. However, a subpopulation of IgA deficient patients has been identified who appear to have an increased susceptibility to respiratory and gastrointestinal infection[9] and, interestingly, some of these patients do not secrete IgM[10].

The nasopharyngeal entry site is maintained at a lower temperature than that required for replication of most viruses (34°C compared with 37°C). Rhinoviruses have adapted to use this lower temperature as the optimum for their replication, which may help them to occupy this environmental niche. The respiratory tract has local collections of lymphoid tissue, in the larger airways, which may be important in inducing local immunity to respiratory pathogens, particularly as they contain a high frequency of IgA specific B cells. In addition, the epithelium of the larger airways is heavily infiltrated with lymphocytes, including γδ T cells. Further down the respiratory tract, there are specialised reticuloendothelial cells such as alveolar macrophages. These cells dominate in alveolar fluid (80–90%), with T cells making up the next most prevalent population[11]. These mechanisms function to ensure that alveolar fluid in the normal lung is largely free of bacteria, but it is probable that these mechanisms eliminate many respiratory viral pathogens.

VIRUS INFECTION OF RESPIRATORY EPITHELIAL CELLS

Having bypassed the mucociliary barrier, a virus must infect an epithelial cell to establish the focus of infection. Virus tropism is determined in part by the binding of viral proteins to host cell receptor proteins to allow virus entry to the cell; these cellular receptors have been identified for some respiratory viruses (Table 16.1). Viruses infecting epithelial cells also have to overcome host cell polarisation; epithelial cells have an apical and a basolateral aspect. Most respiratory viruses are directed to the apical surface (e.g. influenza[12,13]). This predilection for one side of a polarised epithelial cell may be inherent in the structure of the viral envelope glycoproteins; even a single amino acid change in the case of influenza haemagglutinin may affect its selective polarity during subsequent infection[14,15]. Furthermore, virus particles infecting an apical surface will insert glycoproteins during membrane fusion and these later serve to direct newly formed particles to bud from that surface[16]. A change in the polarity of virus release may have considerable impact on the pathogenesis of infection. Sendai virus, which normally binds to the apical surface of bronchial epithelial cells, can have its host cell range extended and virulence enhanced by a change to its polarity of infection[17].

Viruses in the respiratory tract also utilise host factors to allow efficient infection of the respiratory epithelium. Influenza virus haemagglutinin uses sialic acid residues as its cell surface receptor, but then requires a proteolytic cleavage of the haemagglutinin, to expose a domain to allow virus–cell membrane fusion. This cleavage is mediated by furin, a proteinase located in the trans-Golgi, if an amino acid motif of Arg–X–Lys or Arg–Arg is present in the haemagglutinin molecule. Most human influenza strains contain only a single Arg residue at this site and are probably cleaved by a Factor Xa-like proteinase; it is possible that influenza strains which possess furin sensitive cleavage sites may be more virulent[18]. Proteinase inhibitors can block this cleavage and prevent virus infection[19,20]. Once the haemagglutinin HA2 domain is exposed by proteolytic cleavage, it is stabilised by the low pH present in the endosomal compartment[21]. The stable, exposed hydrophobic domain then allows membrane fusion to occur and the virus genome is released into the cytoplasm. Haemagglutinin is not the only surface envelope protein which has virulence determinants. The degree of glycosylation of the neuraminidase glycoprotein also influences the virulence of influenza[22]. Local virulence factors may therefore operate at all levels of virus infection of the epithelial cell, and these are often a consequence of the interplay between viral proteins and host cell determinants.

However, there are other host cell factors which can affect the process of entry, uncoating, and initial viral transcription. Enhancer regions in the virus genome interact with host cell transcription and translation factors to allow full replication only in certain cells, and often only at certain stages of cellular differentiation. Human cytomegalovirus (HCMV) is a herpesvirus that has a temporally regulated cascade of virus gene expression, and is critically dependent on viral transactivators to initiate the lytic cycle of virus replication. It has been found that HCMV can enter embryonic human cell lines, but will fail to express the immediate early gene products that are the important transactivators for further viral gene expression. However, if the cell is induced to differentiation by retinoic acid, this repression is removed and a full virus replicative cycle ensues. This *in vitro* observation has an *in vivo* counterpart; HCMV is found in human monocytes[23], but it does not produce a full lytic cycle of infection in such cells. Monocytes are infected at the stage of precursor cells in the bone marrow[24]. If monocytes from asymptomatic, persistently infected subjects are allowed to mature *in vitro* by prolonged culture or *in vivo* when monocytes mature to tissue specific macrophages (e.g. alveolar macrophages), virus release is observed. This last observation is of particular importance in the context of HCMV pneumonia (see below).

It is commonly held that virus infection inevitably progresses to destruction of the infected cell. Although this is certainly the case for many of the common acute respiratory pathogens—viral infection inhibits cell division and host cell macromolecular synthesis, redirecting the host cell machinery to virus encoded protein synthesis—some infections can be non-cytopathic, allowing an equilibrium to be established between the virus and the host. This often results in a persistence of the virus infection[25] in the respiratory tract (e.g. adenovirus), allowing the virus to be shed for prolonged periods, whilst producing minimal damage to the host.

IMMUNE RESPONSES AGAINST VIRUS INFECTION

If the initial physical barrier of the respiratory tract is penetrated by a virus, the immune system is activated to clear the focus of infection. Initial non-specific mechanisms may provide an element of local control of virus infection before an antigen specific response can be generated. Cytokines such as interferons (type 1 alfa/beta (IFNα, IFNβ) are important in the control of virus infection; inhibition of interferon action with antibody[26] or by targeted disruption of the IFNα/β receptor[27], enhances susceptibility to experimental virus infection. Coupled with early cytokine release is the activity of natural killer (NK) cells that recognise virus infected cells, although this is not through the recognition of virus encoded proteins[28,29]. The effectiveness of this non-specific immune response is well characterised in murine cytomegalovirus (CMV) infection[30]. In man, NK deficiency is associated with an increased susceptibility to herpesvirus infections[31], but no excess of respiratory viral infections has been observed.

Viral antigens are complex and exhibit several important differences compared with simple model antigens. First, viruses multiply in the host, hence the antigen load not only has a compartmental distribution, but also provides a variable qualitative and quantitative antigen load. Second, viruses have an interactive relationship with the immune response, in that the immune response can exert a selective pressure on the virus, yet the virus can also interfere with the immune response. Third, some viral antigens can be important for elimination from the host (e.g. neutralising determinants), whilst others behave as model antigens and responses directed against most viral proteins may not influence clearance of infection[32].

ANTIVIRAL ANTIBODIES

The antibody response to viruses is T cell dependent. Most classes of antibody are produced, with their characteristic functional differences. Most attention has focused on the neutralising antibodies. These are the primary protective mechanism against picornavirus infection, in which the epitopes have been mapped to specific regions of rhinoviruses[33], and in the antihaemagglutinin response against influenza[34]. From these studies, it is clear that the neutralising response is conformationally dependent; indeed, neutralisation can be disrupted by a single amino acid change in the epitope, resulting in virus escape[34].

T CELL RESPONSES — ANTIGEN PRESENTATION

T cell responses require proteolytic processing of antigen and the presentation of linear peptides in the context of major histocompatibility complex (MHC) class I and II molecules on the surface of the infected cell[35,36] (Fig. 16.1). These two pathways have probably evolved to ensure that intracellular (MHC class

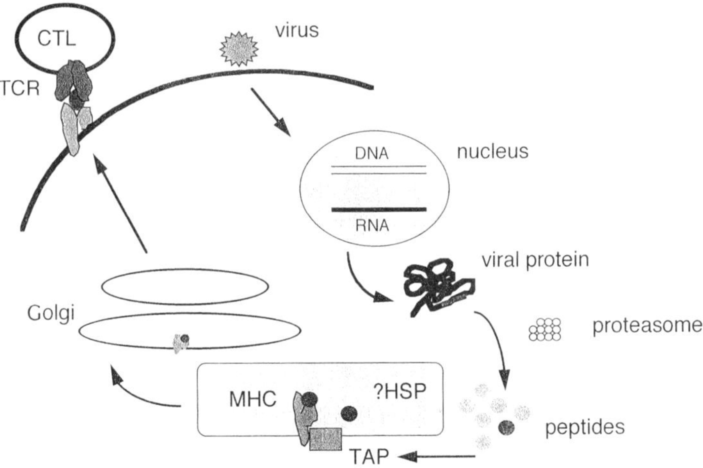

Figure 16.1. Major histocompatibility complex (MHC) class I antigen presentation to CD8+ cytotoxic T cells. CTL = Cytotoxic T lymphocyte; TCR = T cell receptor; HSP = heat shock protein; TAP = transporter associated with antigen presentation

I and II) and extracellular (MHC class II) antigens are efficiently presented in order to generate appropriate immune responses. However, by the nature of virus infection, some crossover between the two pathways has been identified[37]. The detailed aspects of presentation through these pathways is considered elsewhere (see Chapter 11), but viruses, as complex replicating antigens, can inhibit these mechanisms (Fig. 16.2) (see below).

CD4 Mediated Responses

Classical immunity mediated by cluster of differentiation (CD)4 T cells results in the release of cytokines after activation of the lymphocyte. CD4 cells are grouped into two major functional types: Th1 cells and Th2 cells. Th1 cells secrete interleukin (IL)-2, IFNγ and lymphotoxin, which promote cytotoxic T cell and delayed type hypersensitivity and are of particular importance in the clearance of intracellular organisms. Th2 cells secrete IL-4, IL-5, IL-6, IL-10 and IL-13, and enhance allergic and B cell responses. A third intermediate type, Th0, has been identified. At present, the role of these functional subsets in virus infection remains to be defined, but a dominance of one type of response has been observed in bronchial lavage material in viral infections such as respiratory syncytial virus (RSV) infection.

Clearly, CD4 T cells have a pivotal role in regulating appropriate antiviral responses. In this context, it is interesting that viruses may subvert this role by secreting cytokine or receptor homologues that may divert the immune response in such a way to favour persistence: Epstein-Barr virus (EBV) and IL-10[38], vaccinia and tumour necrosis factor/IL-1 receptor[39].

CD8 Mediated Responses

Cytotoxic T lymphocytes (CTLs) are important in the clearance of acute infections and in the maintenance of the virus–host equilibrium during virus persistence. The majority of CTLs are restricted through MHC class I (that is, they express CD8) and kill by the insertion of a pore forming protein, perforin—contained in CTL cytoplasmic granules—into the infected cell membrane[40]. Through this channel, other factors pass, to induce apoptosis of the infected cell. Although a proportion of CD4 cells also mediate cytolysis, they do so largely by the non-perforin or Fas–ligand mechanism of lysis[41,42]. The relative importance of these two cell types has been shown in mice in which the perforin gene is disrupted: these mice have an enhanced susceptibility to lymphocyte choriomeningitis virus (LCMV) infection and tumours[43], even though Fas mediated lysis is retained. The ability of CTLs to clear infection is evident in certain experimental virus infections. Murine CMV and LCMV infections are cleared by CTLs, and immunisation with CTL epitopes in a vaccinia recombinant, which can only induce specific CD8 CTL immunity, will protect mice against subsequent murine CMV or lethal LCMV[44] challenge.

In man, CTLs have an important role in herpesvirus infections. Adoptive transfer of HCMV specific CTLs may protect against the development of disease in bone marrow transplant recipients[45], and CTLs against the other herpesviruses that have specificity for input or immediate early non-structural antigens are becoming recognised. In the case of EBV induced lymphoproliferative disease occurring in transplant recipients, the adoptive transfer of CTLs can clear such virus induced tumours in man[46]. However, CTLs rarely provide protective immunity against initial contact with virus, especially if this is through mucosal routes. Influenza specific CTLs are cross reactive between the common influenza A subtypes, as they recognise internal virus proteins and not the surface haemagglutinin and neuraminidase at which most antigenic variation is observed. Even in the presence of this CTL response, influenza A infection could be established, although clinical and virological clearance was faster in those subjects with CTLs[47]. CTLs against many viruses producing lower respiratory tract infection have been described, but their relative contribution to host protection or immunopathology in man remains to be established (see below).

VIRAL EVASION OF IMMUNE RESPONSES

In order to survive the selective pressures of the immune response, viruses have evolved a number of evasive strategies.

INDUCTION OF IMMUNOSUPPRESSION

Viruses may directly infect those cells producing immune effector mechanisms to eliminate them. A whole range of viruses can infect immunocompetent cells, perhaps the most noteworthy example being that of HIV infection. Among the important human respiratory pathogens, CMV infects alveolar macrophages, measles and mumps viruses infect and inhibit T and B cell function, RSV and influenza can infect monocytes and lymphocytes, and group C adenoviruses infect T, B and "null" lymphocytes[48].

EVASION OF ANTIBODY RESPONSES

Antibodies that neutralise virus infection pose a major challenge for most respiratory pathogens. Influenza has adapted to this selection pressure by the high rate of mutation possible in RNA genomes using the virally encoded RNA polymerase. Provided that virus viability is retained by a continued ability of the mutated haemagglutinin to bind virus receptor, the presence of neutralising antibody would give the mutant virus a selective advantage. This has been termed antigen drift, and the mutations that arise are closely localised to the haemagglutinin–sialic acid binding site[34]. This process underlies the minor epidemics of influenza A that are observed annually. However, the major pandemics of influenza A that are observed periodically, arise as a more dramatic "antigenic shift". Influenza is maintained in the environment by having multiple hosts other than man, notably birds. As influenza has a segmented genome, if two strains of influenza infect the same cell it is possible for segments of both viruses to exchange. If this exchange involves the major glycoprotein, the reassortant virus would be able to evade the antibody responses in the natural host (man), enabling pandemics such as that in 1919 to occur.

In vivo persistence of virus infection results in the downregulation of all virus surface proteins, so that any circulating specific antibodies would be unable to recognise the cell as infected. This is most vividly seen in Herpes simplex virus (HSV) latency in dorsal root ganglia neurones, when no HSV proteins are expressed. Their expression may be inhibited by specific transcripts that restrict expression of lytic cycle proteins.

EVASION OF CTL RESPONSES

Recognition of a virus infected cell by CD8 CTL requires the presentation of linear viral peptide in association with MHC class I molecules on the surface of the infected cell. The infected cell can be recognised with as few as 200 virus peptide–MHC class I complexes on the surface[49]. In order to load MHC class I molecules with peptide, *de novo* synthesis of class I is required; viruses can interfere with this pathway (Fig. 16.2). Viruses such as HCMV downregulate MHC class I expression by enhancing breakdown of MHC class I complexes[50], whereas other viruses may inhibit transport of the complex to the cell surface[51].

Just as variation in epitope structure can allow evasion of antibody mediated immunity, so can variation in the linear peptides recognised by CTLs[52]. However, the importance of this effect may be mitigated by the observation that most individuals possess CTLs that recognise more than one virus protein or peptide–MHC complex during infection[53]. Possibly more significant is the observation that minor differences in the peptide structure may still allow peptide to bind to MHC class 1, but, if it does not trigger the full lytic cascade in CTLs, such a peptide may act as an antagonist to block further CTL function. Initially recognised with model antigens, this observation has been extended to human virus specific CTLs[54].

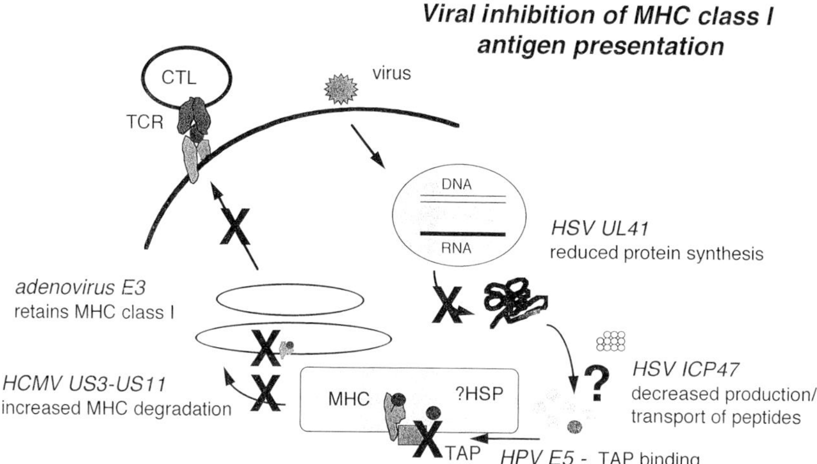

Figure 16.2. Viral evasion of major histocompatibility complex (MHC) class I restricted cytotoxic T cells by disruption of the antigen presentation pathway in the infected cell. CTL = Cytotoxic T lymphocyte; TCR = T cell receptor; HSV = Herpes simplex virus; HCMV = human cytomegalovirus; HSP = heat shock protein; TAP = transporter associated with antigen presentation; HPV = human papilloma virus

INDUCTION OF IMMUNOPATHOLOGY

The responses considered in relation to virus infection have focused on the protective effect of the immune response. However, viral infection can also induce immunopathology, and this may have a variable role in a number of respiratory infections (see below). Again, this aspect is well demonstrated during experimental infection with LCMV or Aleutian mink disease, when immune complex mediated disease may occur. In man the phenomenon is well described with hepatitis B and subsequent autoimmune liver disease. This aspect of the immunopathology that follows virus infection can be extended, as viruses are often considered triggers of autoimmune responses[55].

Viral infection followed by interaction with the immune system may therefore produce a range of clinical presentations that could be indicative of virus clearance and recovery at one end of the spectrum, to the induction of virus induced cytopathology or a consequence of an overaggressive immune reaction at the other extreme. In this context, we will consider some specific examples of viral disease affecting the human respiratory tract.

HUMAN RESPIRATORY VIRUS INFECTIONS
Human Cytomegalovirus Infection

Clinical Observations

Cytomegalic inclusion disease of the fetus is caused by CMV infection *in utero*. There is widespread infection involving the central nervous system, but the lung can also be affected. Such symptomatic disease is usually associated with primary maternal infection rather than reactivation of the virus in the mother[56]. However, 90% of children with congenital CMV infection are asymptomatic at birth and in most there are no adverse effects, although nerve deafness and intellectual impairment may occur lates in life[57].

Outside the neonatal period, it is in immunocompromised individuals, particularly those with acquired immunodeficiency syndrome (AIDS) and recipients of solid organ and bone marrow transplants, that CMV produces a severe and sometimes fatal illness. CMV infection occurs in almost all seropositive recipients of renal, liver[58], heart, lung[59] and bone marrow allografts[60], but it is with CMV pneumonia that serious adverse effects of this infection occur. High fatality rates are found, despite the use of antiviral drugs and CMV immunoglobulin.

Immunological Responses to Human Cytomegalovirus Infection

After CMV infection, a large number of antibodies specific for various viral determinants are generated, but they probably have a minor protective role in immunosuppressed patients. Antibodies are directed against the virion, whereas cell mediated responses, including CTLs and NK cells are directed against the virus infected cell. CMV specific CTLs were found at 1 in 5000–20 000 peripheral blood T cells from normal seropositive subjects, which require non-structural virus gene products[61,62]. The specificity of these CTLs was against the immediate early-1 (IE-1) and glycoprotein B (late) proteins: 23–68% of CTL clones were specific for the IE-1 gene product[63].

More recently, McLaughlin-Taylor *et al*[64] identified the CMV matrix protein, pp65, as a major target antigen for CD8+ class I MHC-restricted CMV-specific CTLs derived from the peripheral blood of normal seropositive individuals. In most individuals, the frequency of pp65 CTLs is greater than that of IE-1 specific CTLs. The protein pp65 is interesting, as it enters the cell with the input virus and can be redirected to MHC class 1 processing without *de novo* virus protein synthesis. Therefore pp65 specific and IE-1 specific CTLs may provide an important effector mechanism to limit CMV infection, as both are expressed before virus DNA replication in the infected cell.

Studies of CMV specific CTLs have also been undertaken in immunosuppressed patients. The development of a CTL response correlated with a favourable outcome after CMV infection in transplant recipients[65,66]. Reusser *et al.*[67] studied the CMV specific CTL response in 20 recipients of bone marrow transplants from CMV seropositive donors using peripheral blood mononuclear cells stimulated *in vitro* with CMV infected, donor derived fibroblasts. All 20 donors demonstrated cytolytic activity, but CMV specific CTLs were present in only 10 of 20 patients after transplant, none of whom developed CMV pneumonia, whereas six of 10 patients without a detectable CMV specific CTL response died with CMV pneumonia.

Immunopathology of CMV Pneumonia

The histopathological features of CMV pneumonia are of "owl's eye" intranuclear and granular cytoplasmic inclusions in association with a diffuse viral alveolitis[68]. However, it is also recognised that immunosuppressed patients may have asymptomatic shedding of CMV from the lung, detectable by bronchoalveolar lavage, in the absence of pneumonia or an alveolitis on lung biopsy. Evidence of the specific acute inflammation which occurs in the lung during CMV pneumonia is provided by studies in lung transplant recipients, which revealed the concentrations of tumour necrosis factor and IL-6 in bronchoalveolar lavage fluid to be increased in patients with CMV pneumonia compared with patients experiencing acute rejection[69].

It has been suggested that lung damage associated with CMV pneumonia is due to the cell mediated immunopathological process rather than direct cytopathic effects of the virus[70]. AIDS patients have an impaired ability to mount a T cell response and a high incidence of CMV disease (eye and gastrointestinal tract), yet deaths from CMV pneumonia are rare, and antiviral therapy is effective. This is in contrast with bone marrow transplant recipients, in whom CMV pneumonia is associated with the development of graft versus host disease and in whom antiviral agents, while reducing the titre of CMV in the lungs, do not prevent death. In this context it is suggested that CMV pneumonia should be treated with immunosuppressive therapy. This hypothesis is at variance with the interpretation by Reusser *et al.*[67], who suggested that adoptive transfer of CMV specific CTL clones might protect immunocompromised patients from severe CMV disease. The peak incidence of CMV disease in bone marrow transplant recipients is in the first 3 months after transplant and is related to profound immunosuppression. The association between graft versus host disease and CMV pneumonia is attributed to the delayed restoration of cellular immunity associated with graft versus host disease *per se* and the immunosuppression used to treat it. In heart–lung transplant recipients, Smyth *et al.*[71] have observed that rates of CMV pneumonia were significantly increased when treatment with augmented immunosuppression had been given in the preceding 30 days.

In lung transplant recipients, while primary, donor acquired CMV infection in seronegative recipients is a risk factor for CMV pneumonia, there appears to be no additional risk associated with a CMV seropositive donor in CMV seropositive recipients[71]. Indeed, studies of the restriction enzyme digest profiles of CMV isolates from lung transplant recipients have implied that seropositive patients may reactivate an endogenous CMV strain which can infect the transplanted lungs from seronegative donors[72]. In murine CMV the lungs are an important site of CMV latency[73], and if this is also true in man it may explain why the lungs are the site of most severe end organ damage from CMV infection, although at present immunopathology cannot be excluded.

Herpes simplex Virus

Compared with CMV pneumonia, HSV pneumonia is unusual even in immunocompromised patients, although seropositivity rates within populations are similar for the two herpes viridae. In the neonate, infections acquired perinatally are responsible for a high morbidity and mortality and about 50% of such infections will become disseminated to multiple organs, including the lungs.

Reactivated HSV infection in the transplant recipient most commonly involves the mouth. It is generally believed that involvement of the middle and lower respiratory tracts occurs by contiguous spread from the upper respiratory tract, causing first a necrotising tracheobronchitis and then pneumonia[74]. The characteristic histological findings in HSV pneumonia are of "ground glass" intranuclear inclusions, cellular degeneration and focal parenchymal necrosis in association with a viral alveolitis[75].

The occurrence of HSV pneumonia in heart–lung transplant recipients appears to be related to the degree of immunosuppression. In one series, six episodes of HSV pneumonia were reported in five patients, of whom one died. All episodes occurred within the first 2 months after transplantation and within 30 days of augmented immunosuppression[75].

While there is still debate about the site of latency of CMV, the site and mechanisms of latency of HSV have been well described. The virus replicates at the site of primary infection and either the intact virion or the nucleocapsid is transported via axons to neuronal bodies in sensory or autonomic ganglia, where latency is established[76]. There is a growing body of evidence which implicates the CTLs in the control of HSV infection. Studies using depletion and adoptive transfer of selected populations of CD4+ and CD8+ T lymphocytes, NK cells and macrophages demonstrated protection against HSV. Suppression of non-HSV specific and anti-HSV specific cellular immune responses can predispose the host to severe HSV infection. It may be that differences in mechanisms of latency between CMV and HSV, rather than the nature of the immune response to these viruses, may account for the much less frequent occurrence of HSV pneumonia in immunocompromised patients.

Respiratory Syncytial Virus

RSV bronchiolitis is one of the most important causes of death and morbidity in infants younger than 6 months. Seroepidemiological studies have shown that RSV infection is very prevalent in young children and almost all have been infected with RSV by the age of 2 years. However, the proportion of those showing serological evidence of infection who develop any symptoms is unknown. In older children and adults, RSV infection is known to cause symptoms of the common cold[77]. However, in the immunocompromised patient[78], or the elderly[79], it has been implicated as the cause of life-threatening pneumonias. Studies of urban populations[80] have estimated that 25 in 1000 infants will develop RSV bronchiolitis severe enough to require hospital admission, and about 3% of these develop respiratory failure and require artificial ventilation. Although there is evidence that factors such as pre-existing cardiopulmonary disease, prematurity, parental smoking and atopy may predispose to severe bronchiolitis and death from RSV infection, the mechanisms by which this occurs are not understood.

There is some evidence that RSV bronchiolitis may be an immunopathological condition and that it is the host response to the infecting organism, rather than viral load or virulence, which determines the severity of the illness. In the 1960s, young children were vaccinated with formalin inactivated RSV and developed an augmented lower respiratory tract disease during subsequent natural infection.

Those who died showed complicated pathological changes which included an influx of eosinophils into the lung[81]. This concept of RSV bronchiolitis as an immunopathological condition, possibly mediated by eosinophils, T cells, or both, has been supported by experimental studies in BALB/c mice[82] in which passive transfer of CD4+ and CD8+ cell lines into animals that were subsequently infected with RSV caused them to become ill and lose weight. Both cell lines reduced the lung titres of RSV (CD4+ more than CD8+), but increased the severity of their lung pathology. In addition, recipients of CD4+ cells developed a striking pulmonary eosinophilia.

Wheezing is an important clinical sign of bronchiolitis and children who have had bronchiolitis show an increased incidence of asthmatic symptoms, even some years after recovery[81,83]. The eosinophil is intimately associated with the pathophysiology of asthma, and blood eosinophilia correlates with reactivity to bronchoconstrictive agents[84]. Eosinophil efflux into bronchoalveolar lavage fluid is a feature of the allergen induced late phase asthmatic reaction. Although no direct measurements of bronchoalveolar eosinophils have been made in children with bronchiolitis, the concentrations of the toxic granule protein produced by eosinophils, (eosinophil cationic protein) have been measured in the nasopharyngeal secretions of children with RSV infection and have been found to correlate with the severity of their illness[85]. Controversy surrounds the question of whether the injury to the airways which occurs during bronchiolitis increases the susceptibility to subsequent wheezing, or whether infants of an atopic disposition who become infected with RSV are predisposed to developed bronchiolitis.

REFERENCES

1. Gerone P J, Couch R B, Keeter G V, *et al*. Assessment of experimental and natural viral aerosols. *Bacteriol Rev* 1966; **30:** 576–584.
2. Knight V, Gilbert B E, Wilson S L. Airborne transmission of virus infections. In: Fields B, Martin M, Kamely K, eds. *Genetically Altered Viruses and the Environment.* Cold Spring Harbor NY: Cold Spring Harbor Laboratory, 1985; 73–94.
3. DeJong J G, Winkler K C. The inactivation of polioviruses in aerosols. *J Hyg* 1968; **66:** 557–565.
4. Hemmes H H, Winklerk K C, Kool S M. Virus survival as a seasonal factor in influenza and poliomyelitis. *Nature* 1960; **188:** 1107–1115.
5. Tyler K L, Fields B N. Pathogenesis of viral infections. In: Fields BN, Knipe DM, Howley PM, eds. *Fundamental Virology*, 3rd edn. Philadelphia: Lippencott-Raven Publishers, 1996; 161–206.
6. Dang Γ, Bang B, Foard M. Responses of upper respiratory mucosa to drugs and viral infections. *Am Rev Respir Dis* 1966; **93** (suppl): 5142–5149.
7. Brownstein D. Resistance/susceptibility to lethal Sendai virus infection is genetically linked to a mucociliary transport polymorphism. *J Virol* 1987; **61:** 1670–1671.
8. Burks A W J, Steele R W. Selective IgA deficiency. *Ann Allergy* 1986; **57:** 3–10.
9. Ammann A J, Hong R. Selective IgA deficiency: presentation of 30 cases and a review of the literature. *Medicine (Baltimore)* 1971; **50:** 223–236.
10. Mellander L, Bjorkander J, Carlsson B, *et al*. Secretory antibodies in IgA deficient and immunosuppressed individuals. *J Clin Immunol* 1986; **6:** 284–291.
11. Reynolds H Y. Immunologic system in the respiratory tract. *Physiol Rev* 1991; **71:** 1117–1133.
12. Rodriguez-Boulan E, Prendergast M. Polarised distribution of viral envelope proteins in the plasma membrane of infected epithelial cells. *Cell* 1980; **20:** 45–54.

13. Roth M G, Compans R W, Giusti L, *et al.* Influenza virus haemagglutinin expression is polarised in cells infected with recombinant SV40 viruses carrying cloned haemagglutinin. *Cell* 1983; **33:** 435–442.

14. Nayak D P, Jabbar M A. Structural domains and organisational conformation involved in sorting and transport of influenza virus transmembrane proteins. *Annu Rev Microbiol* 1989; **43:** 465–501.

15. Brewer C B, Roth M G. A single amino acid change in the cytoplasmic domain alters the polarised delivery of influenza virus haemagglutinin. *J Cell Biol* 1991; **114:** 413–422.

16. Owens R J, Dubay J W, Hurter G, *et al.* Human immunodeficiency virus envelope protein determines the site of virus release in polarised epithelial cells. *Proc Natl Acad Sci USA* 1991; **88:** 3987–3991.

17. Tashiro M J, Seto J T, Choosakul S, *et al.* Budding site of Sendai virus in polarised epithelial cells is one of the determinants for tropism and pathogenicity in mice. *Virology* 1992; **187:** 413–422.

18. Klenk H D, Garten W. Host cell proteases controlling virus pathogenicity. *Trends Microbiol* 1994; **2:** 39–43.

19. Zhirnov O, Ovcharenko A, Burinskaya A. Suppression of influenza virus replication in infected mice by proteinase inhibitors. *J Gen Virol* 1984; **65:** 191–196.

20. Tashiro M, Klenk H D, Rott R. Inhibitory effect of a protease inhibitor, leupeptin, on the development of influenza pneumonia mediated by a concomitant bacteria. *J Gen Virol* 1987; **68:** 2039–2041.

21. Bullough P A, Hughson F M, Skehel J J, *et al.* Structure of influenza haemagglutinin at the pH of membrane fusion. *Nature* 1994; **371:** 37–43.

22. Li S, Schulman J, Itamura S, *et al.* Glycosylation of neuraminidase determines the neurovirulence of influenza A/WSN/33 virus. *J Virol* 1993; **67:** 6667–6673.

23. Taylor-Weideman J, Sissons J G P, Borysiewicz L K, *et al.* Monocytes as a major site of persistence of human cytomegalovirus in peripheral blood monounclear cells. *J Gen Virol* 1991; **72:** 2059–2064.

24. Minton E J, Tysoe C, Sinclair J H, *et al.* Human cytomegalovirus infection of the monocyte/acrophage lineage in bone marrow. *J Virol* 1994; **68:** 4017–4021.

25. Ahmed R, Morrison L A, Knipe D M. Persistence of viruses. In: Fields B N, Knipe D M, Howley P M, eds. *Virology*, 3rd edn, Vol 1. Philadelphia: Lippencott-Raven Publishers, 1996; 219–250.

26. Gresser I. Role of interferon in resistance to viral infection *in vivo*. In: Vilcek J, Maeyer E D, eds. *Interferon*, Vol 2. Amsterdam: Elsevier Science, 1984; 221–247.

27. Muller U, Steinhoff U, Reis L F L, *et al.* Functional role of type I and type II interferons in antiviral defence. *Science* 1994; **264:** 1918–1921.

28. Borysiewicz L K, Rodgers B, Morris S, *et al.* Lysis of human cytomegalovirus infected fibroblasts by natural killer cells: demonstration of an interferon-independent component requiring expression of early viral proteins and characterisation of the effector cells. *J Immunol* 1985; **134:** 2695–2710.

29. Karre K. Express yourself or die: peptides, MHC molecules and NK cells. *Science* 1995; **267:** 978–979.

30. Bukowski J F, Warner J F, Dennert G, *et al.* Adoptive transfer studies demonstrating the antiviral effect of natural killer cells *in vivo*. *J Exp Med* 1985; **161:** 40–52.

31. Biron C A, Byron K S, Sullivan J L. Severe herpesvirus infections in an adolescent without natural killer cells. *N Engl J Med* 1989; **320:** 1731–1735.

32. Zinkernagel R M. Immunity to viruses. In: Paul W E, ed. *Fundamental Immunology*, 3rd edn. New York: Raven Press, 1993; 1211–1250.

33. Colonno R J, Callahan P L, Leippe D M, *et al.* Inhibition of rhinovirus attachment by neutralising monoclonal antibodies and their Fab fragments. *J Virol* 1989; **63:** 36–43.

34. Wiley D C, Wilson I A, Skehel J J. Structural identification of the antibody-binding sites of Hong Kong influenza haemagglutinin and their involvement in antigenic variation. *Nature* 1981; **289:** 373–378.

35. Townsend A, Bodmer H. Antigen recognition by class I-restricted T lymphocytes. *Annu Rev Immunol* 1989; **7:** 601–624.

36. Germain R N, Margulies D H. The biochemistry and cell biology of antigen processing and presentation. *Annu Rev Immunol* 1993; **11:** 403–450.

37. Long E O, Jacobson S. Pathways of viral antigen processing and presentation to CTL: defined by the mode of virus entry? *Immunol Today* 1989; **10:** 45–48.

38. Suzuki T, Tahara H, Narula S, *et al*. Viral interleukin 10 (IL-10), the human herpesvirus 4 cellular homologue, induces local anergy to allogeneic and syngeneic tumours. *J Exp Med* 1995; **182:** 477–486.

39. Alcami A, Smith G L. Cytokine receptors encoded by poxviruses: a lesson in cytokine biology. *Immunol Today* 1995; **16:** 474–478.

40. Liu C-C, Walsh C M, Young J D-E. Perforin: structure and function. *Immunol Today* 1995; **16:** 194–201.

41. Berke G. The binding and lysis of target cells by cytotoxic lymphocytes: molecular and cellular aspects. *Annu Rev Immunol* 1994; **12:** 735–774.

42. Griffiths G M. The cell biology of CTL killing. *Curr Opin Immunol* 1995; **7:** 343–348.

43. Kagi D, Vignaux F, Ledermann B, *et al*. Fas and perforin pathways as major mechanisms of T cell-mediated cytotoxicity. *Science* 1994; **265:** 528–530.

44. Whitton J L, Sheng N, Oldstone M B A, *et al*. A "string of beads" vaccine, comprising linked minigenes, confers protection from lethal dose virus challenge. *J Virol* 1993; **67:** 348–352.

45. Riddell S R, Greenberg P D. Principles for adoptive T cell therapy of human viral diseases. *Annu Rev Immunol* 1995; **13:** 545–586.

46. Rooney C M, Smith C A, Ng C Y C, *et al*. Use of gene-modified virus specific T lymphocytes to control Epstein-Barr-virus-related lymphoproliferation. *Lancet* 1995; **345:** 9–13.

47. McMichael A, Gotch F, Noble G R, *et al*. Cytotoxic T-cell immunity to influenza. *N Engl J Med* 1983; **309:** 13–17.

48. Whitton J L, Oldstone M B A. Immune response to viruses. In: Fields B N, Knipe D M, Howley P M, eds. *Fundamental Virology*, 3rd edn. Philadelphia: Lippencott-Raven Publishers, 1996; 311–340.

49. Christinck E R, Luscher M A, Barber B H, *et al*. Peptide binding to class I MHC on living cells and quantitation of complexes required for CTL lysis. *Nature* 1991; **352:** 67–70.

50. Warren A P, Ducroq D H, Lehner P J, *et al*. Human cytomegalovirus-infected cells have unstable assembly of major histocompatibility complex class I complexes and are resistant to lysis by cytotoxic T lymphocytes. *J Virol* 1994; **68:** 2822–2829.

51. Cox J H, Bennink J R, Yewdell J W. Retention of adenovirus E 19 glycoprotein in the endoplasmic reticulum is essential to its ability to block antigen presentation. *J Exp Med* 1991; **174:** 1629–1637.

52. Phillips R E, Rowland-Jones S, Nixon D F, *et al*. Human immunodeficiency virus genetic variation that can escape cytotoxic T cell recognition. *Nature* 1991; **354:** 453–459.

53. Carmichael A, Jin X, Sissons J G P, *et al*. Quantitative analysis of the human immunodeficiency virus Type 1 (HIV-1)-specific cytotoxic T lymphocyte (CTL) response at different stages of HIV-1 infection: differential CTL responses to HIV-1 and Epstein–Barr virus in late disease. *J Exp Med* 1993; **177:** 249–256.

54. Meier U-C, Klenerman P, Griffin P, *et al*. Cytotoxic T lymphocyte lysis inhibited by viable HIV mutants. *Science* 1995; **270:** 1360–1362.

55. Weetman A P, Borysiewicz L K. Viruses and autoimmunity. *Autoimmunity* 1990; **5:** 277–293.

56. Stagno S, Pass R F, Sworsky M E, *et al*. Congenital cytomegalovirus infection. The relative importance of primary and recurrent maternal infection. *N Engl J Med* 1982; **306:** 945–949.

57. Peerce P M, Pearl K N, Peckham C S. Congenital cytomegalovirus infection. *Arch Dis Child* 1984; **59:** 1120–1126.

58. Singh N, Dummer S, Ho M, *et al*. Infections with cytomegalovirus and other herpesviruses in 121 liver transplant recipients: transmission by donated organ and the effects of OKT3 antibodies. *J Infect Dis* 1988; **158:** 124–131.

59. Wreghitt T G, Hakim M, Gray J J, *et al*. Cytomegalovirus infections in heart and lung transplant recipients. *J Clin Pathol* 1988; **41:** 660–667.

60. Meyers J D, Flournoy N, Thomas E D. Risk factors for cytomegalovirus infection after human marrow transplantation. *J Infect Dis* 1986; **153:** 478–488.

61. Borysiewicz L K, Morris S, Page J D, *et al*. Requirements for *in vitro* generation of human cytomegalovirus specific cytotoxic T cell lines. *Eur J Immunol* 1983; **13:** 804–809.

62.	Borysiewicz L K, Graham S, Hickling J K, *et al*. Human cytomegalovirus-specific cytotoxic-T-cells: their precursor frequency and stage specificity. *Eur J Immunol* 1988; **18:** 269–275.

63.	Borysiewicz L K, Hickling J K, Graham S, *et al*. Human cytomegalovirus specific cytotoxic T cells recognise the 72kD immediate early protein and glycoprotein B in recombinant vaccinia viruses. *J Exp Med* 1988; **168:** 919–931.

64.	McLaughlin-Taylor E, Pande H, Forman S J, *et al*. Identification of the major late human cytomegalovirus matrix protein pp65 as a target antigen for CD8+ virus specific cytotoxic T lymphocytes. *J Med Virol* 1994; **43:** 103–110.

65.	Quinnan G V, Kirmani N, Rook A H, *et al*. Cytotoxic T cells in CMV infection. *N Engl J Med* 1982; **307:** 7–13.

66.	Smyth R L. Susceptibility to pulmonary infection in heart–lung transplant recipients [Thesis]. Cambridge: University of Cambridge, 1993.

67.	Reusser P, Riddell S R, Meyers J D, *et al*. Cytotoxic T-lymphocyte response to cytomegalovirus after human allogeneic bone marrow transplantation: pattern of recovery and correlation with cytomegalovirus infection and disease. *Blood* 1991; **78:** 1373–1380.

68.	Crawford S W, Bowden R A, Hackman R C, *et al*. Rapid detection of cytomegalovirus pulmonary infection by bronchoalveolar lavage and centrifugation culture. *Ann Int Med* 1988; **108:** 180–185.

69.	Humbert M, Roux-Lombard P, Cerrina J, *et al*. Soluble TNF receptors (TNF-sR$_{55}$ and TNF-sR$_{75}$) in lung allograft recipients displaying cytomegalovirus pneumonia. *Am J Respir Crit Care Med* 1994; **149:** 1681–1685.

70.	Grundy J E. Virologic and pathogenic aspects of cytomegalovirus infection. *Rev Infect Dis* 1990; **12:** S711–719.

71.	Smyth R L, Scott J P, Borysiewicz L K, *et al*. Cytomegalovirus infection in heart–lung transplant recipients: risk factors, clinical associations and response to treatment. *J Infect Dis* 1991; **164:** 1045–1050.

72.	Smyth R L, Sinclair J, Scott J P, *et al*. Infection and reactivation with cytomegalovirus strains in lung transplant recipients. *Transplantation* 1991; **52:** 480–481.

73.	Balthesen M, Messerle M, Reddehase M J. Lungs are a major organ site of cytomegalovirus latency and recurrence. *J Virol* 1993; **67:** 5360–5366.

74.	Ramsey P G, Fife K H, Hackman R C, *et al*. Herpes simplex pneumonia: clinical, virological and pathologic features in 20 patients. *Ann Int Med* 1982; **97:** 813–820.

75.	Smyth R L, Higenbottam T W, Scott J P, *et al*. Herpes simplex virus infection in heart–lung transplant recipients. *Transplantation* 1990; **49:** 735–739.

76.	Lancet T. Herpes simplex latency. *Lancet* 1989; **1:** 194–195.

77.	Hamre D, Procknow J J. Viruses isolated from natural common colds in the USA. *BMJ* 1961; **2:** 1382–1385.

78.	Hall C B, Powell K R, Macdonald N E, *et al*. Respiratory syncytial virus infection in children with compromised immune function. *N Engl J Med* 1986; **315:** 77–81.

79.	Vikerfors T, Gandien M, Olcen P L. Respiratory syncytial virus infection in adults. *Am Rev Respir Dis* 1987; **136:** 561–564.

80.	Stott E J, Taylor G. Respiratory syncytial virus. Brief review. *Arch Virol* 1985; **84:** 1–52.

81.	Kim H W, Canchola J G, Brandt C D, *et al*. Respiratory syncytial virus disease in infants despite prior administration of antigenic inactivated vaccine. *Am J Epidemiol* 1969; **89:** 422–434.

82.	Alwan W H, Record F M, Openshaw P J M. CD4 T cells clear virus but augment disease in mice infected with respiratory syncytial virus. Comparison with the effects of CD8 cells. *Clin Exp Immunol* 1992; **88:** 527–536.

83.	Murray M, Webb M S C, O'Callaghan C, *et al*. Respiratory status and allergy after bronchiolitis. *Arch Dis Child* 1992; **67:** 482–487.

84.	Durham S R, Kay A B. Eosinophils, bronchial hyper-reactivity and late phase asthmatic reactions. *Clin Allergy* 1985; **15:** 411–414.

85.	Garofalo R, Kimpen J L L, Welliver R C, *et al*. Eosinophil degranulation in the respiratory tract during naturally acquired respiratory syncytial virus infection. *J Pediatr* 1992; **120:** 28–32.

17

Helminth Infections

D. I. PRITCHARD

University of Nottingham, Nottingham, UK

R. A. WILSON

The University of York, York, UK

INTRODUCTION

The human lung is an important staging post in the life cycles of many helminth pathogens of man. Parasites enter either via the microvasculature or from the peritoneum, and either parasitise the lung or transit to continue their life cycle in another anatomical location. Fig. 17.1 illustrates the sites of entry and exit of many of these human pathogens. It can be seen from the figure that the range of parasites coming into contact with lung tissue is extensive. As large metazoan foreign bodies, their effects on the human lung can be very damaging, from both a physical and an immunological standpoint.

It is not the purpose of this review to cover all aspects of parasitic infection, but to concentrate on immune reactions that occur in the lung in response to selected helminths. To do this, the biological distinction of "helminths" needs to be clarified. Phylogenetically, they can be divided into nematodes (roundworms), trematodes (the flukes) and cestodes (tapeworms). This classification forms the framework within which the events that take place following human infection with the range of parasites shown in Fig. 17.1 will be described.

NEMATODES (ROUNDWORMS)

NECATOR AMERICANUS (THE HUMAN HOOKWORM)

The human hookworm has a direct life cycle, in which fertilised ova are released into the small intestine after the copulation of the adult worms in this same anatomical location. The eggs are deposited in faecal material onto the ground where, in hot and humid conditions, they develop within 10 days into infective L3

Pulmonary Defences. Edited by Robert A. Stockley.
© 1997 John Wiley & Sons Ltd.

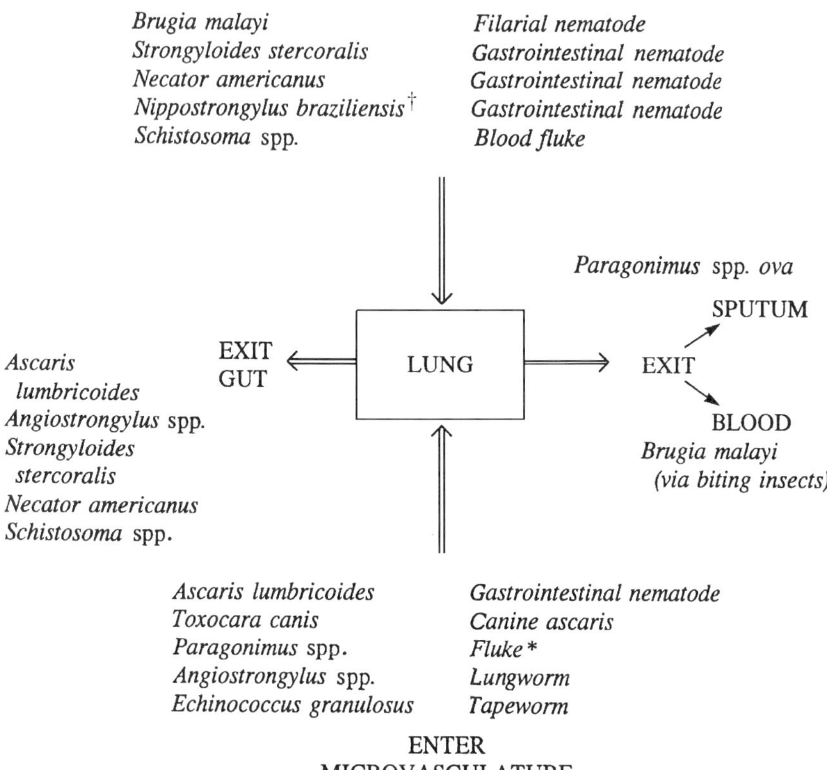

Figure 17.1. Pulmonary pathways for helminth infections. *Enters lung from gut via peritoneum. †Rodent model

stage larvae. These larvae infect the host percutaneously, entering the microvasculature to be carried to the lungs. Breaking through the alveolar wall, they enter the bronchioles, migrate up the trachea, down the oesophagus and into the small intestine. This migration completes the life cycle.

Pathology and Immunology

Asthma and bronchitis occurring during hookworm migration through the lungs have been reported, and small alveolar haemorrhages and eosinophilic infiltration would appear to occur[1,2]. However, little else is known about pulmonary responses to hookworms in man, although a systemic T helper 2 (Th2)-type response has recently been implicated in protective immunity in humans[3]. In a study in a laboratory model of necatoriasis in mice, Wells and Behnke[4,5] concluded that reinfected mice have the capacity to trap migrating larvae, although the immune response responsible was not identified.

Another animal model, *Nippostrongylus braziliensis* infection in the rat, has provided the greatest amount of information about pulmonary responses to migrating nematode larvae. Migration of the larvae in a primary infection is very rapid, before an immune response has time to develop, and pulmonary inflammation is consequently mild. However, a distinct mastocytosis has been recorded, which persists for many weeks[6]. In contrast, the arrival of larvae in the lungs of a previously primed rat elicited a marked exudative leucocytic infiltration of the alveolar, peribronchial and perivascular tissues[7]. There was a lasting effect on the cellular content of pulmonary tissues, with residual lymphocyte, eosinophil and plasma cell populations, and some larvae became surrounded by granulomatous reactions involving eosinophils and giant cells. There is, indeed, every indication that larvae are trapped and killed by the interstitial responses[7,8]. The immune responses underlying this cellular activity have been explored to some extent. Local synthesis of specific IgA has been reported[9] and, after *N. braziliensis* infection, activated macrophages express the appropriate Fc receptors, so that they may be armed by antibodies of this class. In addition, site specific compartmentalisation of the lymphocyte and IgE response in the lung has been suggested, although the functional significance of these dynamic changes in lymphocyte subsets remains to be identified[10,11].

The nature of the responses described above correlates well with the recorded Th2 cell activity in this model system[12], in which interleukins 4 and 5 are the predominant cytokines produced.

STRONGYLOIDES STERCORALIS

The life cycle of this gastrointestinal nematode parasite is considerably more complex than that described for *Necator americanus*. Eggs are again deposited in the small intestine, but hatch immediately into male and female rhabditiform larvae, which pass out in the faeces to continue an *external* sexual cycle. Here, in the soil, the larvae can develop into free living adults which in turn can produce infective filariform larvae, which enter the human host percutaneously. These larvae then transit the lungs as described for *Necator*. Autoinfection can also occur, when larvae hatched in the intestine transform into filariform larvae and enter the tissues to migrate to the lungs. This process may become important, even life-threatening, when individuals with a cryptic infection are immunosuppressed[13]. In some cases, adults can develop in the bronchial epithelium and produce progeny.

Pathology and Immunology

The symptomatology of *S. stercoralis* infection is similar to that already described for *N. americanus*, except that in cases of heavy infection, symptoms of bronchopneumonia with associated Loeffler's type hypereosinophilia (see *Ascaris lumbricoides*) can also occur. The adult respiratory distress syndrome has also been documented in patients with *Strongyloides* hyperinfection[14].

Once again, the human immune response has been poorly studied. In rats infected with *Strongyloides ratti*, pulmonary reactions are severe on challenge infection, with a pronounced eosinophilia in peribronchial and perivascular tissues[15]. However, leucocytes are not seen to make contact with migrating larvae, suggesting a parasite-evasion strategy. The balance of evidence would suggest that *Strongyloides* spp. are eliminated in the gut, but the possibility that irreversible damage occurs in the lung is worthy of consideration and has been reviewed elsewhere[16].

ASCARIS LUMBRICOIDES

This nematode causes one of the commonest and most widespread human infections. Infection follows the ingestion of eggs from contaminated soil, usually by children. Eggs hatch in the gut, and damage to the lungs occurs during the migration of larvae on route to the intestine (cf. hookworms).

Pathology and Immunology

A characteristic Loeffler's syndrome[17] occurs, and is accompanied by a pronounced eosinophilia in both the blood and the sputum (associated with larvae entering the airways), fever, cough and asthma. Immediate hypersensitivity would appear to have a large part to play in the development of these symptoms and, accordingly, *Ascaris suum* infection of primates is one of the commonest and most valuable models used for the development of antiallergic pharmaceuticals[18,19]. Indeed, the major *Ascaris* allergen (ABA-1) is one of the best characterised nematode allergens[20,21].

Investigations of immunopathology in animal models of ascariasis have provided some information on pulmonary responses. In primary infections, reactions are proportional in intensity to the numbers of migrating larvae. In pigs there is a progressive influx of eosinophils accompanying peripheral eosinophilia as migration proceeds, but mastocytosis develops after larvae have passed through the lungs (L. Eriksen, Proceedings of the Congress of the International Pig Veterinary Society, 1980). After a secondary exposure, overall pulmonary responses may be lower, probably as a result of larvae being arrested in the gut wall or liver, before they can reach the lungs[22,23]. However, at points where larvae enter the alveoli in primed animals, there is an early, intense leucocytic infiltrate which could indicate deployment of an anamnestic response. The involvement of the lungs and draining lymphoid tissue in the induction of a protective response is unclear, although in guineapigs a sequential response has been reported in mesenteric, hepatic and mediastinal lymph nodes, coincident with the different phases of larval tissue migration[24,25]. It is notable that IgE antibody was particularly prominent in the mediastinal lymph nodes draining the lungs of infected animals.

It is, nevertheless, not clear whether these responses contribute a protective response against the larvae in the lungs and, again, little is known of responses in man. Experiments in pigs infected with *Ascaris lumbricoides* seem to indicate that larvae must undertake a pulmonary migration to stimulate a protective immune response. However, immunological elimination of the infection would appear to take place in the liver, reinforcing the point that irreversible immunologically mediated damage in the lungs may be an important prerequisite.

FILARIAL NEMATODES

The adult stages of the filarial nematodes *Wuchereria bancrofti* and *Brugia malayi* are tissue dwelling. From this anatomical location, living larvae called microfilaria are produced. They frequently show periodicity in the peripheral blood, because the microfilariae have a tendency to remain in the arterioles of the lungs during the day, to emerge at night when the disease vectors (night-biting mosquitoes) are most active. The microfilariae undergo three stages of development in the insect host to form infective larvae, which are then reinjected into the human host.

Pathology and Immunology

The presence of microfilariae in lung arterioles appears to be well tolerated by the majority of infected individuals. However, in fewer than 1% of individuals with filariasis, a clinical condition called tropical pulmonary eosinophilia (TPE) occurs[26], characterised by bouts of night time (non-productive) coughing, accompanied by breathlessness and chest pain. Circulatory levels of IgE and eosinophilia are extremely high in these patients. Bronchoalveolar lavage of individuals with acute TPE reveals an intense alveolitis in which eosinophils are dominant. The concentration of these leucocytes in alveolar epithelial lining fluid greatly exceeds that of blood, implying their selective concentration in the lungs[27]. Ultrastructural examination of eosinophils from the lungs of patients with TPE suggests they are in an activated state, and this may relate to the immunological hyperresponsiveness to microfilarial antigens[28]. High levels of parasite specific antibodies have been detected in the lavage fluid from patients with TPE, and in their circulation[29].

The major allergen of *Brugia malayi* is expressed mainly in the microfilarial stage, and is composed of two molecules (23 and 25 kDa, referred to as Bm 23–25). The allergen is capable of inducing T cell proliferation, and IgE production from peripheral blood mononuclear cells from infected patients. The bronchoalveolar fluid of patients with TPE contained IgE that recognised Bm 23–25 strongly, implicating the allergen in the pathogenesis of the TPE syndrome[30].

Clearance of microfilariae would appear to be accomplished by adherent leucocytes after opsonisation with antibody[31,32]. Filariasis has been described as a spectral disease, with differential immune responsiveness associated with different clinical manifestations. It now seems to be accepted that asymptomatic patients, previously described as immunosuppressed with respect to their ability to produce a proinflammatory Th1 response, are fully responsive to parasite antigens but produce anti-inflammatory Th2 mediated effects. The factors which determine whether TPE develops in a minority of patients await discovery. It has been suggested that the onset of recognition of microfilarial antigens and the implementation of clearance mechanisms in the lung is related to the onset of TPE[33,34].

Unless treated, TPE is slowly progressive with increasing fibrosis, scarring, and diminished lung function[35]. The eosinophils that accumulate in the lungs are probably the chief agents of this pathology. The interaction of filarial antigens in the lungs with abundant specific antibody, possibly bound to eosinophils via Fc receptors, may well activate these cells. This would lead to their degranulation, as noted above[27], with release of cytotoxic granule proteins and generation of toxic radicals.

ZOONOTIC PULMONARY DIROFILARIASIS

Dirofilaria immitis, better known as the dog heartworm[37], can be transmitted to man by biting insects. Patients with histologically confirmed pulmonary dirofilariasis have recently been used to develop a specific and sensitive serological test for infection[37].

ANGIOSTRONGYLUS CANTONENSIS

This is normally a parasite of rats, but man can become infected by eating molluscs or crustaceans containing infective larvae[38]. The larvae pass from the stomach to enter the bloodstream, and then congregate in the central nervous system. Further development (usually in the anterior cerebrum) produces a young adult, which migrates to its definitive site, the pulmonary artery. Eggs produced here hatch into larvae which break into the respiratory tract, to be eventually swallowed and transmitted to the mollusc or crustacean in the faecal material.

Pathology and Immunology

The presence of adult worms in the pulmonary arterioles appears to be of little consequence. However, the eggs which embolise in the lungs, and the larvae which hatch from them, provoke granulomatous lesions in the pulmonary interstitium[39]. Plasma cells are abundant in the cellular infiltrates, suggesting local antibody production. Deposits of immunoglobulin and complement factors have also been observed, suggesting that immune complexes may contribute to granuloma formation[40]. The end result for the lungs is a progressive increase in fibrosis, emphysema and pulmonary insufficiency in dogs infected with *Angiostrongylus vasorum*[41]. Whether or not these pulmonary immune responses are host protective remains unclear[42], although recent work with immunosuppressed rats suggests that the overall immune response to *A. cantonensis* can reduce the parasite burden[43].

TOXOCARA CANIS

This parasite causes toxocariasis in man, a disease which is the result of infection with the canine ascarid, *Toxocara canis*. The life cycle is similar to that already described for *Ascaris lumbricoides*, except that the life cycle is not completed in man, and larvae are destroyed in a number of anatomical locations. Pulmonary infiltrates are found in more than 30% of patients, and airway disorders have been described[44]. Desowitz[45] linked IgE antibodies to *T. canis* with an increased prevalence of asthma. T cell clones derived from humans previously exposed to *Toxocara* larvae have Th2 characteristics[46]; this T helper phenotype would account for the allergic features of the disease in man, namely peripheral eosinophilia and increased serum IgE (although in most individuals infection is silent). Laboratory mice have served as experimental models for toxocariasis, and bronchoalveolar lavage has revealed eosinophil rich infiltrates in the lungs peaking 11 days after ingestion of eggs[47]. The infiltrating cells may aggregate into foci or granulomata around larvae in the lungs. The successful adoptive transfer of this hypersensitivity to naive recipients using lavaged lymphocytes suggests a cellular rather than a humoral basis[48]. Diagnosis is by enzyme linked immunosorbent assay, and the serological prevalence of toxocariasis ranges from 2% to 10%, depending on the demography of the population under study. Toxocariasis has recently been fully reviewed elsewhere[49].

TREMATODES (FLUKES)

SCHISTOSOMES

Schistosome ova are passed in the faeces or urine, and the newly hatched larval stages utilise freshwater snails as intermediate hosts before infecting man. This infective stage, the cercaria, rapidly loses its means of propulsion (its tail) as it penetrates the human skin to become a schistosomulum. Once inside the body, schistosomula reach the lungs via the pulmonary artery. This is followed by a period of development lasting about 4 days[50]. The parasite is then ready for intravascular migration to the hepatic portal system, where it will mature to a fecund adult. However, this can be a prolonged process[51] lasting for up to 20 days, at least in the murine host.

Pathology and Immunology

An allergic larval pneumonitis can occur during the phase of migration of schistosomula through the lungs, and this is associated with a peripheral eosinophilia. Verminous pneumonitis is also seen after the embolisation of dead or dying worms in the lung as a result of chemotherapeutic intervention.

Should ova (or adult worms) escape from the portal system in established hepatosplenic schistosomiasis and reach the systemic venous system, they become embolised in the pulmonary arterioles (embolisation of eggs is common; translocation of adults is a rarer phenomenon). If this process is prolonged and considerable accumulation of eggs occurs, pulmonary hypertension and cor pulmonale ensue.

In an immunological sense, schistosomiasis is perhaps the best studied of parasites that transmigrate the pulmonary tissues. Work with *Schistosoma mansoni* in mice has revealed that the majority of unsuccessful parasites are eliminated in the lungs. It would appear that parasites are literally "off loaded" into the alveoli (alveolar extrusion) as a result of mechanical damage during passage through the capillary bed. These schistosomula have a limited ability to re-enter the microcirculation, and die as a consequence, either in the lungs or in other anatomical locations[52].

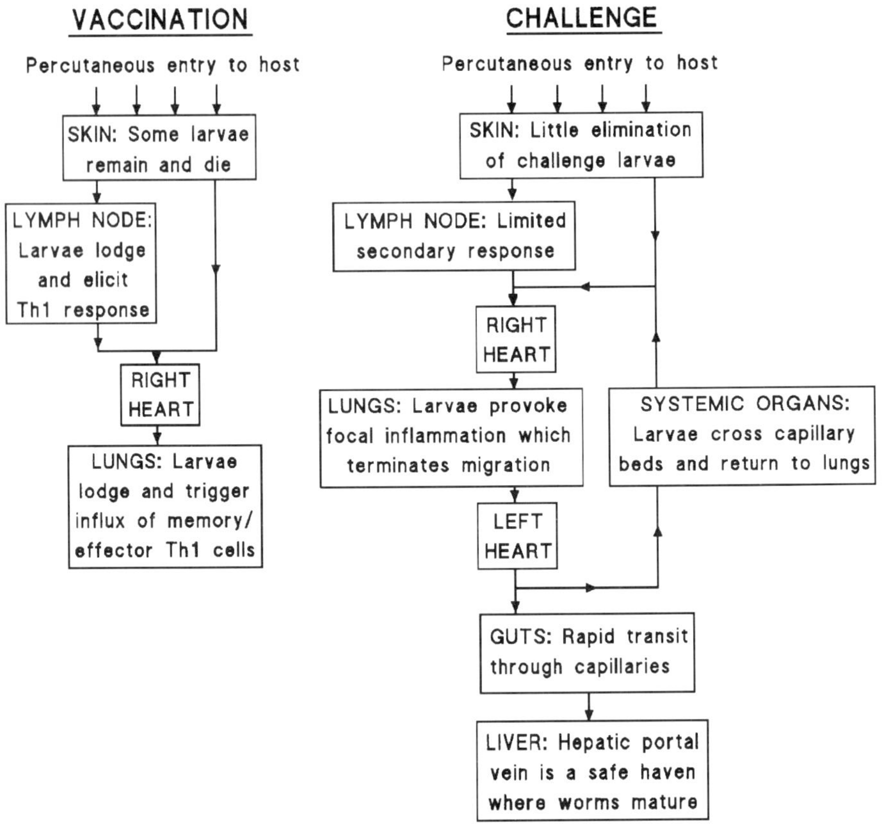

Figure 17.2. Immunological events associated with migration of schistosomes in mice after exposure to irradiated cercaria vaccine (left) and challenge of vaccinated mice with normal cercaria (right). Arrows indicate direction of migration

Many laboratory hosts can be protected against *S. mansoni* infection by exposure to radiation attenuated cercariae, as summarised in Fig. 17.2. For ethical reasons, the vaccine has not been tested in man, but it is known to be effective in primates[53]. The relevance of this vaccine to pulmonary immunity is that, in mice at least, a proportion of the attenuated, vaccinating larvae are trapped in the lungs. Here they recruit a persistent leucocyte infiltrate rich in cluster of differentiation 4 positive (CD4+) T cells of the Th1 subset. These lymphocytes have an effector/memory phenotype and may arm the lungs against the arrival of challenge larvae[54,55].

The arrival of challenge larvae in a primed lung triggers the development of compact inflammatory foci, that appear to function by trapping migrating larvae (Fig. 17.3). Interferon gamma (IFNγ, a Th1 cytokine) appears to be of central importance to focus formation[56]. Administration of antibodies to IFNγ coincident with larval migration through the lungs virtually abolishes protective immunity and markedly alters the composition of focal infiltrates[57]. These are

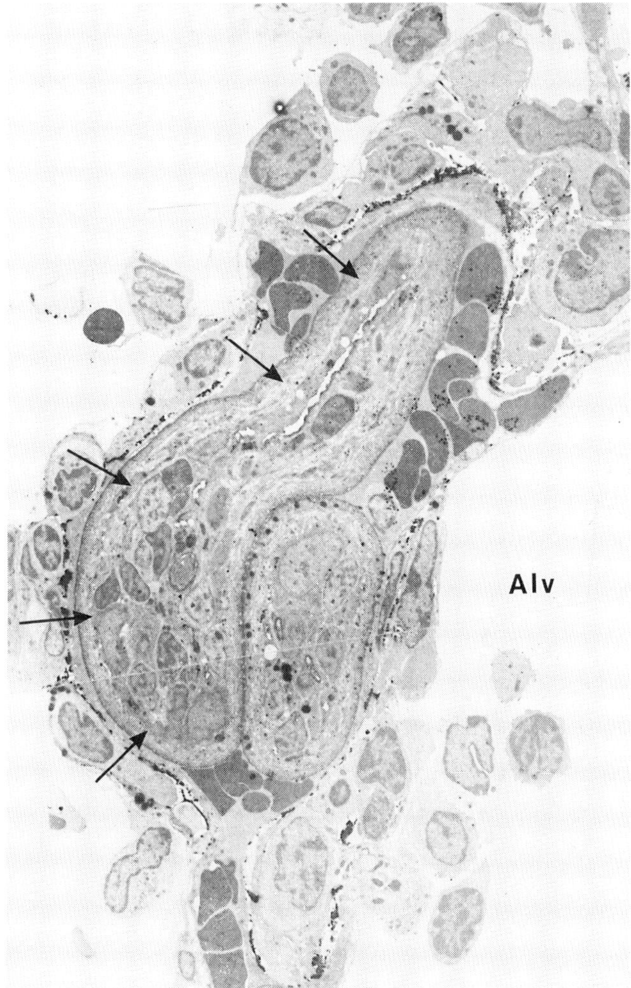

Figure 17.3. Schistosomulum of *S. mansoni* (arrowed) in the lungs of a vaccinated mouse 7 days after challenge. Numerous macrophages and lymphocytes are seen in the alveolus (ALV) and interstitium

larger and looser, contain many eosinophils, and appear to have a reduced ability to trap migrating larvae. Induction of a Th1 response may thus be crucial to the development of protective immunity. It therefore appears paradoxical, on initial consideration, first that schistosome eggs are potent inducers of a Th2 response[58,59]. However, this response may be beneficial to the parasite, as it aids translocation of eggs across the intestinal wall to the lumen.

Conversely, the egg induced Th2 response has important consequences for pathogenesis. The inflammatory foci which develop around eggs deposited in the lungs or other tissues rapidly become fibrotic, and much surrounding tissue is destroyed. CD4+ T cells and their cytokines are central to this process of granuloma formation, which initiates the chain of pathological events referred to above. The situation is rendered more complex by the suggestion that protective immunity in man, which takes several years to develop, may also be mediated by the Th2 arm of the immune response (reviewed elsewhere[60]). Precisely which parasite stage is the target of this immunity, and where in the body it operates, remain to be determined.

These eggs are destined to reach the intestinal tissues, from where they will be deposited in faecal material into the water supply. However, some break free and are carried either to the liver or, via portal–systemic collaterals, to the lung. Egg induced granulomas develop at each site, apparently mediated by Th2 CD4+ T cells and their cytokines[58,59].

The antigens responsible for generating these different spectra of the immune response are currently under active investigation[61,62], and for a recent review of this complex area, the reader is referred to Pearce and Simpson[60].

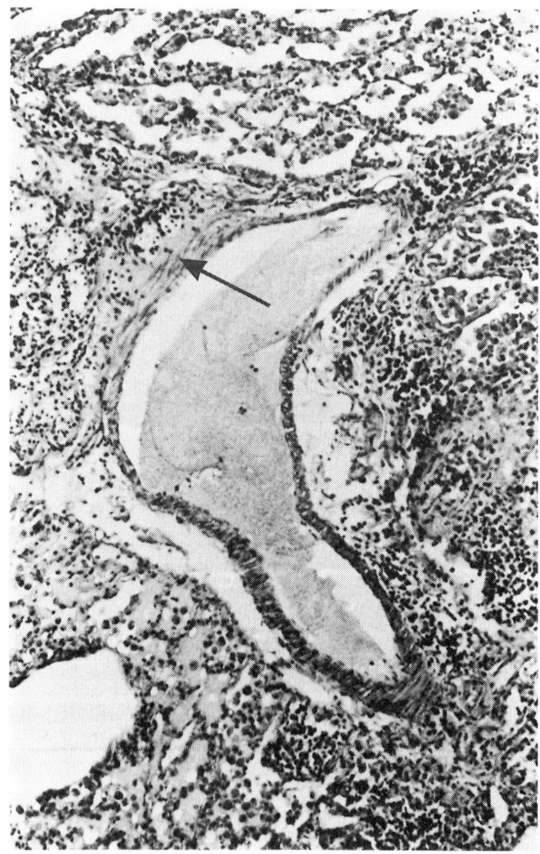

Figure 17.4. Adult *P. westermania* within a fibrous capsule (arrow) in the lung periphery

PARAGONIMIASIS

More than 10 species of *Paragonimus* are reported to cause human disease. The adult flukes encyst in the lung, and ova are expectorated in sputum, or swallowed and passed in the faeces. The ova embryonate in water, and hatch within 3 weeks, to invade an intermediate snail host in which further development occurs. Cercariae released by the snail penetrate crustaceans and encyst in their tissues, to develop into infective metacercariae. Man is infected after the ingestion of undercooked crustaceans. The metacercariae excyst in the gut and penetrate the intestinal wall to reach the abdominal cavity. They enter the pleural cavity across the diaphragm as young flukes, and burrow into the pulmonary parenchyma (Fig. 17.4), where they can reside for up to 30 years.

Pathology and Immunology

Young flukes in the lung cause haemorrhage, and an inflammatory response which results in the encystment of the parasite in a fibrous capsule. The fluke matures in about 6 weeks, produces eggs, and the cyst swells and bursts to release its contents into the bronchiole. The cyst contents are then expectorated in the sputum.

The clinical picture of chronic paragonimiasis is mild, with symptoms of chronic cough and respiratory discomfort. A "rusty cough" results from the production of gelatinous, blood tinged sputum, which contains parasite ova, necrotic tissue and occasional eosinophil derived Charcot-Leyden crystals. The immunology of this disease is poorly understood, as most early work was carried out in rats and dogs[63,64]. However, immunological studies in humans[65,66] seem to indicate that total antibody production in the lungs may be important to immunity or pathology, and that certain parasite antigens may be important for diagnosis.

CESTODES (TAPEWORMS)

ECHINOCOCCUS GRANULOSUS

Echinococcus or hydatidosis is a somatic infection, caused by the accidental ingestion of ova from the adult stages of tapeworms resident in carnivores. When ingested by an intermediate host, the activated ovum or oncosphere penetrates the intestinal mucosa, to be distributed to various anatomical sites by the circulatory system. Some reach the lungs, where post-oncosphere development results in the formation of a fluid filled hydatid cyst containing protoscolices. These develop into adult tapeworms when tissue containing cysts is fed to, or eaten by, carnivores.

The so called "pastoral" life cycle through man involves sheep and sheep dogs in circumstances in which the dogs are fed infected sheep offal and subsequently pass their ova to humans.

Pathology and Immunology

Hydatid cysts in the lung compress lung tissue and depress lung function. They can normally be found by X-ray, but specific imaging using antibodies raised specifically to cyst antigens has been suggested as a more reliable diagnostic probe. The main danger from hydatid infection is the rupture of the cyst, either naturally or during exploratory or remedial surgery. This can lead to "daughter cyst" formation by dissemination, or anaphylactic shock following the release of potent allergens from the cyst fluid.

SUMMARY

Pulmonary defences against helminths seem to be relatively limited. This partly reflects our lack of knowledge of immunological responses to parasitic infection in the *human* lung, resulting from the difficulties associated with working in this subject area under tropical conditions. However, it would appear that immunological defence mechanisms, once triggered, may themselves lead to the development of pathological damage, particularly if the incorrect immunological spectrum of responses is initiated. For example, in schistosomiasis, a Th1 response at the outset (as induced by the irradiated vaccine) would probably be highly protective. The problem, after a normal schistosome infection, is that egg deposition subverts the reaction, towards a Th2 response. It then appears to take several years before the Th2 mediated switch to IgE production (without blocking IgG4) is strong enough to have an impact on the schistosome worm burden. Meanwhile, the pathological consequences of chronic infection must be endured.

It should be recognised also that the generation of an otherwise protective response in an inappropriate location such as the lung could have serious consequences with respect to this organ. For example, Th2 responses (proallergic) appear to be important in controlling human hookworms[3], and an active Th2 response in the lung could result in secondary pathological changes. Nevertheless, this may be the price that has to be paid for the regulation of human parasitic infection, and could explain why, as reviewed elsewhere[67], people in the tropics with an allergic phenotype appear to be protected against some helminth infections.

REFERENCE

1. Muhleisen J P. Demonstration of pulmonary migration of the causative organism of creeping eruption. *Ann Int Med* 1953; **38**: 595–600.

2. Kalmon E H. Creeping eruption associated with transient pulmonary infiltrations. *Radiology* 1954; **62**: 222–226.

3. Pritchard D I, Quinnell R J, Walsh E A. Immunity in humans to *Necator americanus*: IgE, parasite weight and fecundity. *Parasite Immunol* 1995; **17**: 71–75.

4. Wells C, Behnke J M. The course of primary infection with *Necator americanus* in syngeneic mice. *Int J Parasitol* 1988; **18**: 47–52.

5. Wells C, Behnke J M. Acquired resistance to the human hookworm *Necator americanus* in mice. *Parasite Immunol* 1988; **10**: 493–505.

6. Arizono N, Koreto O, Nakao S, *et al.* Phenotypic changes in mast cells proliferating in the rat lung following infection with *Nippostrongylus brasiliensis*. *Virchows Arch B* 1987; **54**: 1–7.

7. Ramaswamy K, De Sanctis G T, Green F, *et al.* Pathology of pulmonary parasitic migration: morphological and bronchoalveolar cellular responses following *Nippostrongylus brasiliensis* infection in rats. *J Parasitol* 1991; **77**: 302–312.

8. Love R J, Kelly J D, Dineen J K. *Nippostrongylus brasiliensis:* effects of immunity on the pre-intestinal and intestinal larval stages of the parasite. *Int J Parasitol* 1974; **4:** 183–191.

9. Salman S K, Brown P J. A study of the pathology of the lungs of rats after subcutaneous or intravenous injection of active or inactive larvae of *Nippostrongylus brasiliensis. J Comp Pathol* 1980; **90:** 447–455.

10. Ramaswamy K, Befus D. Pulmonary inflammation and immune responses during the course of *Nippostrongylus brasiliensis* infection: lymphocyte subsets in bronchoalveolar lavage fluids of rats. *Parasite Immunol* 1993; **15:** 281–290.

11. Ramaswamy K, Befus D. IgE antibody responses in bronchoalveolar spaces of rats infected with *Nippostrongylus brasiliensis. Exp Parasitol* 1993; **76:** 23–31.

12. Urban J F, Madden K B, Svetic A, *et al.* The importance of Th-2 cytokines in protective immunity to nematodes. *Immunol Rev* 1992; **127:** 204–220.

13. Morgan J S, Schaffner W, Stone W J. Opportunistic strongyloidiasis in renal transplant recipients. *Transplantation* 1986; **42:** 518–524.

14. Cook G A, Rodriguez H A, Silva H, *et al.* Adult respiratory distress secondary to strongyloidiasis. *Chest* 1987; **6:** 1115–1116.

15. Moqbel R. Histopathological changes following primary, secondary and repeated infections of rats with *Strongyloides ratii*, with special reference to tissue eosinophils. *Parasite Immunol* 1980; **2:** 11–27.

16. Wilson R A. Pulmonary immune responses to parasites. In: Behnke J M, ed. *Parasites: Immunity and Pathology* London: Taylor and Francis, 1990; 208–248.

17. Loeffler W. Transient lung infiltrations with blood eosinophilia. *Int Arch Allergy Appl Immunol* 1956; **8:** 54–59.

18. Richards I M, Eady R P, Jackson D M, *et al.* Ascaris-induced bronchoconstriction in primates experimentally infected with *Ascaris suum* ova. *Clin Exp Immunol* 1983; **54:** 461–468.

19. Johnson H G, Stout B K. Late phase bronchoconstriction and eosinophilia as well as methacholine hyperresponsiveness in *Ascaris* sensitive rhesus monkeys were reversed by oral administration of U-83836E. *Int Arch Allergy Immunol* 1993; **100:** 362–366.

20. Christie J F, Dunbar B, Kennedy M W. The ABA-1 allergen of the nematode *Ascaris suum:* epitope stability, mass spectrometry, and N-terminal sequence comparison with the homologue in *Toxocara canis. Clin Exp Immunol* 1993; **92:** 125–132.

21. Spence H J, Moore J, Brass A, *et al.* A cDNA encoding repeating units of the ABA-1 allergen of *Ascaris. Mol Biochem Parasitol* 1993; **57:** 339–344.

22. Eriksen L, Nansen P, Roestorff A, *et al.* Response to repeated inoculations with *Ascaris suum* eggs in pigs during the fattening period. *Parasitol Res* 1992; **78:** 241–246.

23. Urban J F, Alizadeh H, Romanowski R D. *Ascaris suum:* development of intestinal immunity to infective second-stage larvae in swine. *Exp Parasitol* 1988; **66:** 66–77.

24. Khoury P B, Soulsby E J L. *Ascaris suum:* immune response in the guinea pig. 1. Lymphoid cell responses during primary infections. *Exp Parasitol* 1977; **41:** 141–159.

25. Khoury P B, Soulsby E J L. *Ascaris sum:* lymphoid cell responses during secondary infections in the guinea pig. *Exp Parasitol* 1977; **41:** 432–445.

26. Ottesen E A. Immunological aspects of lymphatic filariasis and onchocerciasis in man. *Trans R Soc Trop Med Hyg (Suppl)* 1984; **78:** 9–18.

27. Pinkston P, Vijayan V K, Nutman T B, *et al.* Acute tropical pulmonary eosinophilia. *J Clin Invest* 1987; **80:** 216–225.

28. Ottesen E A, Nutman T B. Tropical pulmonary eosinophilia. *Annu Rev Med* 1992; **43:** 417–424.

29. Nutman T B, Vijayan V K, Pinkston P, *et al.* Tropical pulmonary eosinophilia: analysis of antifilarial antibody localized to the lung. *J Infect Dis* 1989; **160:** 1042–1050.

30. Lobos E, Ondo A, Ottesen E A. *et al.* Biochemical and immunologic characterization of a major IgE-inducing filarial antigen of *Brugia malayi* and implications for the pathogenesis of tropical pulmonary eosinophilia. *J Immunol* 1992; **149:** 3029–3034.

31. Weiss N, Tanner M. Studies on *Dipetalonema viteae* (Filarioidea). 3. Antibody-dependent cell-mediated destruction of microfilariae *in vivo. Trop Parasitol* 1979; **30:** 73–80.

32. Piessens N F, Mackenzie C D. Immunology of lymphatic filariasis and onchocerciasis. In: Cohen S, Warren K S, eds. *Immunology of Parasitic Infections* Oxford: Blackwell, 1982; 622–653.

33. Ottesen E A. Infection and disease in lymphatic filariasis: an immunological perspective. *Parasitology* 1992; **104:** S71–S79.

34. Williams J F, Mackenzie C D, El Khalifa M. Onchocerciasis and lymphatic filariasis. In: Kierszenbaum F, ed. *Parasitic Infections and the Immune System.* London: Academic Press, 1994; 225–247.

35. Udwadia F E. Tropical eosinophilia: a review. *Respir. Med* 1993; **87:** 17–21.

36. Tanaka K I, Atwell R B. Immunohistological observations on pulmonary tissues from dogs infected with *Dirofilaria immitis. Vet Res Commun* 1993; **17:** 109–117.

37. Akao N, Kondo K, Fujita K. Immunoblot analysis of *Dirofilaria immitis* recognised by infected humans. *Ann Trop Med Parasitol* 1991; **85:** 455–460.

38. Shih S L, Hsu C H, Huang F Y, *et al. Angiostrongylus cantonensis* infection in infants and young children. *Pediatr Infect Dis J* 1992; **11:** 1064–1066.

39. Takai A. Immunopathological studies of rats infected with *Angiostrongylus cantonensis.* 1. Circulatory immune complexes and deposition of the immune complexes in tissues. *Acta Med Biol* 1983; **30:** 105–123.

40. Kanbara T, Ohmomo N, Umemura T, *et al.* Local antibody production and immune complex formation in rats experimentally infected with *Angiostrongylus cantonensis. Am J Trop Med Hyg* 1988; **39:** 353–360.

41. Caruso J P, Prestwood A K. Immunopathogenesis of canine angiostrongylosis: pulmonary effects of infection. *Comp Immun Microbiol Infect Dis* 1988; **11:** 85–92.

42. Yoshimura K, Aiba H, Hirayama N. *et al.* Acquired resistance and immune responses of eight strains of inbred rats to infection with *Angiostrongylus cantonensis. Jap J Vet Sci* 1979; **41:** 245–259.

43. Kamis A B, Ahmad R A, Badrul-Munir M Z. Worm burden and leukocyte response in *Angiostrongylus malaysiensis* infected rats: the influence of testosterone. *Parasitol Res* 1992; **78:** 388–391.

44. Taylor M R H, O'Connor P, Keane C T, *et al.* The expanded spectrum of toxocaral disease. *Lancet* 1988; **26:** 692–695.

45. Desowitz R S, Rudoy R, Barnwell J W. Antibodies to canine helminth parasites in asthmatic and non-asthmatic children. *Int Arch Allergy Appl Immunol* 1981; **65:** 361–366.

46. Del Prete G F, De Carli M, Mastromauro C, *et al.* Purified protein derivative of *Mycobacterium tuberculosis* and excretory–secretory antigen(s) of *Toxocara canis* expand *in vitro* human T cells with stable and opposite (type 1 T helper or type 2 T helper) profile of cytokine production. *J Clin Invest* 1991; **88:** 346–350.

47. Kayes S, Jones R E, Omholt P E. Use of bronchoalveolar lavage to compare local pulmonary immunity with the systemic immune response of *Toxocara canis*-infected mice. *Infect Immun* 1987; **55:** 2132–2136.

48. Kayes S, Jones R E, Omholt P E. Pulmonary granuloma formation in murine toxocariasis: transfer of granulomatous hypersensitivity using bronchoalveolar lavage cells. *J Parasitol* 1988; **74:** 950–956.

49. Lewis S N, Maizels R M, eds. *Toxocara and Toxocariasis. Clinical, Epidemiological and Molecular Perspectives* London: Institute of Biology and British Society for Parasitology, 1993.

50. Crabtree J E, Wilson R A. A scanning electron microscope study of the developing schistosomulum. *Parasitology* 1980; **81:** 553–564.

51. Wilson R A, Coulson P S. *Schistosoma mansoni:* dynamics of migration through the vascular system of the mouse. *Parasitology* 1986; **92:** 83–100.

52. Dean D A, Mangold B L. Evidence that both normal and immune elimination of *Schistosoma mansoni* take place at the lung stage of migration prior to parasite death. *Am J Trop Med Hyg* 1992; **47:** 238–248.

53. Yole D S, Pemberton R, Reid G D F, *et al.* Protective immunity to *Schistosoma mansoni* induced in the olive baboon *Papio anubis* by the irradiated cercaria vaccine. *Parasitology* 1996; **112:** 37–46.

54. Coulson P S, Wilson R A. Pulmonary T helper lymphocytes are CD44^{hi}, CD45RB$^-$ effector/memory cells in mice vaccinated with attenuated cercariae of *Schistosoma mansoni. J Immunol* 1993; **151:** 3663–3671.

55. Ratcliffe E C, Wilson R A. The role of mononuclear-cell recruitment to the lungs in the development and expression of immunity to *Schistosoma mansoni*. *Parasitology* 1992; **104:** 299–307.

56. Mountford A P, Coulson P S, Pemberton R M, *et al.* The generation of interferon-gamma-producing T lymphocytes in skin-draining lymph nodes, and their recruitment to the lungs, is associated with protective immunity to *Schistosoma mansoni*. *Immunology* 1992; **75:** 250–256.

57. Coulson P S, Smythies L E, Wilson R A. Pulmonary granulomatous type sensitivity: cell-mediated responses to embolised schistosome larvae and eggs. *Reg Immunol* 1993; **5:** 165–173.

58. Lukacs N W, Boros D L. Utilization of fractionated soluble egg antigens reveals selectively modulated granulomatous and lymphokine responses during murine *Schistosomiasis mansoni*. *Infect Immun* 1992; **60:** 3209–3216.

59. Chensue S W, Terebuh P D, Warmington K S, *et al.* Role of IL-4 and IFN-gamma in *Schistosoma mansoni* egg-induced hypersensitivity granuloma formation: orchestration, relative contribution, and relationship to macrophage function. *J Immunol* 1992; **148:** 900–906.

60. Pearce E J, Simpson A J G. Schistosomiasis. In: Kierszenbaum F, ed. *Parasitic Infections and the Immune System*. London: Academic Press, 1994; 203–223.

61. Langley J G, Dunne D W. (1992). Temporal variation in the carbohydrate and peptide surface epitopes in antibody-dependent, eosinophil-mediated killing of *Schistosoma mansoni* schistosomula. *Parasite Immunol* 1992; **14:** 185–200.

62. Reynolds S R, Shoemaker C B, Harn D A. T and B cell epitope mapping of SM23, an integral membrane protein of *Schistosoma mansoni*. *J Immunol* 1992; **149:** 3995–4001.

63. Choi N-Y, Lee O-R, Jin Y-K. Lung findings in experimental paragonimiasis. *Korean J Parasitol* 1979; **17:** 132–146.

64. Lee O-R. A histopathologic study of the lungs infected with *Paragonimus westermani* in the dog. *Korean J Parasitol* 1979; **17:** 19–44.

65. Ikeda T, Oikawa Y, Owhashi M, *et al.* Parasite-specific IgE and IgG levels in the serum and pleural effusion of *Paragonimiasis westermani* patients. *Am J Trop Med Hyg* 1992; **47:** 104–107.

66. Maleewong W, Wongkham C, Pariyanonda S, *et al.* Analysis of antibody levels before and after praziquantel treatment in human paragonimiasis heterotremus. *Asian Pac Allergy Immunol* 1992; **10:** 69–72.

67. Pritchard D I. Parasites and allergic disease. In: Moqbel R, ed. *Allergy and Immunity to Helminths* London: Taylor and Francis, 1992; 38–50.

18

Antigens and Allergens

P. HOWARTH AND V. A. VARNEY*

Southampton General Hospital, Southampton, UK

INTRODUCTION

A wide variety of macromolecules originating from plant products, foods and drugs can be harmful to some individuals. These macromolecules are generally inert, yet may induce hypersensitive or "allergic" immune responses that cause tissue damage. The basis of this reaction is the immunological recognition of antigenic molecular protein structures within these macromolecules which are capable of provoking an immune response. A complex protein may have many different antigens over its surface, and collectively these may provoke a harmful allergic immune response and are therefore called allergens[1].

AIRBORNE ALLERGENS AND THE RESPIRATORY TRACT

Airborne allergens such as house-dust mite, animal dander and grass pollen are the main agents inducing allergic inflammation of the respiratory tract. Such inflammation produces the clinical picture of allergic rhinitis and asthma in susceptible individuals. The respiratory tract normally affords protection against inhaled allergens by means of a number of mechanisms acting in synergy. On inhalation, air is filtered by the nose and nasopharynx to remove large particles such as pollens. As a result of aerodynamic factors, moderate sized particles which escape this filter are deposited in the large airways, where they are trapped and expelled by the mucociliary escalator. Tight junctions between epithelial cells usually limit permeability and access of the particles to the immune system. Phagocytic cells in the small airways with the mucociliary escalator clear remaining particles. In reality, these barriers are never absolute, and small amounts of inhaled allergens

---

* Present address: St Helier Hospital, Carshalton, UK

are able to pass into the peripheral blood. In normal individuals, a process of tolerisation rather than sensitisation to small amounts of antigen occurs, and their deposition in the lung does not activate an immune response.

Allergens (especially pollens) that are deposited on mucosal surfaces of the airway can rapidly release water soluble allergenic components. With other allergens, especially animal danders, the process of allergen release into the mucus is much slower and requires the particle to dissolve. Pollen allergens are large and easily trapped by the nasal airway, causing allergic rhinitis, which is the

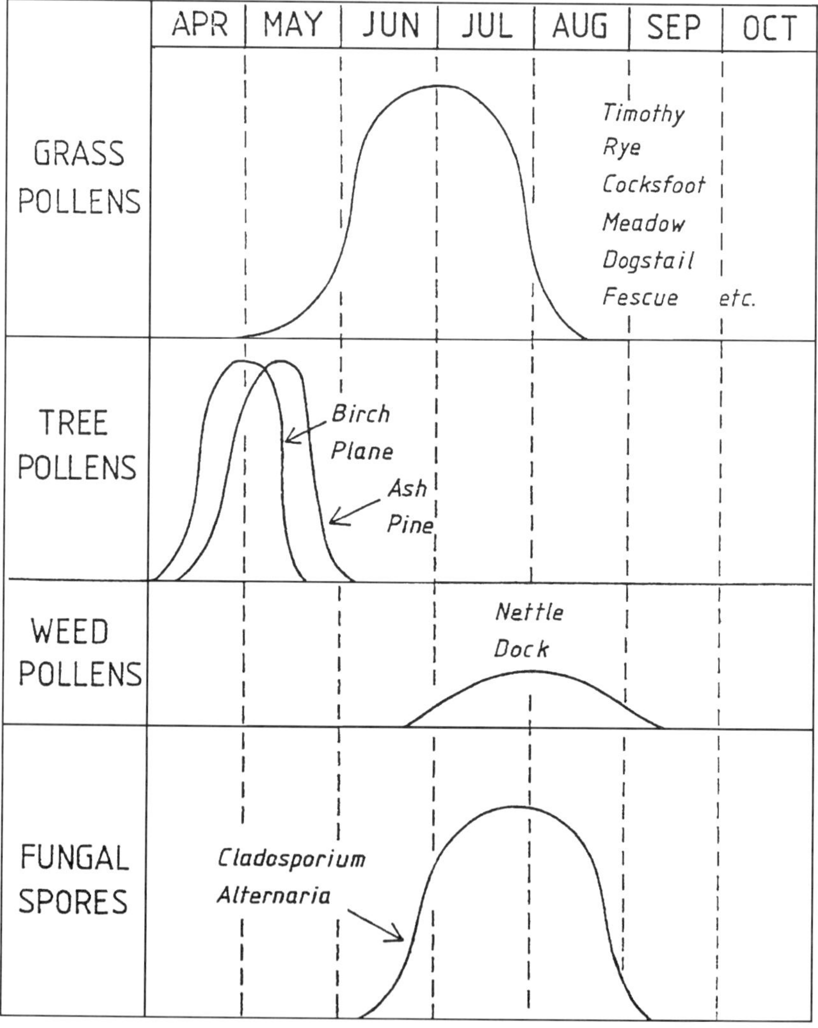

Figure 18.1. Calendar of common seasonal aeroallergens in the United Kingdom. (Courtesy of Professor A. B. Kay, Department of Allergy and Immunology, Royal Brompton Hospital, London)

commonest pollen induced symptom and shows a relevant seasonal variation (Fig. 18.1). In contrast, house-dust mite and mould spores are much smaller particles, which more easily gain access to the bronchus, producing asthma.

PROTEOLYTIC ENZYME PROPERTIES OF ALLERGENS

Effort has been devoted to the characterisation of common aerial allergens such as house-dust mites. Examination of immunochemical, biochemical and molecular characteristics demonstrates that many important allergens are proteolytic enzymes[2].

In mites, amylases are secreted by the salivary glands and stomach to aid digestion of starch and glycogen, derived from food such as skin scales, fungi and bacteria. These enzymes have been shown to be allergenic and to include cysteine proteases, chymotrypsin and lysozymes. Similar evidence exists for moulds, and even for occupational agents such as papain (in meat tenderisation) and the causative agents of baker's allergy. The biological effects of these enzymes may enhance epithelial permeability and induce a persistent allergic response. Other mechanisms may exist, such as enzyme interactions with protease inhibitors which could influence the presentation and processing of antigen; for example, antigens coupled to the protease inhibitor, α_2 macroglobulin, have been shown to increase proliferative responses of T cells. Further studies in this area are in progress.

ALLERGIC DISEASE OF THE RESPIRATORY TRACT

Allergic rhinitis and asthma may be seasonal when pollens and moulds are involved, or perennial when house-dust mite and animal danders are responsible. A combination of seasonal and perennial allergy is relatively common, and in individuals thus affected, chronic exposure to allergens will produce daily symptoms interspersed with acute seasonal exacerbations.

Current statistics show allergic rhinitis to affect 15–20% of the population, with grass pollen allergy predominant[3]. Medical consultations for hayfever have increased from 5.1 per 1000 population in 1955–56 to 10.6 per 1000 in 1970–71 and 19.8 per 1000 in 1981–82[4]. In the case of asthma, 4–10% of the UK population are affected, with an estimated 2000 deaths per year[5]. In children, 90% are allergic with an identifiable allergen, commonly house-dust mite[6], although this figure falls to 50% in adults.

ATOPY

Allergic response to common environmental allergens is described as atopy[7]. Atopic individuals appear to have a genetic predisposition to generate immunoglobulin E (IgE) antibodies in response to these innocuous substances. Atopy is characterised by increased levels of serum IgE antibodies and positive skin prick tests for these common allergens (Fig. 18.2). Atopic disease includes asthma, eczema, rhinitis and urticaria, and approximately 30% of the population are atopic[8]. Atopy is a risk factor for the development of asthma, which is the

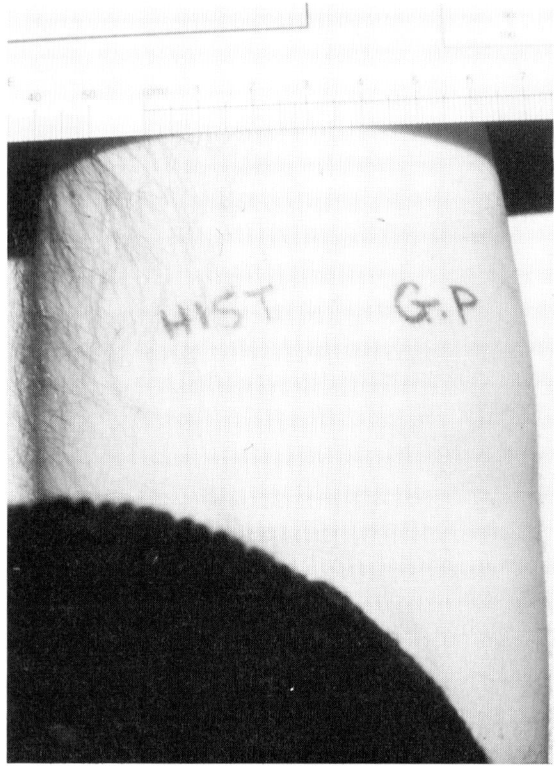

Figure 18.2. Positive skin tests to histamine (HIST) and grass pollen (G.P.) at 15 min, demonstrating weal and flare reaction from IgE mediated histamine release in the skin

most serious atopic disease because of its disabling chronicity and the risk of death in severe cases[9].

THE ALLERGEN INDUCED INFLAMMATORY STATE

The symptoms developing immediately after exposure to allergen represent the interaction of allergen with specific IgE bound to mast cells in the respiratory tract[10] (Fig. 18.3). Here, cross linking of the IgE molecule by allergen triggers the release of mast cell mediators. These mediators have been recognised by the techniques of nasal[11] and bronchial lavage and comprise two main types[12]:

(i)   Preformed mediators (histamine, heparin, chymase and tryptase) (Table 18.1).

(ii) Rapidly formed products of phospholipid metabolism (prostaglandin D_2, platelet activating factor, leukotrienes C_4, D_4, E_4) (Table 18.2).

These mediators quickly produce an increase in vascular permeability, smooth muscle contraction, goblet and glandular secretion, and stimulate irritant

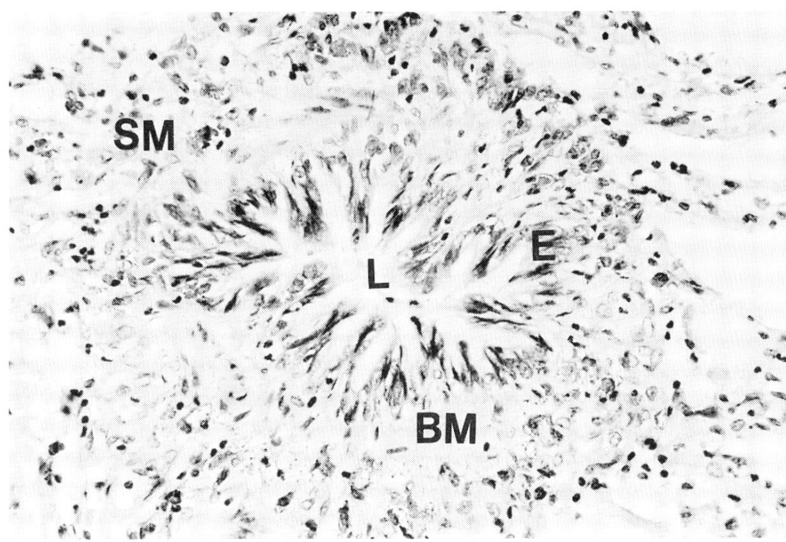

Figure 18.3. Cross section of a small bronchus taken at postmortem examination, from a mild asthmatic patient whose death was unrelated to asthma. Mast cells are shown as brown staining cells located in the epithelium and submucosa. AA1 monoclonal antibody directed against mast cell tryptase and developed with streptavidin biotin peroxidase was used, courtesy of Andrew Walls. L = Lumen; E = epithelium; BM = basement membrane; SM = submucosa. (Photograph courtesy of Dr Miroslav Synek, University Medicine, Southampton General Hospital)

Table 18.1. Preformed mast cell mediators and their functions

Mediator	Function
Histamine	Contracts smooth muscle Increases mucus secretion Stimulates irritant receptors
Heparin	Anticoagulant, anticomplement activity
Tryptase and chymase	Complement and kinin activation Degrades ground substance Basement membrane thickening
Neutrophil chemotactic factor(s)	Recruits and activates neutrophils
Eosinophil chemotactic peptide(s)	Recruitment and activation of eosinophils

receptors. As a result, bronchospasm, bronchorrhoea and cough are produced in the lung, and sneezing and rhinorrhoea in the nose.

These mediators are rapidly degraded, and are believed not to produce a significant inflammatory component on a single exposure to allergen. In reality, allergic disease of the respiratory tract is usually the result of continuous exposure to allergen, and asthma is attributed to a pronounced underlying inflammation in the lung. Such findings suggest a more complex mechanism than IgE dependent mast cell degranulation alone.

Table 18.2. Rapidly formed mast cell mediators and their functions

Mediator	Function
Platelet activating factor	Platelet activation and aggregation Neutrophil and eosinophil recruitment and activation Mucus secretion Smooth muscle contraction Vasomotor depression
Prostaglandin D_2	Contracts smooth muscle Increases mucus secretion Vasomotor depression Increases neutrophil migration
Leukotrienes C_4, D_4, E_4	Prolongs contraction of smooth muscle Increases vascular permeability Vasodilatation

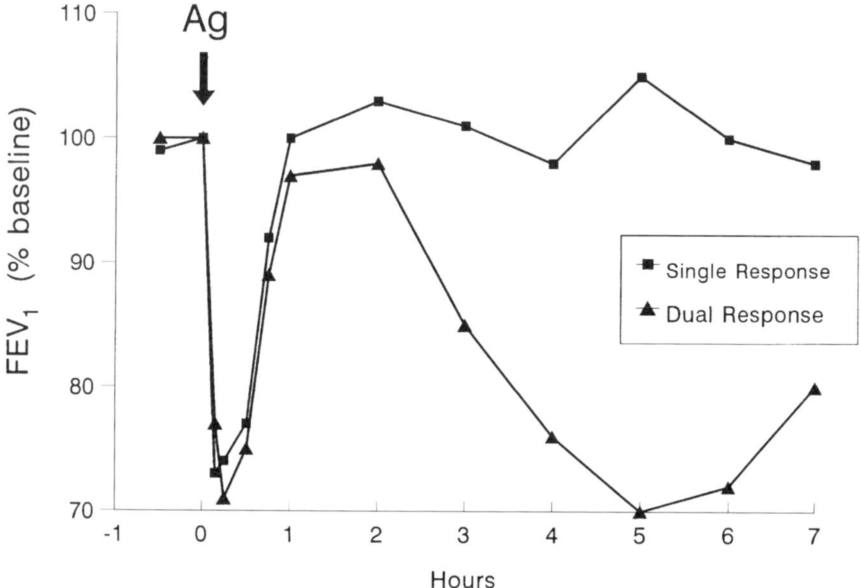

Figure 18.4. Immediate asthmatic reaction to allergen (Ag) showing transient decrease in forced expiratory volume in 1 sec (FEV$_1$) and late asthmatic reaction dual responses induced by a larger allergen challenge

LATE ALLERGIC REACTIONS

It is now appreciated that, if exposure to allergen is sufficient, all sensitised subjects develop a delayed asthmatic reaction or late phase reaction[13]. This late asthmatic reaction occurs 3–12 h after the initial mast cell response (Fig. 18.4), and is associated with heightened airway reactivity and bronchial inflammation[14].

This inflammation involves mucosal infiltration predominantly by eosinophils and T lymphocytes, but basophils and other granulocytes are also present. Identical responses can arise on nasal challenge[15].

The late phase response to allergen is associated with pulmonary function changes and air trapping in the lung. It resembles naturally occurring disease by its responsiveness to antiasthma treatment. It can be prevented by oral and inhaled steroids, but because corticosteroids do not inhibit mast cell degranulation, and diminish IgE concentrations only when given in high doses for long periods, a second steroid dependent mechanism for allergen induced inflammation is required.

MAST CELLS AND INTERLEUKINS

After years of controversy, the central role of the mast cell in allergic inflammation has now resurfaced. This has followed the recognition that mast cells are a source of cytokines, which may attract eosinophils, neutrophils and T cells to the allergen challenged site[16]. Northern hybridisation analysis (performed on mast cells stimulated through their IgE receptors) identified messenger RNA transcripts for interleukins IL-3, IL-4, IL-5 and IL-6. Mast cell cytokine production may therefore be mediated through mast cell stimulation, but remain distinct from that which stimulates degranulation[17]. This suggests a second pathway for mast cell activation, and a possible mechanism for its involvement in the late asthmatic response and inflammation (Fig. 18.5). The cytokines identified, are those which attract and support an eosinophilic inflammation typical of allergic conditions[18]. The outcome of exposure to allergen may therefore depend on whether IgE cross linking results in degranulation alone, or in association with cytokine production. This second event may explain why the interaction of allergen with the mast cell does result in local tissue destruction and inflammation, as observed in naturally occurring allergic disease.

HYPER-REACTIVITY OF THE RESPIRATORY TRACT

Nasal and bronchial hyperreactivity are a consequence of allergen induced inflammation of the respiratory tract[19] and are manifest by heightened reactivity to non-specific stimuli such as cold air, exercise, histamine and methacholine, all of which can induce bronchospasm more readily in asthmatic subjects. Disruption of the respiratory epithelium with exposure of airway nerve endings through inflammatory effects may be the reason for this increased reactivity. Certainly, epithelial cell numbers in bronchial lavage do correlate with the severity of hyperreactivity, which supports this concept.

T CELLS AND EOSINOPHILS

T lymphocytes are present in bronchial biopsy specimens and do exhibit increased activation in asthma[20]. These T cells are predominantly of the T helper subset (cluster of differentiation (CD) 4+). Two different CD4+ T subsets are now recognised, termed Th1 and Th2[21]. The difference has been determined by

                P. Howarth and V. A. Varney

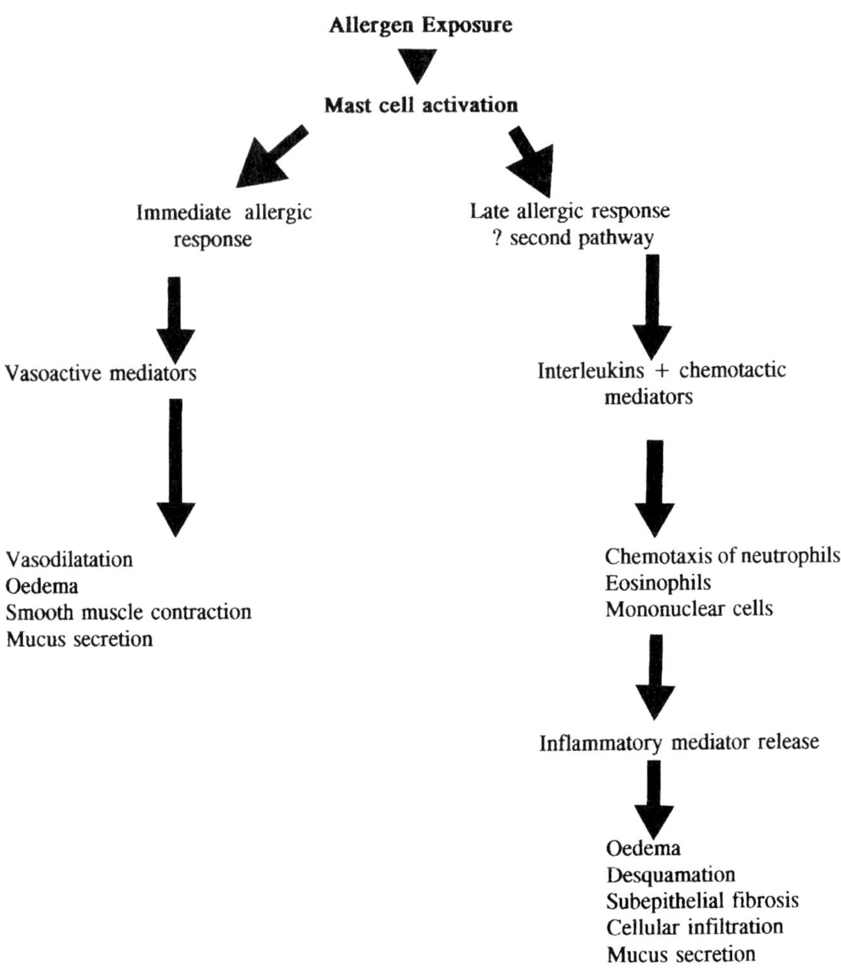

Figure 18.5. Possible inflammatory mechanisms in allergy

the cytokines produced, Th2 characteristically secreting IL-4, IL-5, and IL-6, whereas Th1 cells secrete IL-2 and interferon gamma. Examination of CD4+ T lymphocytes in allergic tissue of the nose, bronchi and skin confirms a predominant Th2 type subset that secretes cytokines which support allergic inflammation. Messenger RNA for IL-2, IL-4 and IL-5 has been demonstrated in T cells recovered from bronchial lavage[22]. Eosinophils are also important, and release proinflammatory mediators involved in the pathogenesis of asthma[23]. The movement of eosinophils into allergen challenged sites is clearly the result of the actions of chemoattractant cytokines[24]. Their survival in the tissues is increased by the cytokines IL-3, IL-5 and granulocyte macrophage colony stimulating factor, the origins of which may include mast cells, T cells and macrophages[25].

PATHOLOGY

ASTHMA

The asthmatic lung at autopsy is hyperinflated as a result of the presence of tenacious and viscous mucus plugs in the airway[26]. Clusters of columnar cells (creola bodies) and Charcot-Leyden crystals (a precipitated eosinophil enzyme product) can be seen in the sputum. The epithelium is desquamated and the bronchi are characterised by oedema, an increase in goblet cells, basement membrane thickening, and smooth muscle hypertrophy. Mast cells, T lymphocytes and large numbers of eosinophils are present in the subepithelial layer (Fig. 18.6). Evidence for granulocyte activation comes from eosinophil secreted major basic protein and neutrophil elastase at sites of epithelial damage.

Biopsy specimens from patients with chronic stable asthma show milder forms of this histological picture, although basement membrane thickening is disputed and subepithelial fibrosis demonstrated even in mildly asthmatic patients[27].

RHINITIS

In allergic rhinitis, a similar picture of submucosal oedema and infiltration by eosinophils, neutrophils and T cells is seen but, unlike the conditions in asthma, the mucosa remains intact, without evidence of epithelial injury[28]. Mast cell

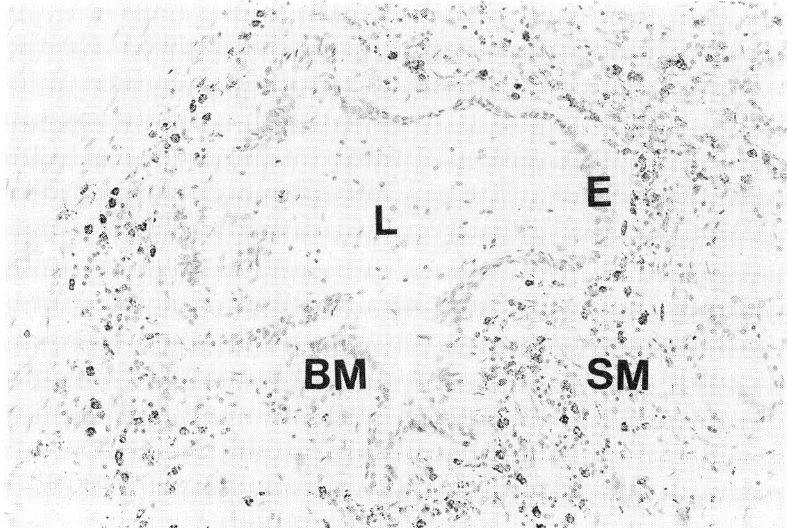

Figure 18.6. Cross section of medium size bronchus taken at postmortem examination, from a patient who died from an asthmatic attack. Eosinophils are shown as dark staining cells using EG2 monoclonal antibodies (Pharmacia Supsala, Sweden), developed with streptavidin biotin peroxidase. The lumen is heavily occluded by mucus secretions and shed epithelial cells. A marked eosinophilic infiltrate is present in the submucosa. L = lumen; E = epithelium; BM = basement membrane; SM = submucosa. (Photograph courtesy of Dr Miroslav Synek, University Medicine, Southampton General Hospital)

numbers in the nasal mucosa increase during continuing exposure to allergen, and some appear to move into the epithelial compartment after 4–5 days. There is evidence of granulocyte activation as described for the lung.

ALLERGEN SENSITISATION AND ASTHMA

The economic cost of asthma in the UK in terms of Health Services, Sickness Benefit and loss of productivity was £950 000 per year in the mid 1990s. Related diseases such as allergic rhinitis add to this morbidity. In the majority of asthmatic individuals, the most important aetiological factor in the development of asthma is sensitisation to allergens, particularly to house-dust mite[29]. Worldwide, there appears to have been an increasing prevalence of allergic disease in the past 30 years, particularly in industrialised countries[30]. The exact magnitude of this increase is difficult to assess accurately, but reports estimate it to be by a factor of 4. This cannot be explained easily as an increasing genetic susceptibility. It is therefore important to determine which factors could influence allergen sensitisation, as appropriate intervention could offset the development of allergic disease. Studies so far suggest that susceptibility to allergen sensitisation depends upon:

- The level of genetic susceptibility
- Pre- and post-natal factors
- Exposure to relevant allergen
- Exposure to adjuvant factors

GENETICS OF ATOPY

Thirty-five percent of children with an atopic parent develop allergy. Such familial clustering of atopic diseases encouraged research into genetic factors. From these studies, a gene transmitting atopy has been recognised on chromosome 11q from linkage studies[31]. This gene appears to transmit atopy through the maternal line, explaining why its inheritance is greater for children with atopic mothers than those with atopic fathers, although genes of paternal origin have also been recognised. Studies now suggest a "dose–response" effect of polygenetic inheritance, with dominant and recessive genes[32]. This could explain the greater than predicted incidence of atopy in offspring from two affected parents. Studies in monozygotic (identical) twins show a concordance for atopy of only 60%[33], which indicates a role of additional factors determining IgE responses and disease.

PRE-AND POST-NATAL FACTORS

Before birth, cord blood IgE levels are significantly greater in babies with atopic mothers[34]. In addition, smoking increases cord blood IgE concentrations yet further, in a dose dependent fashion. This effect is also seen in non-atopic mothers who smoke, and is reversible. There is no evidence that the IgE is directed against tobacco allergens and it would appear more likely that tobacco affects the regulation of the synthesis of immunoglobulin in response to other antigens. However,

70% of new born babies with increased cord blood IgE will develop allergic symptoms before the age of 18 months[35].

Smoking during pregnancy is one factor responsible for low birth weight babies. Studies show that prematurity, low birth weight and increased IgE levels all carry increased risk for early house-dust mite sensitisation, although the reasons for this are unclear. Immaturity of the immune system with transient IgA deficiency, allowing allergen penetration and sensitisation, has been suggested[36]. In the neonatal period generally, there is a deficiency in humoral and cellular immune responses that is reported to be more marked in infants with a positive family history for atopy[37].

EXPOSURE TO RELEVANT ALLERGENS

It would appear that the initial encounter with an individual allergen, especially in the first few months of life, may determine sensitisation in those genetically predisposed, although identification of the factors which influence this is difficult. The only reliable methods of determining causation between environmental factors and allergy are randomised controlled interventions. Most epidemiological studies are cross sectional in design, and examine allergic disease and possible risk factors without proving causation. Despite this, there is mounting evidence that allergic sensitisation is greatly influenced by early exposure to allergen[38].

Studies of house-dust mite allergy show a relationship between levels of exposure and the likelihood of sensitisation. Atopic individuals sleeping in beds with mite allergen concentrations greater than $2000\,\text{ng·g}^{-1}$ dust have very high levels of specific IgE against mites, compared with those subject to lower exposure[39]. Other have found asthmatic symptoms likely to occur when mite concentration exceeded $10\,000\,\text{ng·g}^{-1}$ dust[6]. When mite levels are reduced in the bedroom, symptomatic improvement can be demonstrated[40] (Fig. 18.7).

The month of birth demonstrates that susceptible infants born just before a high allergen season such as the grass pollen season are more likely to develop atopy, compared with those born at other times[41]. Similarly, exposure to dog and cat allergens in the first year of life is more likely to sensitise than if introduced after the first year of life[42].

Although infancy represents a vulnerable period, sensitisation can occur at any age if the stimulus is strong enough.

EXPOSURE TO ADJUVANT FACTORS

Environmental pollutants such as sulphur dioxide, nitrogen dioxide, diesel fumes and smoking may increase mucosal permeability and enhance allergen penetration. Diesel exhaust particles are powerful adjuvants for IgE production. Airborne particles less than 1 μm in diameter are easily inhaled, and show an adjuvant effect on sensitisation in experiments with low dose antigen exposure[43] a situation likely to be reproduced in the environment. Certainly, the increase in allergic rhinitis and asthma over the past three decades has paralleled an increase in air pollution and car exhaust fumes. Similarly, tobacco smoke may also increase

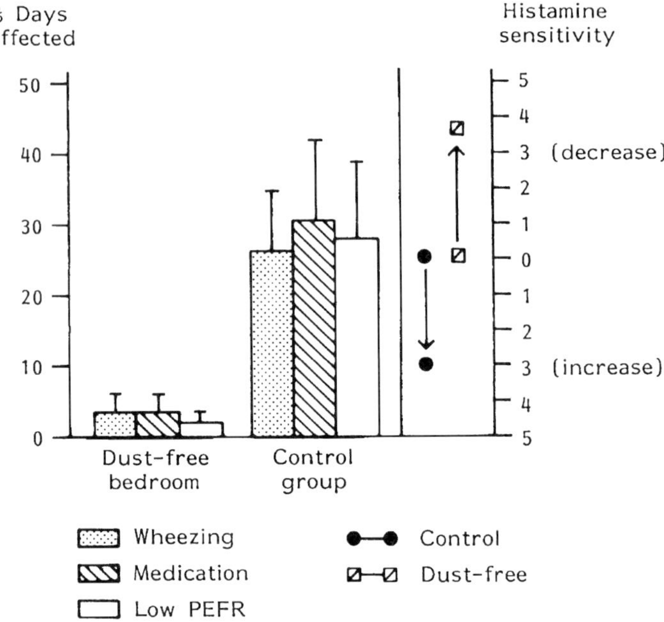

Figure 18.7. Dust free bedrooms as treatment for asthma. In children with house-dust mite allergy and asthma, reductions in dust reduced symptoms and bronchial hypersensitivity to histamine[40]. PEFR = Peak expiratory flow rate

mucosal permeability and hence sensitisation, which may explain why adult smokers develop "new" allergies, especially in response to exposure to occupational allergens. The increase in the numbers of females who smoke over the past 30 years could, in part, account for the increased prevalence of allergic disease observed in children born since the 1960s[44], as a result of a "sidestream" effect.

The effects of viral infections on allergen sensitisation have not been clearly defined in man. Studies in animals suggest an enhancing effect on sensitisation and IgE production in mice and dogs[45]. In man, some studies suggest that household acquired infection resulting from contact with older children protects against allergic disease, whereas in others, allergen sensitisation has been observed after viral infections[46].

CONCLUSION

The evidence to date supports the view that allergen induced disease of the respiratory tract is increasing. Our knowledge of these allergic reactions has grown. Clearly, genetic factors are important, but they appear to be significantly influenced by environmental allergens and adjuvants. Our understanding of antigens, allergens and adjuvants may be the key to limiting allergic disease of the respiratory tract in future.

REFERENCES

1. Ada G, Skehel J S. Are proteins good antigens? *Nature* 1985; **316:** 764–766.
2. Editorial. Mite allergens groups I–VII. A catalogue of enzymes. *Clin Exp Allergy* 1993; **23:** 350–353.
3. Ayres J G. Trends in asthma and hayfever in general practice in the UK 1976–1983. *Thorax* 1986; **41:** 111–116.
4. Fleming D M. Prevalence of asthma and hay fever in England and Wales. *BMJ* 1987; **296:** 279–283.
5. Burr M L, Butland B K, King S, *et al.* Changes in asthma prevalence: two surveys 15 years apart. *Arch Dis Child* 1989; **64:** 1452–1456.
6. Sporik R, Chapman M D, Platt Mills T A E. Housedust mite exposure as a cause of asthma. *Clin Exp Allergy* 1992; **22:** 897–906.
7. Burrows B, Martinez F D, Halonen M, *et al.* Association of asthma with serum IgE levels and skin reactivity to allergens. *N Engl J Med* 1989; **320:** 271–277.
8. Roberts D M. The incidence of atopy in a working population. *J Soc Occup Med* 1987; **37:** 106–110.
9. Ninan T K, Russel G. Respiratory symptoms and atopy in Aberdeen school children: evidence from two surveys 25 years apart. *BMJ* 1992; **304:** 873–875.
10. Pipkorn U, Coran K, Enerback L. The natural response of the human allergic mucosa to allergen exposure. *J Allergy Clin Immunol* 1988; **82:** 1046–1050.
11. Naclerio R M, Meier H L, Kagey-Sabotka A, *et al.* Mediator release after nasal airway challenge with allergen. *Am Rev Respir Dis* 1983; **128:** 597–602.
12. Oertel H L, Kaliner M. The biologic activity of mast cell granules: purification of inflammatory factors of anaphylaxis responsible for causing late-phase reactions. *J Immunol* 1981; **127:** 1398–1402.
13. Durham S R, Lee T H, Cromwell O. Immunologic studies in allergen-induced late-phase asthmatic reactions. *J Allergy Clin Immunol* 1984; **74:** 49–60.
14. Bhagat R G, Strunk R C, Larsen G L. The late asthmatic response. *Ann Allergy* 1985; **54:** 297–301.
15. Buscom R, Pipkorn U, Lichtenstein L M. The influx of inflammatory cells into nasal washings during the late response to allergen challenge. *Am Rev Respir Dis* 1988; **138:** 406–411.
16. Frew A J, Kay A B. Eosinophils and T-lymphocytes in late-phase allergic reactions. *J Allergy Clin Immunol* 1990; **85:** 533–539.
17. Plaut M, Piece J A, Watson C J, *et al.* Mast cell lines produce lymphokines in response to cross-linkage of FCeR1 or calcium lonophores. *Nature* 1989; **339:** 64–67.
18. Gleich G J, Flavahen N A, Fujisawa T, *et al.* The eosinophil as a mediator of damage to the respiratory epithelium. *J Allergy Clin Immunol* 1988; **81:** 776–781.
19. Boushy H A, Holtzman M J, Sheller J R *et al.* Bronchial hyper-reactivity. *Am Rev Respir Dis* 1980; **121:** 389–413.
20. Azzawi M, Bradley B, Jeffery P K, *et al.* Identification of activated T-lymphocytes and eosinophils in bronchial biopsies in stable atopic asthma. *Am Rev Respir Dis* 1990; **142:** 1407–1413.
21. Lamb J R, Faith A, Higgins J, *et al.* Clonal analysis of CD4 mediated accessory function on the effector activity of human CD4+ T-cell subsets. *Clin Exp Allergy* 1995; **25:** 839–847.
22. Robinson D, Harid Q, Bentley A, *et al.* Activation of CD4+ and T-cells, increased TH$_2$-type cytokine MRNA expression, and eosinophil recruitment in bronchio-alveolar lavage after allergen challenge in patients with atopic asthma. *J Allergy Clin Immunol* 1993; **92:** 313–324.
23. Djukanovic R, Wilson J, Britten K, *et al.* Quantitation of mast cells and eosinophils in the bronchial mucosa of symptomatic atopic asthmatics and healthy control subjects using immunohistochemistry. *Am Rev Respir Dis* 1990; **142:** 863–871.
24. Warringa R A, Schweizer R C, Maikoe T, *et al.* Modulation of eosinophil chemotaxis by interleukins. *Am J Respir Cell Mol Biol* 1992; **7:** 631–636.
25. Brodie D H, Paine M M, Firestein G S. Eosinophils express interleukin 5 and granulocyte macrophage - colony - stimulating factor mRNA at sites of allergic inflammation in asthmatics. *J Clin Invest* 1992; **90:** 1414–1424.

26. Houston J C, De Nava Squez S, Trouce J R. A clinical and pathological study of fatal cases of status asthmaticus. *Thorax* 1953; **8:** 207–213.

27. Dunnill M S. The pathology of asthma with special reference to changes in the bronchial mucosa. *J Clin Pathol* 1960; **13:** 27–33.

28. Connell J T. Quantitative intranasal pollen challenge. Effect of a daily pollen challenge, environmental pollen exposure and placebo challenge in the nasal membrane. *J Allergy* 1968; **41:** 123–139.

29. Hill A B. The environment and disease: association or causation? *Proc R Soc Med* 1965; **58:** 295–300.

30. Bousquet J, Burrey P. Evidence for an increase in atopic disease and possible causes. *Clin Exp Allergy* 1993; **23:** 484–492.

31. Cookson W, Young R P, Sandford A J, *et al*. Maternal inheritance of atopic IgE responsiveness on chromosome 11_q. *Lancet* 1992; **340:** 381–384.

32. Solter D. Differential imprinting and expression of maternal and paternal genomes. *Annu Rev Genet* 1988; **22:** 127–146.

33. Bazara M, Orgel H A, Hamburger R N. Genetics of IgE and allergy in twins. *J Allergy Clin Immunol* 1974; **54:** 288–304.

34. Michel F B, Bousquet J, Greillier P, *et al*. Comparison of cord blood IgE concentration and maternal allergy for the production of atopic disease in Infancy. *J Allergy Clin Immunol* 1980; **65:** 422–30.

35. Magnusson C G M. Maternal smoking influences cord serum IgE and IgD levels increase the risk for subsequent infant allergy. *J Allergy Clin Immunol* 1986; **78:** 898–904.

36. Holt P G, McNenamin C, Nelson D. Primary sensitisation to inhalant allergens during infancy. *Pediatr Allergy Immunol* 1990; **1:** 3–13.

37. Holt P G, Clough J B, Holt B J, *et al*. Genetic risk for atopy is associated with delayed post natal maturation of T-cell competence. *Clin Exp Allergy* 1992; **22:** 1093–1099.

38. Rugtveit J. Environmental factors in the first month of life and the possible relationships to later development of hypersensitivity. *Allergy* 1990; **45:** 154–156.

39. Lau S, Falkenhorst G, Weber H, *et al*. High mite allergen exposure increases risk of sensitisation in atopic children and young adults. *J Allergy Clin Immunol* 1989; **84:** 718–725.

40. Brostoff J, Scadding G. Allergic disorders. In: Brostoff J, Scadding G, Male D, *et al*., eds. *Clinical Immunology*, chapter 17, London: Gower Medical Publishing, 1991.

41. Bjorksten F, Suoniemi I. Dependence of immediate hypersensitivity on month of birth. *Clin Allergy* 1976; **6:** 161–171.

42. Arshad H. Pets and atopic disorders in infancy. *Br J Clin Pract* 1991; **45:** 88–89.

43. Muranaka M, Suzuki S, Koikumikk K, *et al*. Adjuvant activity of diesel-exhaust particulates for the production of IgE antibody in mice. *J Allergy Clin Immunol* 1986; **77:** 616–623.

44. Murray A B, Morrison B J. The effect of cigarette smoke from the mother on bronchial responsiveness and severity of symptoms in children with asthma. *J Allergy Clin Immunol* 1986; **77:** 575–581.

45. Frick O L. Effect of respiratory and other virus infections on IgE immunoregulation. *J Allergy Clin Immunol* 1986; **78:** 1013–1018.

46. Cogswell J J, Halliday D F, Alexander J R. Respiratory infections in the first year of life in children at risk of developing atopy. *BMJ* 1982; **284:** 1011–1013.

Index

Note: page numbers in italics refer to figures and tables.